HEALING THE DISTRESS OF PSYCHOSIS

Healing the Distress of Psychosis

LISTENING WITH PSYCHOTIC EARS

Shannon Dunn, PhD, LCSW, CRADC
CLINICAL ASSOCIATE PROFESSOR OF SOCIAL WORK
UNIVERSITY OF SOUTHERN CALIFORNIA
SUZANNE DWORAK-PECK SCHOOL OF SOCIAL WORK

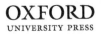
OXFORD
UNIVERSITY PRESS

OXFORD
UNIVERSITY PRESS

Oxford University Press is a department of the University of Oxford. It furthers
the University's objective of excellence in research, scholarship, and education
by publishing worldwide. Oxford is a registered trade mark of Oxford University
Press in the UK and certain other countries.

Published in the United States of America by Oxford University Press
198 Madison Avenue, New York, NY 10016, United States of America.

Library of Congress Cataloging-in-Publication Data
Names: Dunn Shannon, author.
Title: Healing the distress of psychosis : listening with psychotic ears / Shannon Dunn.
Description: New York, NY : Oxford University Press, [2018] |
Includes bibliographical references and index.
Identifiers: LCCN 2018003489 (print) | LCCN 2018004319 (ebook) |
ISBN 9780190858766 (updf) | ISBN 9780190858773 (epub) | ISBN 9780190858759 (paperback : alk. paper)
Subjects: | MESH: Psychotic Disorders—therapy
Classification: LCC RC480 (ebook) | LCC RC480 (print) | NLM WM 200 | DDC 616.89/1—dc23
LC record available at https://lccn.loc.gov/2018003489

9 8 7 6 5 4 3 2 1

Printed by WebCom, Inc., Canada

To Missy and Morgie
You are my sources of joy and purpose.
May you always have deep love, unconditional support,
inspiration, personal satisfaction, and generosity for others.

Contents

Preface: Everything You Need to Know to Navigate This Book

EXPERIENCES OF PSYCHOSIS, including hallucinations, delusions, and disorganized thinking, and rates of disability from it are higher than ever, despite the availability of mental health treatment, especially promising antipsychotic medications. More government money is spent on the use of psychotropic medications than any other treatment modality. Given these increasing disability numbers, it appears that these medications are being used as a method of socially controlling and silencing individuals who live with symptoms of severe mental illness (SMI), especially psychosis. There must be a better way for people who live with symptoms of mental illness and psychosis to live and flourish! The philosophy of *Listening with Psychotic Ears* is a fresh and accessible way to accurately understand the expressions of a person whose brain is communicating under the influence of psychosis and facilitate a self-determined life worth living.

READER POPULATION

Reader audience for this book is threefold: mental health professionals, individuals with lived psychotic experiences, and their family members and loved ones. All three perspectives need a strong and accurate voice that validates the past and present disappointments in mainstream public mental health treatment and delivers hope in creating a secure and thriving self-determined life worth living.

Mental health professionals who will most benefit from the information in this book are those who do not solely rely on psychotropic medications for the treatment of psychosis but also see the value in building an authentic therapeutic relationship by entering the subjective world of individuals who experience symptoms of psychosis. In the context of this book, the term "mental health professional" refers to anyone in a professional healing role, including, but not limited to, case managers, social workers, psychologists, art therapists, peer counselors, occupational therapists, psychiatrists, lawyers, and nurses. This book gives permission and structure to enter the subjective world of the person who experiences psychotic symptoms and delivers the necessary language to do so. This book includes numerous diverse cases in which clinical skills are applied, illustrating unique nuances and effectiveness. The main intention of this book is not wholly to disparage psychotropic medication administration, as ethical administration can and does offer stabilizing results for some individuals. Instead, the primary intention of this book is to find successful methods to accurately understand and effectively communicate with individuals who are actively experiencing psychosis for the purpose of increasing their quality of life.

Individuals who live with psychotic experiences can benefit from this book. This audience has given the most resoundingly positive reactions to the information in *Listening with Psychotic Ears*. It is hoped that this information and diverse case stories will validate the bizarre, dehumanizing, and dark experiences one has received from the mainstream public mental health treatment system. Beyond validation, the philosophical values and concrete skills of *Listening with Psychotic Ears* will be an invitation to the living, hope for creating a secure and thriving existence that is full of creative energy, meaningful connectedness, flourishing spiritual energy, and exceeding personal potentials.

Finally, loved ones of those who experience psychosis can benefit from the information in this book. The information and cases in this book can give accurate insights into the previously misunderstood subjective psychotic world and associated misunderstood communications of individuals who experience symptoms of psychosis. *Listening with Psychotic Ears* philosophy gives opportunities for families to be in accurate communication and enjoy closer interpersonal relationships, which will result in increased quality of life for them and their loved ones. Whereas clinical terminology is used in this book, these concepts are also explained for nonclinician consumption.

The River

Some rivers have a strong undercurrent that is seemingly impossible to resist. Despite any effort to stay on a desired course, this overpowering undercurrent can easily pull an object or person under the water, causing lifeless submission. Without a fight, this object is taken down the river's path, sometimes showing up miles down the passageway in a dilapidated condition that is very different than its entry point. Ultimately, the object or person may be so battered and beat down that there is no hope for life.

The River is the chosen metaphor for mainstream public mental health treatment system. On paper and according to those towing the *party line*, the *River* treatment pathway is intended to expedite the recovery process in the person seeking mental health services. However, in both subtle and powerful means, these *River* practices can silence the person's faith in himself or herself and any hope of real recovery and swiftly crush any means for a self-determined quality of life. These overt spirit-crushing *River* messages include the following:

- "All psychotic symptoms are caused by the misworkings of brain tissue and neurotransmitters and are minimized by the consistent use of psychotropic medications."
- "Stress causes functional decompensation. Work causes stress. You are disabled and unable to earn an income. You must be given money to meet your basic needs. You should be able to provide for your basic needs with a monthly fixed income. You are being done a fiscal favor to not be expected to work."
- "You should make friends with other disabled people like you. You all have similar needs and can be dealt with more efficiently in a group."
- "A resourceful case manager can link you with charity programs that will meet all your unmet needs."
- "Psychotic disorders render you like a child. You should not be left to think/ act for yourself, else tragedy is imminent."

Most people who receive treatment for psychosis in the mainstream public mental health system hear these messages over and over again. While these statements are well intentioned, they become a philosophical mantra that comes to be believed by many clients and cause them to have low self-expectation beliefs and self-sabotaging underachieving behaviors.

New to and having hope and trust in the mainstream public mental health treatment system, individuals will often submit to *The River* treatment pathway for many years. With the passing of time, individuals who have a spiritual awakening and are released from the grip of *The River* find themselves in a drastically impaired state that is different from their point of entry. This impaired state can include severe depression, brain and other vital organ damage, severe weight gain, metabolic and cardiovascular disease, little to no personal direction, social marginalization, isolation, disempowerment, extreme poverty, emotional numbness, and self-sabotaging indulgences as desperate attempts to feel alive, such as excessive drug use (including tobacco), with the ultimate offense for these individuals being early death. In fact, there is a 25-year premature death rate for people with mental illness, mainly caused by three factors (Hartz et al., 2014): (1) the use of psychotropic medications creates such a hardship on other organs and weakens the body's internal structure that the stage is set for chronic or life-threatening health problems or diseases; (2) the amount of weight commonly gained when taking these medications can lead to heart complications and the development of diabetes, as well as other complications; and (3) the stigma of psychosis often creates an atmosphere where people experiencing symptoms are not taken seriously when expressing concerns about a physical health condition or seem undeserving of medical advances or life-saving procedures. As one becomes emotionally numb and disconnected from himself and his world, he loses hope for his future well-being, and psychogenic or spiritual death ensues. This myopic *mainstream public mental health treatment pathway* metaphor, *The River*, is referred to throughout this book.

On an administrative level and working backward, we can understand the origins of *The River*. Individuals who experience symptoms of psychosis do, for a fact, experience unique thoughts and behaviors compared with those without psychosis. Things that are different are sometimes feared. Over the years, there have been many varied and unsuccessful attempts to *cure* unwanted symptoms of psychosis. A cure for such a devastating illness has not been discovered and, as a result, scientists, religious leaders, and society consciously or unconsciously experience despair. Since the brain functions more efficiently when it experiences positive emotions, emotions such as despair, especially if unconscious, may not be fully attended to. When we do not talk about a particular experience, it stays underdeveloped, and as a result, the potential for change is limited.

The administration of psychotropic medications has become the *central* focus of mainstream public mental health treatment for the remedy of psychotic symptoms for several reasons. One important reason is this: as the cause of psychotic symptoms settles on neurophysiology—the inner workings of the brain—other viable explanations, such as trauma, are not entertained. As this reductionist reasoning becomes a more certain conclusion, further explanations are not even considered. Pharmaceutical companies have taken both scientific advances and reductionist conclusions and asserted that all symptoms of psychosis are caused by neurophysiology. Additionally, they assert that psychotropic medications are the most efficient and humane way to fix these symptoms. Colossal wealth has allowed pharmaceutical companies to leverage their massive power to indoctrinate their mantra to medical schools and health insurance companies, thereby indoctrinating everyone. This pervasive indoctrination by pharmaceutical companies has left society with millions of individuals who suffer an unnecessarily low quality of life and spiritual death.

Occasionally and miraculously, some individuals are lucky enough to be spontaneously released by *The River*'s grip, resulting in an existential spiritual awakening. *River* messages and interventions are questioned and protested by this individual. This individual will look back on his life and his mental health treatment career and be filled with a variety of emotions, including loss, sadness, disillusionment, and sometimes rage. This existential awakening is a life-or-death process. There are pockets of available supports for this individual, but the miracle is in their veridical (truthful) human connections and sustainability in these relationships and other life forces.

Now, some readers might wonder whether this argument is too dramatic and too idealistic. As evidenced by the numerous psychiatric survivor narratives, some included in this book, creating a self-determined life worth living for people who live with psychosis *is* an extreme life-and-death situation. Improving wellness options for these individuals is going to require a heavy dose of idealism, even more than what this single book can offer. Our mainstream public mental health system is broken and must be reconsidered and reconstructed with client well-being as the main priority. The author acknowledges those individuals who do experience the benefits from well-meaning mainstream mental health treatment services, including the ethical and conscious use of psychotropic medications. The philosophy of *Listening with Psychotic Ears* is intended for those individuals, families, and clinicians who are still seeking a model with strategies for creating a self-determined life worth living and sustainable healing from the distress of living with psychosis.

ETHICS OF PROFESSIONAL OBLIGATION

All mental health treatment professionals are bound by the ethics of professional obligation, and each discipline has its specific code of ethics. There are four principles that compose ethical practice: (1) respect for autonomy (the patient has the right to choose and refuse treatment); (2) justice (fairness and equality in the distribution of scarce resources); (3) beneficence (the practitioner will act in the patient's best interest); and (4) nonmalfeasance (first, do no harm) (Gillon, 1994). While most interventions, especially medical ones, carry their risks for ethical practice to be achieved, the intervention benefits have to outweigh the resulting harm.

The person must ultimately decide for himself which treatment course holds the most benefits and risks—in this case, the psychotic symptoms or the list of harms that are caused by the treatments, especially when using psychotropic medications. In the case of mainstream public mental health treatment for psychosis, several important ethical questions are asked: (1) Is the individual presented with a *full range of effective treatment* options? (2) Is the patient given *full freedom* to choose the best course of action? (3) Are these individuals given *full disclosure of the potential harms* of the proposed course of treatment, especially when psychotropic medications are presented? The information in this book argues that individuals who interface with mainstream public mental health are not given the full story on available and effective treatment options, are coerced into the *River* treatment pathways, and are not adequately advised of the potential harms of the treatments they are administered.

MEANING OF *LISTENING WITH PSYCHOTIC EARS*

Every individual perspective is constructed from a variety of influences that we use to interpret our experiences and communicate with the world around us. The meaning of *Listening with Psychotic Ears* is explained with the following example.

A native English-speaking, bilingual woman is standing in the grocery line waiting for her turn to pay for her items. The line is stalled for an unknown reason. She notices that the checkout clerk and the customer are speaking to one another. At first, listening with her English ears, she does not understand them or why the line is stalled. However, she notices that they are speaking in Spanish and she tunes in to their conversation with her Spanish language and cultural ears. Listening with the language that is being spoken, she is able to accurately understand what they are saying, understand why the line is stalled, and consider an effective resolution to their barrier.

Because of the neurological and existential impacts on the brain and mind, people who experience symptoms of psychosis have unique neurological and existential experiences that cause them to communicate in distinctive ways. When we listen and communicate outside of this unique culture, accurate understanding and effective communication are not probable. As a result, many conclude that these psychotic communications are mysterious, bizarre, and incomprehensible. Accessing their unique methods of communication *is* possible and vital for accurate understanding and effective communication with individuals who experience symptoms of psychosis.

When encountering a person who is experiencing psychosis, we are able to enter their subjective world by accessing their cultural experiences and language by *listening with our psychotic ears*, just as the bilingual woman listened differently with her *Spanish ears* to the language and cultural context at hand. We tune in to the distinctive metaphorical speech patterns and consider the person in his or her cultural context, using imagination and empathy to accurately understand what is being communicated. By doing so, we are afforded more opportunities for accurate understanding and effective communication with the person who is experiencing psychosis. Furthermore, this ethical and effective communication method and attitude is the foundation for healing the distress of psychotic experiences and creating a self-determined life worth living.

AUTHOR'S BACKGROUND

For the majority of my life, I have chosen to work with individuals and their families who experience SMI. I have been most drawn to those who experience symptoms of psychosis, leaving them socially marginalized, living in poverty, and desperately accessing methods (including drug misuse and homelessness) to keep their dying spirits afloat. My work has taken me to almost every available level of care, including long-term state psychiatric hospitals, inpatient acute psychiatric hospitals, residential treatment centers, emergency crisis centers, outpatient mental health centers, intensive outpatient day hospitals, and private practices. I have witnessed the results of both the medical model and the recovery model and observed individuals and their families both flourish and perish as a result of the ideas I have shared here in *Listening with Psychotic Ears.* My authority on this topic comes from my 36 years of hands-on work and education in the mental health field.

During these years of immersion in the mainstream public mental health treatment delivery system, I found myself naturally using my intuitive clinical skills to understand and communicate with people who experience symptoms of psychosis. As a social worker, I have not relied on psychotropic medication as an intervention and naturally developed my own attitude and effective methods and strategies. With these methods and no psychotropic medications, within the very conversation, I have regularly witnessed clients spontaneously come out of their psychotic experiences and be involved in linear and meaningful conversations.

Even at the beginning of my professional career, I have relied on a passionate attitude of connecting with the strengths and spirit of others. Right there is the essence of the effectiveness of this philosophy and model. When I first began talking about these clinical skills, students would look at me, consistently, with simultaneous expressions of skepticism, inspiration, and hope. They would return in subsequent weeks, telling story after story of how these skills were applied in their clinical internships and had positive results. Students relayed clients' reports of deeply feeling heard and accurately understood, and to their surprise, the students could therapeutically communicate with the individuals who were actively experiencing psychosis. The students, year after year, encouraged me to write so others might have access to these skills. Over the years and around the globe, I received enormous encouragement from mental health clinicians, students, and most of all, people who have lived experiences of psychosis, either personally or within families. Based on all the encouragement that I received, this book was realized.

SUMMARY OF CHAPTERS

This book is organized in three units: (1) "Traditional Treatment Approaches for Healing Psychosis"; (2) "New Discoveries About the Causes and Healing Approaches for Psychosis"; and (3) "Ethical and Professional Obligations Impact Micro, Mezzo, and Macro Levels of Treatment Delivery." Diverse case examples are offered throughout the book to illustrate both the unique dynamics and effective skills of this philosophy. Further, it's worth noting that many of the resources used within this book are older, and this decision was consciously made for two reasons: (1) I wanted to go back and revive the original works concerning these issues from the authors who introduced them, and (2) these issues are not discussed or examined to the depth they once were and have, to some extent, become lost within the framework of ethical practice. The following paragraphs narrate the purpose of each unit and its chapters.

Unit I—"Traditional Treatment Approaches for Healing Psychosis"—addresses how the mainstream public mental health treatment delivery system has been tainted with a long and dark history of misunderstandings, abuses, and unethical and ineffective treatment practices. These practices have been endorsed by pervasive myths about people who experience psychosis. We must reflect on these mistreatments and misunderstandings to avoid repeating the same or worse mistakes. Finally, in Unit I, we explore historical and pioneering individuals, groups, and communities who have exercised more effective and humane relational mental health treatments and highlight how these methods have not been visible in the mainstream public mental health system.

Unit II—"New Discoveries About the Causes and Healing Approaches for Psychosis"—addresses new discoveries about accurate understandings and effective and ethical treatments for healing experiences of psychosis. The convincing evidence between early and severe trauma and the development of psychotic symptoms is explored. In an effort to illustrate the varied causes of psychotic symptoms, neurobiological manifestations of psychotic symptoms are surveyed.

Unit III—"Ethical and Professional Obligations Impact Micro, Mezzo, and Macro Levels of Treatment Delivery"—explores the professional obligation for accurate understanding and effective interventions grounded in an ethical treatment philosophy of building a therapeutic relationship in which the client's world can be entered and accurately understood. The historical and contemporary underpinnings of the recovery movement are illustrated, showing how members of the consumer/ psychiatric survivor/ex-patient (C/S/X) movement have gone public with psychiatric iatrogenic treatment stories to empower slow and sporadic changes in the mainstream mental health system. Common existential experiences and related terminology are proposed as tools to assist the reader in further understanding and exploring an individual's psychotic inner world. Clinical strategies of *Listening with Psychotic Ears* are offered. Not everyone is readily reachable and a unique attitude and methods are necessary for working with these unique individuals who live with more complex traumatic experiences and relying on maladaptive coping styles to survive. Families and loved ones hold an essential place in the caregiving recovery story, therefore, essential survivor and self-care skills for families and clinicians are proposed.

Finally, Unit IV—"Conclusions and Future Remarks"—asserts essential conclusions of the *Listening with Psychotic Ears* philosophy and interventions, namely that effective and ethical mental health treatment is of urgent importance for helping to heal the symptoms and distress of psychosis. Additionally, future effective and humane macro and micro change efforts are named.

The appendices of this book list a wide range of resources that can be accessed to support individuals who live with psychosis, their loved ones, and clinicians with the intention to empower, support, and facilitate creating lives worth living.

Acknowledgments

THE PROCESS OF writing this book has truly taught me that no one does big things in isolation. I wish to express my deep gratitude for those who helped me to complete this book.

I thank my mentor and friend Dr. Thomas Meenaghan, beginning back when we met at Loyola University of Chicago, where he was the dean and I was an MSW student. Thank you for our mentoring meetings then and for all your guidance throughout my career. I especially thank you for all of our conversations during which you guided me through this book writing process from the very beginning to the very end. I could not have done this without your mentoring and inspiration!

I thank David Follmer for being so flexible with my timeline and encouraging words over the years.

Charli Englehorn is the most amazing and aberrant wordsmith. I thank you for your skilled editing work, writing guidance, laughing with me through my anxieties and helping me to linearly organize my thoughts that were all over the place. I could not have done this work without you!

I thank Dr. Shelley Levin for offering recovery-oriented resources, inspiration, and emotional support, especially during moments of panic. Thank you for always asking, "How is the book coming along?"

I thank University of Southern California Master of Social Work students who, over the years, shared your most mysterious and bizarre stories of "unreachable" individuals who were actively experiencing psychosis. I especially was inspired when you told me that you had not ever heard this *Listening with Psychotic Ears* content before in your academic education and when you tried it, you enthusiastically reported back successful stories in which you accurately understood and communicated with your clients. It is my hope that you now have skills to continue this healing work, language to discuss the effective and humane therapeutic process, and the confidence to talk about this process with all health and mental health professionals.

I thank Meggan Thompson for sharing stories and inspiration to keep going.

I thank Tosha Sweet for our straight-up conversations that spoke directly to my spirit when it felt small and making me laugh to shake off the stress. I am forever grateful for your encouragement!

I thank Guyton Colantuono and Malia Javier for connecting me with peer groups and feedback about how this information is perceived by people with lived psychotic experiences. It is these groups from which I have received the most enthusiastic feedback.

I thank Dr. Kimberly Finney for the neurobiology references and our many encouraging conversations. You are an angel in this world.

I thank Sally Zinman for sharing your resources, inspiration, and passion to help in the active efforts to "turn this ship around."

I thank Mark Sanders, my first social work supervisor, who taught me how to be the social worker that I am today. Thank you for your generous support and never-ending encouragement.

I thank Jyung Kyung Park for all of your loving support and generous friendship.

To all the people who ask, "How is your book coming along?" It served as encouragement and accountability. I am thrilled to now say that the book is finished and available.

To my family, my parents, Pat and Bob Dunn, for all your generous, loving, and constant encouragement and support for my passions, even when my dreams seem a bit lofty.

And, last but not least, I thank and dedicate this book to my daughters, Missy and Morgie, for all the jingliness, especially when the energy was periodically drying up, and your patience when I had to work and you needed to play. I love you girls with all of my huge heart!

HEALING THE DISTRESS OF PSYCHOSIS

UNIT I

Traditional Treatment Approaches for Healing Psychosis

1

Types of Psychosis and General Intervention Approaches

WHEN REFERRING TO psychosis, what kinds of symptoms are we talking about? Psychotic symptoms encompass a large cluster of mental disorders that have in common serious impairments of the individual's capacity to remain in contact with *typical standards* of reality. Symptoms of psychosis are often accompanied by confusion and disorders in thought and perception, which can find expression as delusional thinking and hallucinatory experiences that manifest in the senses (Jackson & Williams, 1994). Psychotic symptoms can come and go suddenly or pervasively linger.

DEFINITIONS AND POPULATION OF FOCUS

When one refers to psychotic symptoms in clinical terms, it can be in the context of positive symptoms or negative symptoms. *Positive psychotic symptoms* are sensations or beliefs that are present, but should not be. Examples of positive symptoms are hallucinations and delusions. There are many types of hallucinations—sensory experiences where there is significant evidence of nonexistence—including auditory, visual, tactile, olfactory, and gustatory. Auditory hallucinations are the most frequently reported type among people with psychotic disorders. Strong beliefs despite significant evidence of nonexistence are termed "delusions." These delusions can be grandiose, annihilatory, persecutory, or obsessed with religion, or can include thoughts relating to loss of control of mind or body, such as Cotard's syndrome (the belief that one is dead or does not exist), unfounded guilt/sin/self-accusation, and thought insertion, just to name a few (Andreasen, 1979; Frith & Cocoran, 1996).

Many people, with and without diagnoses of severe mental illness (SMI), experience auditory hallucinations of sounds, voices, and bodily sensations. When this experience is frequently repeated, naturally, an explanation of origin is desired, which any person experiencing these events would seek. As a result, auditory and other sensory hallucinations and explanatory delusions will often be paired with the existing facts to seemingly formulate a logical conclusion.

For example, Sara, who was later diagnosed with a psychotic disorder, began to hear sounds of radio static, which transformed into a man coughing, then a man's voice calling her name, and, finally, a man's voice cursing her. Seeking a logical cause and explanation for these intrusive noises, Sara came to conclude that this was her deceased abusive father making attempts to communicate with her.

Negative psychotic symptoms are experiences that should exist but do not. Examples of negative psychotic symptoms include restricted or flat affect (restricted emotional expression), apathy (restricted feelings), anhedonia (restricted capacity to experience pleasure), avolition (restricted initiation of goal-directed behavior), alogia (restriction in the production of thought), and asociality (restriction of the desire to form social relationships) (American Psychiatric Association [APA], 2013).

Many people who have been diagnosed with psychotic disorders experience negative psychotic symptoms. These symptoms often become more severe as a person ages and continues to take antipsychotic medications. The origin of these negative psychotic symptoms is in question: Are these negative psychotic symptoms a result of the psychotic disease or from the impact of years of antipsychotic medications on parts of the brain that drive motivation and affect, especially the feeling of pleasure? Additionally, could these negative psychotic symptoms be the result of extreme depression from years of oppressing the individual's sense of agency? Let us consider this example.

Jack Has Negative Psychotic Symptoms

Jack was diagnosed with schizophrenia and has been taking antipsychotic medications for 23 years, since he was 20 years old. Now, at the age of 43, his days are filled with specific prompts to get out of bed and make sure to attend to his activities of daily living, such as eating, caring for his clothes, and brushing his teeth. Jack's expressionless face and minimal conversations with others illustrate his negative psychotic symptom manifestation. He speaks in a monotonous and soft voice, even when he is excited. He has a part-time job as a file clerk and works slowly.

Jack spends most of his leisure time alone or sharing an infrequent lunch with his sister. While Jack reports that he is content and his work of 15 years is satisfying, he manifests many negative symptoms of psychosis, such as emotional indifference, loss of interest in pleasurable activities, and mental blankness. These negative psychotic symptoms could be caused by brain tissue and neurotransmitter deterioration from the psychotic disorder, long-term use of antipsychotic medication, or the impact of low expectations on his existence, or some of all three.

For the purpose of this book, when referring to psychotic symptoms, symptoms of hallucinations, delusions, and disorganized cognition and speech are indicated. The purpose of focusing mainly on positive psychotic symptoms is that the origin, manifestation, and meaning of these symptoms are very different from that of negative psychotic symptoms, in that the negative symptoms are the consequence of treatment, including psychotropic medications and existential oppression. Additionally, there is some evidence that the negative psychotic symptoms are a product of long-term antipsychotic medications (Kantrowitz & Javitt, 2010; Harrison, 1995), which is not the direct focus of this book.

People who experience episodes of positive psychotic symptoms can be diagnosed with any number of mental disorders such as schizophrenia, schizoaffective disorder, brief psychotic disorder, bipolar disorder, acute or transient psychotic disorder, dissociative identity disorder, and other disorders involving cognitive impairment. Additionally, sometimes people who are in the process of severe drug addiction and misuse and living a life of squalor also experience positive symptoms of psychosis and are all too often misdiagnosed with the previously mentioned mental illnesses, especially schizophrenia. To arrive at an accurate diagnosis, the person's medical context, meaning system, and prescribed and illicit drug history must be taken into consideration. To fully understand the way these positive symptoms evolve within different disorders and for the purpose of arriving at an accurate diagnosis, a detailed look at each of the most prevalent psychotic disorders follows.

This discussion is based on a combination of diagnostic parameters set forth by the APA in the *Diagnostic and Statistical Manual* (DSM) and the World Health Organization (WHO) in the *International Classification of Diseases, Tenth Revision, Clinical Modification* (ICD-10-CM) and the author's clinical experiences with individuals who experience these episodes. The two diagnostic parameters, DSM and ICD, were chosen because these have been the parameters and criteria on which both American and International healthcare settings and researchers have relied. In the DSM and ICD text of each disorder, other illnesses are identified that should be first ruled out, including medical circumstances, drug use, and other mental illnesses that can mimic the named disorder. In the next sections, the most common psychotic disorders are identified, defined, and explored by scope, onset, course of illness and contemporary mainstream treatment options. Given the DSM and ICD inconsistencies, subjectivity, and other criticisms, the author's personal diagnostic impressions are also included.

SCHIZOPHRENIFORM DISORDER
Definition

Schizophreniform disorder is the diagnostic name for possible first-episode schizophrenia. The APA (2013) categorizes this episode as the individual experiencing a combination of positive and negative psychotic symptoms and disorganized speech and behavior. According to the DSM-5 and ICD, symptoms will persist for a time period of more than 1 month and less than 6 months (APA, 2013; WHO, 2017).

To arrive at an accurate diagnosis, it is essential to rule out other possible influences. Illicit drug use that induces psychotic symptoms should be considered. All medical conditions should be considered and ruled out as the symptom origin. The extended time frame of symptom manifestation from 1 month to less than 6 months should be acknowledged for accurate diagnosis (APA, 2013).

Scope

According to Naz, Bromet, and Mojtabai (2003), about a third of individuals who experience symptoms of schizophreniform disorder will recover. The remaining two-thirds of this population will go on to be diagnosed with schizophrenia (Bromet et al., 2011).

Onset and Course of Illness

Schizophreniform disorder manifests during the teen years through the early twenties, and one-third of the individuals will experience a full recovery within 6 months of onset. The other individuals will continue to experience symptoms and eventually transition into schizophrenia or schizoaffective disorder (APA, 2013).

Initially, the individual will unusually spend long periods of time alone in his or her room. During this time, he or she may be involved in exploring a novel idea, such as time travel or finding proof of a particular theory, such as "the government suppressing information about alien life on other planets." His or her hygiene will become altered. The individual may forget to regularly brush teeth. Bathing or showering may be forgotten or even feared. Senses, especially appetite, become altered and explained with "someone is poisoning the food." The individual will then become worried and hypervigilant as "the perpetrator is being discovered and ultimately caught." Additional unusual behaviors will emerge, such as covering all possible openings to his room or electrical sockets and windowpane cracks with plastic trash bags or other "insulator." The circadian rhythm may become opposite, and the individual may sleep during the day and stay awake during the night, disrupting the length and quality of sleep, which further impairs one's mental status. Speech may become difficult to understand as a result of being nonlinear and preoccupied with new ideas and theories.

This prodromal, or extended, episode comes on slowly and will become more extreme with time. As previously stated, one-third of the population will resolve symptoms on their own. The remaining two-thirds of the population, who go on to be diagnosed with schizophrenia, will likely experience symptom severity progression, ultimately arriving at a crisis situation that inevitably involves others. Examples include throwing the television or computer out of the window or causing a public disturbance at a mall. At this point, the person will be taken either to jail or a hospital, where comprehensive medical and mental status evaluations should be conducted.

Treatment Options

Initially, a full comprehensive medical workup is indicated to be able to confidently rule out any drug use or medical problem that may be causing the mental status alterations. Gabbard refers to this battery of tests as First Episode Psychosis and Prodrome Workup (Freudenreich, Schulz, & Goff, 2009). This comprehensive workup may or may not be conducted, depending on the quality of care that is delivered. The decision of whether to conduct these diagnostic tests depends on the patient's financial capacity and the strength of professional ethics of the health service provider.

Treatment options for schizophreniform disorder, or the prodromal phase, are considered low risk and less invasive and include psychoeducation, stress reduction, family therapy, and cognitive-behavioral therapy (CBT) (Gabbard, 2014). In addition to talk therapies, medications will also be prescribed to the individual who is experiencing an episode of schizophreniform disorder. Omega-3 fatty acids have been shown to assist in the reduction of both positive and negative psychotic symptoms and to preserve overall functioning (Gabbard, 2014). When little to no sign of improvement is observed with these interventions, the lowest doses of antipsychotic medications are commonly prescribed.

SCHIZOPHRENIA
Definition

Schizophrenia is considered an SMI that results in *episodes* of acute and intense positive psychotic symptoms (hallucinations and delusions) and lingering negative

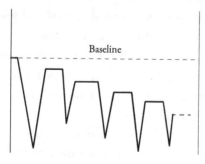

FIGURE 1.1 Schizophrenia Progressive Decompensation.

symptoms (disorganized speech and behavior, lack of motivation, decreased capacity for experiencing pleasure and social interaction, etc.). According to the DSM-5 and ICD-10-CM, symptoms will persist for a time period of more than 6 months, or less if accurately treated (APA, 2013; WHO, 2017).

The distinguishing factor in schizophrenia is the progressive and pervasive decompensation in functioning over the years, with every psychotic decompensation. In other words, with every intense psychotic episode, global functioning decreases. As functioning recompensates, functioning is not restored all the way back up to baseline. As shown in Figure 1.1, over the years and lifetime, with every psychotic decompensation, baseline functioning lowers. This baseline lowering explains why schizophrenia is difficult to diagnose in a young person and fairly straightforward to observe in individuals who have had several psychotic episodes.

This condition is often misdiagnosed for people using illicit drugs; therefore, as with all psychotic disorders, to arrive at an accurate diagnosis, it is essential to rule out this influence and other possible influences. Accurate diagnosis among individuals who use illicit drugs is a huge problem, because drugs do induce positive psychotic symptoms and withdrawal can mimic negative psychotic symptoms. Compounding this problem is that the necessary observation of the person's functioning without illicit drug use is often impossible in the United States, because there is a high frequency of illicit drug use among individuals who experience mental illnesses; thus, clear-headed moments are rare. Additionally, all medical conditions should be considered and ruled out as the symptom origin. Finally, according to the DSM and ICD, the extended time frame of symptom manifestation for more than 6 months should be acknowledged for accurate diagnosis (APA, 2013; WHO, 2017).

Scope

According to McGrath, Saha, Chant, and Welham (2008), approximately 0.3% to 0.7% of the general population will experience schizophrenia. While cases of schizophrenia are observed across all ethnicities and cultures, individuals from certain populations within the United States (e.g., people of color, except Asians but especially African Americans and Latinos), illicit drug users, and those of low socioeconomic status (SES) are overly diagnosed with schizophrenia, suggesting erroneous subjectivity, increased causal factors such as trauma, and lower access to resources, including barriers to receiving high-quality physical and mental healthcare.

According to the DSM-5 (APA, 2013), experiences of early symptoms of schizophrenia are similar in males and females. Men tend to have more frequent and intense episodes, as aggression and drug use cause them to be more visible and, thus, taken into jail or hospital custody. Mental illness, treatments, and criminal justice involvement interferes with male *breadwinner* identity, causing increased distress and the reliance on self-medicating efforts, which further limit one's capacity for independent functionality (APA, 2013).

Women who are diagnosed with schizophrenia tend to manifest more persecutory hallucinations, delusions, and depressive symptoms that are more privately managed and less likely to come to public authority attention. It may appear that women are less frequently diagnosed with schizophrenia and fare better when they do; instead, they may just experience fewer intense crises that come to the attention of public authorities or the general population.

Onset and Course of Illness

Schizophrenia manifests earlier in males than females: males in the midteens to very early twenties; females in the late teens to midtwenties. The onset may or may not be precipitated by a normalized stressful life event, such as a breakup of a close friendship or moving to a new school.

The three phases of schizophrenia are (1) prodromal, (2) active, and (3) remission. Schizophrenia is first manifested by a prodromal phase that can last an extended period of time, as long as 18 months. This first episode, lasting 1 month to 6 months, is diagnosed as schizophreniform disorder. During this time, the young person will often first show signs of social isolation, spending most of his time alone, and suspiciousness. He might be experiencing unusually low energy and may not sleep regularly. As an example, his thoughts might be hypervigilantly focused on proving a theory, such as "finding an apocalyptic theoretical cause for the recent year's extreme weather changes that erode the environment's sustainability." His sensory experiences become altered. His sense of taste is distorted and his explanation for this becomes "that someone is poisoning his food," causing him to eat less and lose weight and have new eating rituals. He may associate the "discovery of the apocalyptic theory to the group of people who want him dead, thus are poisoning his food."

Family members will reluctantly adjust to this new and unusual behavior, simultaneously making attempts to explain it, remedy it, and continue on with their daily lives. Explanations can include a mental health crisis or illicit drug use, among other ideas. Attempts to remedy may include seeing a physician, visiting with a religious leader, going to church more often, or finding alternate explanations through various amateur research methods. Because of the stigmatic nature of these behaviors, family members tend not to openly discuss this process with others, thus limiting incoming information and resources and increasing emotions like sadness, worry, and shame.

While in some cases the unusual behaviors and episodes can be tolerated and managed within the family, most cases ultimately come to the attention of public authority figures. At this crisis point, the individual will be taken to jail, a mental health center, or a hospital and receive a mental health evaluation of varying quality. This is a crucial point in accurate diagnosis and effective treatment delivery to ensure the individual does not blindly enter *The River* (see Preface for full explanation of *The River*).

Accepting the diagnosis of schizophrenia is often quite difficult for any young person, given the socially marginalizing stigma and poor prognosis in mental health settings, which are sustained by the media and social conversations. Often, after the young person is stabilized from the first psychotic episode, he is anxious to involve himself in normalized life as it were, and denial is heavily at play. The young person may turn or return to illicit drug use, especially marijuana, to relieve fear and worry. He will often dispose of the antipsychotic medications, as they cause uncomfortable side effects and are daily reminders of the illness. Resources are often not accessed. With just a little bit of stress, such as an argument, the young unstable person will often quickly experience another psychotic episode. If family is around, there is a good chance that family will know to immediately get the individual to mental health professionals for stabilization. Often, the young person will resist, knowing that psychotropic medication and social isolation are imminent. If behaviors become extreme and dangerous, he may be forcefully taken into custody, which is emotionally difficult on the individual, loved ones, and mental health professionals.

Over the years, the person will likely have psychotic episodes with varying intensity. As the person ages, has additional psychotic episodes, and takes psychotropic medications, negative psychotic symptoms may linger between intense episodes. Among individuals who have psychotic vulnerability, illicit drug use will bring on psychotic symptoms more intensely, rapidly, and frequently. Additionally, stress, disruptions in intimate relationships, medical problems, social isolation, and lack of meaningful purpose increase one's vulnerability for more psychotic episodes (Dunn, 2002).

Treatment Options

Mainstream public mental health treatment agencies focus on the administration of psychotropic medications for the treatment of schizophrenia. Upon the first episode, the lowest doses of psychotropic medications are indicated. Additional resources are strongly encouraged, including application for Social Supplemental Income (SSI) or Social Supplemental Disability Income (SSDI), state financial and medical benefits, supervised housing, supported employment, and a case manager, or point person, to coordinate all these resources. A great deal of *therapeutic* effort is put forth to ensure that the individual takes the psychotropic medication as prescribed (aka, *The River*).

As the person has multiple psychotic episodes, the illness is considered reoccurring or chronic. At this point, quality of care greatly varies, depending on community resources, SES, the individual's physical stature, and ethnicity/race of individual. In my experience, individuals who are identified as low SES, physically large in stature, or of color (especially African Americans and Latinos) receive the poorest prognosis for recovery and the highest doses of the cheapest antipsychotic medications. These medications may or may not be effective. Additionally, as symptom remission is not observed, higher doses and additional medications are almost always prescribed. First- and second-generation antipsychotic medications have serious unwanted side effects, including serious weight gain, sexual dysfunction, emotional numbness, drowsiness, dry mouth, muscle spasms, involuntary movements (tics or tremors), and restlessness. Because of this ineffective treatment pathway, many individuals will desperately seek relief through illicit drug use or even suicide.

Instead, outside of the mainstream public mental health treatment system, there are other effective options for the management of schizophrenia that result in increased quality of life. These options include supported education and employment that deliver an intentional sense of purpose and accomplishment, increased opportunities for socialization with people who may or may not experience mental illnesses, structure, and last but not least, the personal power of money. Many individuals who experience schizophrenia join peer-run empowerment groups, where the goals include peer support, public education, and advocacy. Many pharmaceutical prescribers (i.e., nurse practitioners, psychologists, and psychiatrists) work in close collaboration with their clients and are flexible about prescribing medications, which I term *conscious use of medication*. The ethical, conscious, effective use of medication includes taking into consideration the individual's perspective about which medications and dosages decrease symptoms with the fewest unwanted side effects. Likewise, listening to the individual regarding dose increases when he or she is experiencing higher levels of stress is also important. Individual and group psychotherapy have also shown to have quite favorable effects with individuals who experience symptoms of schizophrenia, and these quality-of-life efforts are further explored in Unit 3—"Ethical and Professional Obligations Impact Macro, Mezzo, and Micro Levels of Treatment Delivery."

SCHIZOAFFECTIVE DISORDER
Definition

Schizoaffective disorder is an SMI that encompasses both severe mood states (depression and/or mania) and experiences of positive psychosis. There are two dynamics that differentiate schizoaffective disorder from schizophrenia or from major depression with psychotic features. In schizoaffective disorder, (1) the symptoms of psychosis come first and *then* the mood severely shifts; and (2) after this decompensation episode, the executive functioning returns closer to baseline, or the previous functioning level, showing only a small amount of decreased functioning with each psychotic episode over the lifetime. Episodes consist of alternating between psychotic and severe mood alteration symptoms. One might think that having both a mood disorder and a psychotic disorder would more severely disrupt stable functioning, but, in reality, the prognosis for individuals with schizoaffective disorder is surprisingly better than for those with schizophrenia.

Scope

The prevalence of schizoaffective disorder is approximately 0.3% and about a third less than schizophrenia (Perälä et al., 2007).

Onset and Course of Illness

Similar to schizophreniform disorder and schizophrenia, the onset of schizoaffective disorder is in late adolescence and early adulthood in both women and men. Even without the use of illicit drugs, schizoaffective episodes can last for several months, upward of 6 months, and are longer than the schizophrenia episodes.

During early onset, the individual may experience more manic mood symptoms and episodes. During midlife and older adult years, the individual may experience more depressive mood symptoms and episodes. Because of the alternating mood and psychotic symptoms, the individual will experience a variety of diagnoses over a lifetime, sometimes being diagnosed with schizophrenia, sometimes bipolar disorder, and sometimes major depressive disorder. The more accurate diagnosis of schizoaffective disorder will not be given until later in life, when the episodic pattern emerges.

Treatment Options

Treatment options for schizoaffective disorder are much the same as for schizophrenia, with the focus primarily on prescribed consumption of psychotropic medications. Family therapy, including psychoeducation, also helps to increase communication and minimize distressing emotions. Thus, for additional quality-of-life efforts for individuals who are diagnosed with schizoaffective disorder, the following should be considered: supported education and employment, peer support and advocacy groups, psychotherapy, and flexible and ethical psychotropic medications administration. Unit III further elaborates on these effective and ethical quality-of-life efforts.

BRIEF PSYCHOTIC DISORDER
Definition

Brief psychotic disorder is the occurrence of psychotic symptoms (usually hallucinations, delusions, and/or disorganized speech and behavior) and persists for 1 day to less than a month. Brief psychotic disorder usually occurs as a reaction to an overwhelmingly stressful event (such as witnessing a fatal automobile accident), but not always.

Scope

Susser and Wanderling (1994) assert that brief psychotic disorder is more common in developing countries than developed countries and twice as common among females as males.

Onset and Course of Illness

Brief psychotic disorder can occur as early as adolescence and across the life span. By definition, following the episode, the individual's functioning will return to his or her premorbid level, and he or she may never experience another episode again, suggesting a favorable prognosis.

Treatment Options

Even for this anomalous disorder, mainstream mental health treatment will focus on the prescription of psychotropic medication. Even though, by definition, the episode will be brief, no one knows that until the termination of the episode. During this occurrence, the individual should be supervised and helped with activities of daily living (i.e., eating, dressing appropriately, etc.) and personal and public safety until stabilization is achieved. Inpatient psychiatric hospitalization may or may not be indicated to prevent self- and/or other harm and for stabilization. Brief talk therapy, where any trauma may be processed, also shows favorable results.

BIPOLAR DISORDER I
Definition

Bipolar disorder I is a psychiatric disorder that causes severe alterations in mood, which can be euphoric, irritable, or a combination. DSM and ICD diagnostic criteria assert that only a manic mood shift is required because if an individual is to experience mania, he or she will also, at some point, experience major or moderate depression. In the case of bipolar disorder I, it is important to note that psychotic symptoms present *only in the severe mood state* that occurs *after* the mood shifts. Additionally, the individual will feel rested after only a few hours of sleep or energetic without any sleep at all. In the manic phase, the individual will experience an increase in rapid and pressured speech, sociability, and goal-directed activity, often engaging in overlapping projects, as energy and creativity are peaked.

Scope

The prevalence of people who meet criteria for bipolar disorder I is approximately 2.4% of the world population and 4.4% in the United States, the highest frequency in the world (Merikangas et al., 2007). Additionally, the prevalence of this mood disorder affects men and women at the same rates, with women experiencing more depressive episodes.

Onset and Course of Illness

Bipolar disorder I manifests in early adulthood. Childhood manifestation is highly questionable and controversial. Mood shifts are episodic, meaning that they occur in a distinct time period, and without intervention, the mood will naturally stabilize over a 6- to 9-week period. The individual will experience shifts in energy level and mood, which can land a person in serious trouble, including disruptions in interpersonal relationships, spending money, sexual promiscuity, civil and criminal law violations, occupational hazards, and even harm to others or the self, especially when grandiosity is confronted. Illicit drug use, especially stimulants and alcohol, can mimic manic or depressive behaviors, causing over- or underdiagnosis. No two individuals will express the same mood shift pattern; however, over time, the individual will likely notice a pattern in his or her episodes. For example, for every three manic episodes, Jacob will then experience one depressive episode. As a result, Jacob has to experience many mood shifts before a repeatable and consistent pattern can be identified.

Treatment Options

Bipolar disorder I is almost unanimously considered a brain chemistry disorder. Mainstream public mental health treatment providers will prescribe mood-stabilizing medications. Many prescribers will assert that this medication must be taken, as prescribed, over the life span, while others state that early mood shift detection and intervention with medication is permissible until stabilization is reached.

Another adjunctive intervention to bipolar disorder I is interpersonal and social rhythm therapy (IPSRT), which has shown favorable prevention and early intervention results (Frank et al., 2005). The IPSRT efforts are to establish and maintain a regular interpersonal and social rhythm so that the brain has every chance to regulate its neurotransmitter metabolization by way of the circadian rhythm cycle.

DISSOCIATIVE IDENTITY DISORDER
Definition

Dissociative identity disorder (DID), formerly known as multiple personality disorder, is the most controversial mental illness that involves psychotic experiences. It is always caused by early, severe, and ongoing trauma or serious threat, almost always involving childhood sexual abuse, during which the child had no escape option (APA, 2013). The individual will have at least two, and likely many more, distinct personalities or alternative identities, known as *alters*, in addition to one main personal identity, known as the *core* or *host* personality. When the alters take over, the host personality will experience this as losing time, meaning, not being able to account for time and behavioral results, such as location, self-harm, environmental changes, and more. Seconds (suggesting transient dissociation) to weeks (suggesting more extreme impairment of DID) can be lost in one single episode (APA, 2013). Each alter has its own race, age, medical phenomena, speech patterns, mannerisms, cognitions, perceptions, and style, which are observable by others and the host personality. As emphasized with all these mentioned psychotic disorders, lost time and behaviors are *not* the result of drug use or medical condition, including seizure disorder. This disorder is very controversial because of the high rate of malingering attempts to decrease social and criminal accountability, suggesting, "the alter made me do it." An additional controversy involves suggestibility by the psychotherapist that may result in false memories. For these and other previously stated reasons, accurate diagnosis is essential.

Scope

Dissociative identity disorder is diagnosed 3–5 times more often in females than in males (Lynn et al., 2012). Also, DID accounts for 1%–3% of the general population and up to 20% in inpatient psychiatric populations (Spiegel et al., 2011).

Onset and Course of Illness

The first dissociative episodes often occur in early childhood, as early as 3 years old, during severe abusive episodes, when the individual adaptively disconnects from her body for physical survival. Common alters include, but are not limited to, stereotypical profiles: innocent and regressed child; rebellious/angry adolescent (aggressive/violent); person of God (nun, preacher, cleric); disabled, sick, or impaired one (blind, diabetic); person of altered gender (lesbian, transgendered); person of different race/ethnicity/culture (African American, French); protector (tough, confident, posturing); and sexually promiscuous (highly sexually active, prostitute), just to include a few. Individuals with DID usually experience impairment in social and intimate relationships, occupation and education disruptions, symptoms of self-harm, interpersonal retraumatization, and sometimes involvement with the legal system. A wide range of accurate diagnosis and effective treatment options exists for individuals who experience symptoms of DID. However, these individuals are often misdiagnosed with a variety of other disorders, including schizophrenia, before being accurately diagnosed with DID and offered effective treatment interventions.

Treatment Options

Most importantly, the treatment for DID is conducted in three phases: (1) safety and stabilization; (2) processing trauma and grieving; and (3) integration, fusion, and reconnection of personality states (Brand et al., 2012). There are no available medications that can treat the splitting off of conscious states. However, there are available psychotropic medications that treat the comorbid symptoms of DID, such as depression, anxiety, obsessive-compulsive symptoms, self-harm, and sleep disturbances. At times, individuals with DID require brief inpatient psychiatric hospitalization for safety and stabilization.

SUBSTANCE-INDUCED PSYCHOSIS
Definition

Some individuals will experience distressing and pervasive psychotic symptoms when illicit drugs are ingested, especially those in the stimulant or amphetamine (i.e., cocaine, crack cocaine, crystal methamphetamine) or hallucinogenic categories (LSD, bath salts, marijuana). By definition, the individual will not have experienced psychotic symptoms before drug ingestion. The individual may experience the psychotic symptoms during intoxication and/or drug withdrawal. Individuals may present themselves to a hospital or clinic for help or be taken into law enforcement custody while behaving uncivilly under the influence of the drug. Often times, when the drug effects wear off, the psychotic symptoms will remit. The individual who has a vulnerability to a psychotic disorder and misuses substances will almost always manifest symptoms of psychosis that can linger after substance misuse.

Scope

Frequency of drug use and misuse is almost impossible to accurately obtain, as individuals may avoid accurate reporting, fearing legal repercussions, resource denial, and social stigma/marginalization. The frequency of co-occurring disordered population varies from 35% to 100%, depending on population and data collection methods.

Onset and Course of Illness

Young people, adolescents, and young adults often turn to substance use and misuse to feel something different from what they are feeling, such as boredom, anger, despair, and loneliness. Illicit drug misuse often results in overall social impairment that impacts education, employment, social relationships (including family), physical health, finances, legal involvement, spirituality, housing, and mental health. The course of drug misuse may be continuous or intermittent with episodes of abstinence. Members of 12-step self-help communities assert that on a continued drug misuse path, one will eventually end up in jail, in institutions (such as physical or mental hospitals), or dead. Whether true or not, many individuals who find themselves misusing drugs and making their way to jails and institutions end up with an inaccurate diagnosis of schizophrenia.

Treatment Options

For an accurate diagnosis to be made, a comprehensive assessment must be conducted. Within that comprehensive assessment, a drug screen is conducted by way of blood or urine. With illicit drugs in the body, an accurate diagnosis is nearly impossible. Hence, without an accurate mental health diagnosis, deciding on a course of effective interventions may also be a significant challenge. In the case of the individual who presents to a clinic, experiencing hallucinations and responding to them, whether drug induced or not, will immediately be evaluated for safety. Some individuals will be legally held against their will, either immediately in the evaluation setting or for an extended period of time on the inpatient hospital unit, until the effect of the drugs abate. Others who do not meet legal hold requirements will be offered addiction and/or mental health treatment, including evaluation for psychotropic medications.

DISCUSSION

Diagnostic errors contribute to the overdiagnosis of schizophrenia. As we have reviewed, many valid scenarios may explain the experience of positive psychotic symptoms. Among those previously outlined in this section, additional valid psychiatric diagnoses that involve psychotic symptoms include borderline personality disorder and post-traumatic stress disorder. Substance overuse and withdrawal are highly representative of positive psychotic symptoms. Unfortunately, all too often, when a young person (less than 40 years old) presents with positive psychotic symptoms to medical and mental health professionals, this person is frequently hastily diagnosed with schizophrenia. Yet, the common treatment modality for schizophrenia is significant and life altering, so, as with any change in mental status, prudent diagnosis is essential.

A diagnosis implies both cause and treatments. If the identifying cause is not accurate, an accurate and effective treatment will not ensue, and the default treatment of psychotropic medications will, again, be pushed. Consequently, if the treatment is not accurate, to what extent will the symptoms be resolved? What iatrogenic symptoms (symptoms caused by treatment-related trauma) will develop as a result of the inaccurate treatments, especially psychotropic medications? Furthermore, when a person is diagnosed with any mental illness, self-identity and functioning are altered, regardless of the disease process and as a result of social interactions that occur based on the impact of mental illness stigma and prejudice. More specifically, when a person is inaccurately diagnosed with schizophrenia, the person may begin to incorporate what he or she believes about the low capacities of people with schizophrenia, often including myths that he or she has learned from the media, society, and mental health professionals. He or she might follow his or her intuition and deny treatment, which might be lifesaving; lower his or her expectations for his or her life and feel entitled to social supports for people with schizophrenia, including SSI, state funding, supportive housing, reduced-fee public transportation cards; and, most importantly, lower his or her own life dreams and accountability. Many people who internalize these low self-standards turn to alcohol and street drugs to numb their existential pain. Low expectations lead to low quality of life, severe depression, and even early death. Beyond these personal reflections of low expectations, common myths held by both some mental health clinicians and the general public perpetuate these negative standards and affect the individual's quality of life.

Common Myths About People Who Experience Symptoms of Psychosis

Common myths exist about people who experience positive symptoms of psychosis. These myths are delivered to the general public through media, family members of people who experience symptoms of psychosis, and, surprisingly, seasoned mental health treatment delivery professionals. This section details some of the most prevalent erroneous myths about psychosis.

Myth 1: People who are psychotic do not know what is going on around them. They are just crazy.

This myth is commonly used to describe many vulnerable populations, including people who experience psychosis, children, and elderly persons. In fact, if the truth is to be known in a family, who is asked? The youngest member is asked because he or she is not yet socialized to keep secrets. How many times has the mother flinched as her toddler loudly and innocently asks, "Mama, why is she so fat?" The elderly person often speaks the truth because, by this age, he or she is no longer attached and guided by interpersonal threats such as shame, dishonor, and excommunication of exposing a family secret. The person with the psychotic disorder will often speak the truth because, for better or worse, the filtering mechanism or repression barrier that edits the conscious and unconscious thoughts is compromised. As a matter of fact, the person with the psychotic disorder is extremely sensitive to what is going on around them. These senses are almost too loud; even smells, temperature, and interpersonal dynamics can be overwhelming. Because of the dynamics of the thought disorder, these sensations may tell the truth, but the conclusions made about the origin of this truth or other impacts may result in an alternative explanation. Let us consider the following examples to further illustrate this point.

You Have Huge Teeth

Deborah, a 34-year-old female, who had been diagnosed with schizophrenia, was sitting in her daily group therapy session at an inpatient psychiatric hospital, where she had been for 7 days. There were two therapists in the group. One therapist was making long-winded attempts to explain a concept but was talking *at* the group members, rather than engaging and interacting with them. When Deborah was called on to share, all she could say was, "Teeth." The second therapist curiously probed, asking Deborah to elaborate. Deborah reported, "She has huge teeth." Upon further exploration, what Deborah really meant to say was this: "The first therapist is talking so much, and I feel alienated. All I experience are her huge teeth smacking together. I feel powerless and chewed up by the first therapist." As anyone might feel when listening to someone drone on and on, Deborah was simply expressing her annoyance in the manner she was able.

A New Kind of Loneliness, All Over Again

A week after the terrorist attacks on the New York City's World Trade Centers, I walked to my office in a bustling area of downtown Chicago. Each time I passed, I saw the same tattered woman, holding a sign reading "Homeless" and a cup, asking for money outside a McDonald's restaurant. Most of the time, this woman seemed *out of it*, as she was introverted and often seemed to be having conversations with herself.

   She was very thin, hunched over, and unkempt. Seeing that every single person in the United States of America was impacted by these terrorist attacks, I wanted to know the impact of 9/11 on *this* woman. Because I have a personal policy of not giving money to people on the street, I purchased a McDonald's meal for her. I gently approached her, respecting her space. I introduced myself and requested her permission to ask a question. I let her know that I was not representing a church or religion and was not trying to push anything on her. I told her that I would like to offer her the McDonald's bag of food to show my appreciation for talking with me. While she listened attentively, she responded by saying, "I don't eat that shit!" She began rambling about megaphones and being "brainwashed by the Popular Party." Sensing that she did not wish to have any further conversation with me, I thanked her for her time and walked away. I got about four steps away when I heard her holler, "Hey you! What was your question anyway?"

   Feeling inspired, I turned around and saw her looking in my direction. I returned to her, explained the basis of my question, and asked her how *she* was impacted by the terrorist attacks. She was engaged and paused with reflection. She said to me, "Look around here. What do you see?" After my own contemplation, I told her that I saw a lot of people hurrying around. She said, "What was the first thing you did when you heard of the attacks?" I told her that I called my family. She said, "That's what I thought. Well, I don't have a family to call. Those attacks made me feel a new kinda loneliness, all over again."

I was stunned at her profound and generous honesty and insight. We talked further, but only just for a moment. I thanked her for sharing with me and said I would watch for her as I came down this street, as I do most days. We shared a brief and meaningful connection. As I got about four steps away again, she hollered out, "Hey! What's in that bag anyway?" She accepted the McDonald's bag of food. I saw this woman many more times, and each time, we knowingly acknowledged one another. She was a woman with psychotic experiences *and* she was also a woman with incredible presence and insight. When acknowledged, this presence and insight was readily accessible, and the only hindrance to her communicating in this way was the way in which she'd been socially marginalized by the outside world.

> Myth 2: People who are experiencing psychotic symptoms do not have the capacity to be involved in meaningful relationships.

This erroneous myth is derived from Freud's psychoanalytic theory, in which he concluded that people who experience psychosis are *untreatable* (Freud, 1914, 1925, p. 59). While flawed, the foundation of Freud's logic was that the operational intervention in psychoanalysis was to resolve the transference reaction. (Transference reactions are when an individual treats another person as though they were someone from their meaningful past, such as a mother who was generously nurturing or a previous coworker who was passive-aggressive). It was erroneously believed that people who experience positive symptoms of psychosis were not capable of meaningful interpersonal relationships; therefore, transference never developed and, consequently, could not be resolved. According to Freud, the ensuing reality would, thus, be that there was nothing to treat.

Fromm-Reichmann asserted that we do not know the capacity of functioning in people with psychosis because the appropriate treatment has not been offered (1960). It is not that people with psychosis are untreatable, as Freud erroneously postulated; rather, the mental health field has not offered accurate and effective treatments. As a result, people with psychotic experiences who have digressed, despite treatment, and continued to feel harsh rejection from family, friends, and society often go inward for self-protection. Additionally, Fromm-Reichmann asserted that people with psychosis are exceptionally sensitive to the dynamics of interpersonal relationships (Fromm-Reichmann, 1960). *Going inward* is a defense mechanism that could easily be viewed and handled as transference, as being guarded with everyone is a prejudice based on negative experiences with one or more persons. What if Freud had recognized this? The truth is that people who experience symptoms of mental illness are exquisitely sensitive to relationships and often become introverted to avoid intrapsychic pain that results from interpersonal rejection. Accurate and effective treatments give hibernated souls a ripe environment in which to become awake and involved in a self-determined life worth living.

> Myth 3: Psychotherapy does not work with people who have severe
> and persistent mental illness.

For what purposes does anyone seek psychotherapy services? Many people seek consultation from a psychotherapist to help connect the psychological dots, which are important early life moments that have impact on and manifest into the conscious and unconscious through symptoms and defenses, such as the dynamic of retreating from trust and collaboration. Another reason people see a therapist is to relieve conscious and unconscious distress from past or current trauma and meaningful losses, to which people who experience psychosis are also subject. Here, the therapeutic relationship welcomes and attends to these strong feelings that may not otherwise be addressed in even close interpersonal relationships, including intense hopelessness and despair, which, among people who experience psychosis, often drastically result in suicide attempts Palmer, Pankratz, & Bostwick (2005). So, if the sharing of these feelings and past traumas is encouraged for those who are not experiencing psychosis, why is this level of sharing and connecting of psychological dots not encouraged, or even accepted, from those who are? Within a therapeutic relationship, an individual, including people who live with psychotic experiences, can learn adaptive coping skills to manage and respond to general and unique life challenges, and both populations should be given the opportunity to do so.

Grace's Boyfriend Is a Government Spy

Grace was a 24-year-old female who was psychiatrically hospitalized because she believed her boyfriend was a spy for a government agency who was trying to kill her. She repeatedly had the feeling that "he was not really who he presented himself to be." As it turned out, her devoted boyfriend was secretly seeing another woman. Grace could sense that his demeanor was different and there was something undisclosed, yet her thought-disordered brain could not logically make sense of her own intuitive thoughts. Her conclusion was that her boyfriend was a spy and trying to kill her.

In the process of psychotherapy, where Grace spoke about her strong intuitive thoughts and brainstormed about possible logical conclusions, she arrived at the idea that her boyfriend, indeed, had another side to him; he was secretly cheating on their committed relationship. While she felt as though this would kill her spirit, it did not. Through psychotherapy and expressing her thoughts and feelings, she realized the accurate truth that was presently occurring and made a choice about what to do. She chose to end the relationship. With this decision and action, she felt incredibly empowered. Psychotherapy was very beneficial in helping Grace arrive at an accurate conclusion about her intuitive senses, and she was supported in her decision to honor herself by ending a relationship with someone who could not be honest with her.

Myth 4: The intimate and emotionally charged conversations that typically occur within a psychotherapeutic relationship should be avoided because they will cause the already vulnerable psychotic person to digress and experience life disruptions.

This myth is common within the clinical realm of mental health treatment. Talking about difficult situations and painful affects can leave any person more psychologically vulnerable to the vicissitudes of his or her emotions. Winnicott (1963) asserted that having a psychotic episode is one of the most authentic experiences a person could have because the true self and true feelings cannot help but to be revealed. Among people whose repression barrier is already thin, as with people who have psychotic experiences, words are said and actions are carried out, for better or worse.

Show Me My Death Certificate

Linda spent her days searching for "proof that she was, indeed, dead." Regularly, she visited the public library and City Vital Records Department to scour the obituaries. Her family insisted that she be evaluated by a mental health professional. As soon as the details of Linda's delusion were gathered in the assessment, no clinician would speak to her about the belief that she was dead for fear it would contribute to her further psychological and functional decompensation. In Linda's situation, emergency medication evaluation became the initial intervention for the purpose of quickly decreasing or removing the delusions.

When Linda stated she was not interested in taking psychiatric medications, everything about her case was dropped because the clinicians assumed she was not interested in mental health treatment. However, Linda was never asked about other types of mental health services, including psychotherapy. No one talked with Linda about what being dead or the method in which she died might mean to her.

Indeed, experiencing oneself as dead is an extremely strong feeling. Upon exploration, Linda would likely have expressed strong emotions, including despair resulting from hopelessness for a better life and rage at the world (and maybe some individuals) for pushing her into this bleak place. Those strong feelings would likely need to be identified, validated, addressed, and worked through over time. It might well be that Linda would need a higher level of support and care, possibly including brief psychiatric hospitalization, while working through these strong emotions. Mainstream mental health clinicians have been overly socialized to avoid psychiatric hospitalization at all costs. Furthermore, there are additional means of higher-level support and supervision than just acute inpatient hospitalization, including more frequent outpatient visits with a mental health clinician and respite care, which is often staffed with some or all peer workers (people with lived experience). Linda might also benefit from support to spiritually revive her spirit in creating a self-determined life worth living, including establishing meaningful relationships, creating meaningful daily structure, and identifying and nurturing some individual dreams for herself. Without addressing Linda's experience of being dead, she is left vulnerable to her delusion and society's rejecting response.

People who experience symptoms of psychosis do indeed have conscious and unconscious distress. However, rarely are these people helped with the strong and distressing feelings they experience; thus, layers of all types of losses accumulate and reoccur, leaving the person more and more vulnerable to dissociation via psychotic episodes. The truth is that these exploratory therapeutic conversations *will* stir a person, with or without psychotic vulnerability. With appropriate support during these important and intimate conversations, growth can transform a person into a state of "weller than well" (Menniger, 1963, p. 406).

Another benefit of traditional psychotherapy, or facilitating sensitive and meaningful conversations, is to facilitate the comprehensive, smooth, veridical (truthful), and linear integration of important events into one's personal meaning system, self-esteem, and identity. Examples of these important and precipitating events include customary developmental milestones, such as transitioning to high school; losses, such as separation of families; or traumatic experiences, such as sexual abuse or witnessing family members in the process of addiction. Without this work, people with psychotic vulnerabilities often take these important personal experiences and manifest these experiences into persecutory hallucinations or delusions. An example of this is the following story.

Not Too Close, I Smell Bad

At the young age of 5, Amy's uncle masturbated to the point of ejaculation on her body. As an adult, Amy has an olfactory hallucination that her body is emitting an offensive smell. Without addressing this hallucination, Amy was left even more vulnerable from the haunting experience and social marginalization, as she would, at all costs, avoid physical and interpersonal contact so that no one would "discover her odor." We can understand Amy's delusion as the experience of being sexually abused being manifested in a psychotic symptom.

If Amy's clinician took her symptom as merely a hallucination stemming from schizophrenia, he or she would simply prescribe psychotropic medication and would likely never understand what the meaning of the smell in Amy's life. If Amy were willing to process this trauma, in time, she could be liberated from it. However, it is noteworthy that not everyone is interested in addressing and revisiting past traumatic situations, no matter how supportive the clinician.

When an individual experiences an acute psychotic episode, at best, mainstream mental health clinicians hope that a psychotic episode will never happen again. And if psychotic symptoms do reemerge, the person is given psychotropic medication for the purpose of quieting or stopping the symptoms. The truth is that psychotherapy can and should be offered to people who experience positive symptoms of psychosis in lieu of, or at least in conjunction with, an accurate dosage of medication. The focus of psychotherapy with people who experience psychosis is really no different than it is with people who do not experience psychosis.

To curb the self-protective act of internal reclusion performed by most persons with psychosis who have been rejected, ensuring that this person has at least one veridical, safe, and trusted relationship will provide him or her with ripe opportunities for coming out of hibernation and fostering a framework for a collaborative professional therapeutic alliance built on trust, respect, compassion, authenticity, and affection. Through the dynamics of this therapeutic relationship, the person is offered the space to reflect, realize, and experience choice in how conscious and unconscious defenses and behaviors impact interpersonal relationships and his or her quality of life, which can reduce future losses and acute psychotic episodes and profoundly increase quality of life.

Myth 5: Psychotic behavior is mysterious and bizarre and is not meant to be understood.

Because of the effects of thought disorder, which are elaborated on in Chapter 7, "The Relationship Between Neurobiology and Psychosis," under the influence of psychosis, language is often communicated in disarray, which is termed *schizophasia* (Berrios, 1999). People who live with psychotic disorders communicate stories that consist of themes including magic, evil, deception, and persecution. Whole conversations are often strung together, connected only by loose associations. Desperate affect punctuates the stories. At first listen, schizophasia is not comprehensible, and as a result, this language is often dismissed. In conversation and in behavior, because of the brain functioning of a person who is experiencing symptoms of psychosis, sometimes the particular desired word cannot be accessed, termed *aphasia*. All language and behavior are attempts to communicate. As such, the person will choose a similar word or phrase instead. Sentence structure is often intact, meaning there is proper use of subjects and verbs. One has to carefully listen and broaden his or her referential thinking to understand what is being said. The truth is, as these clinical skills are applied to the person communicating in *schizophasia*, the person's communications become more decipherable.

The Rabbit Needs a Job

Aaron is a 32-year-old man living in a locked residential psychiatric treatment facility. The groups are often canceled, leaving the disappointed residents with unstructured and purposeless time. Aaron, the energetic man mutters as he paces the halls, "The rabbit needs a job." What is the meaning behind what Aaron is saying? Aaron is saying that he has a lot of energy and motivation, like a rabbit has, and needs a job that results in rewards, such as meaning, purpose, and, possibly, money. To accurately understand Aaron's communications, one could ask him if this is what he meant to say, verifying his communications. At this point, Aaron would have the opportunity to agree or disagree and make the necessary contextual corrections.

Additionally, Sullivan (1947) asserted that when a person who is experiencing psychosis is observed, his or her actions are often only viewed through the current and present environment, which frequently does not explain his or her behavioral and emotional reactions. Instead, Sullivan suggests that the individual be viewed through a lens in which his or her environmental context, including seen and unseen people, places, and situations, is considered to understand his or her current emotional state.

No Privacy

Susan, a 42-year-old woman diagnosed with schizophrenia, was walking down a busy street screaming and gesturing with her arms. After doing a quick visual sweep, it did not appear that anyone was with Susan. In Susan's life earlier that day, she had argued with her roommate and was taking a walk to burn off some steam. She was especially bothered by this argument because it was about her roommate borrowing her belongings from her room without her permission. Also noteworthy is the fact that Susan grew up in a home with two bedrooms and one bathroom that nine people shared. She often experienced a living situation with no privacy, and people were always borrowing her belongings, leaving her frequently feeling frustrated, disappointed, and helpless. Sullivan suggests that if we could redraw Susan's environment system boundary to include even one more layer to include the people and situations in her day-to-day life, we would understand her seemingly bizarre behavior.

Fromm-Reichmann (1960) states that people who experience psychosis feel the same quality of affect that others feel, just bigger. In Susan's example, while some could shake off this conflict, the tension consumed her. She had grown up in an environment where her space, privacy, and resources were always threatened. Her roommate borrowing her things stimulated this deep and long-standing vulnerability. She felt as if her boundaries were exploited and physical integrity and trust were not respected. Susan's experience is easily understood when her story is placed in the context of her early family life and, now, similar living situation with her roommate. Anyone living in this sort of unstable and untrustworthy situation would be frustrated, as well.

Myth 6: Only social supportive interventions should be used with people who experience psychotic symptoms.

This concept has unnecessarily low expectations of the person, is patronizing, and reduces the person to a childlike caricature. Yet, the recovery model suggests that when a person pursues high-risk behavior, such as seeking employment, a high level of support may be needed. Exploring subjective meaning is deeply liberating and can, indeed, be conducted with persons who experience psychosis, especially within the active psychotic episode, when the repression barrier is thinner and the person is in significant emotional distress. The truth is that traditional psychotherapy can and should be offered to and used with people who experience positive psychotic symptoms. Just like any other population, some people want to dig deep, explore, and understand their unconscious motives, whereas others simply are not wired that way and are not prepared to participate in that kind of work. Psychotherapy for people with psychotic experiences should always be offered as an option, and the option to not pursue psychotherapy should also be respected.

Myth 7: People who experience psychosis are violent and dangerous.

This myth has been especially propagated by media stories that highlight mass public gun violence. The certainty of this myth among the American general population has nearly doubled from the 1950s to 1996 and more since then (Link, Phelan, Bresnahan, Stueve, & Pescosolido, 1999).

A small percentage of people who experience persecutory paranoid delusions and auditory hallucinations that command violent behavior do act on these delusions. Very often, the individuals with these daunting psychotic symptoms are additionally under the influence of illicit drugs, such as alcohol, crystal methamphetamine, cocaine, or crack. These individuals are the minority compared with the population of all people who have a mental illness. According to Friedman (2006), "most who are violent are not mentally ill and most people who are mentally ill are not violent" (p. 14).

Studies consistently show that people who experience psychosis are more likely to harm themselves (i.e., suicide) and not others or are the victims and not perpetrators of violent crimes (Hiday, Swartz, Swanson, Borum, & Wagner, 1999; Hiroeh, Appleby, Mortensen, Dunn, 2001; Stuart, 2003). For instance, many people who live with mental illness are more vulnerable to crime because of their limited finances and the necessary housing situations they are forced into, such as transient or poverty-affected neighborhoods. These areas leave people who live with mental illness caught in scenarios where they are the victims of criminal or violent behavior or the unintentional perpetrators of hazardous behavior or acts of crime toward others.

Myth 8: Only psychotropic medication can decrease psychotic behavior.

This concept exemplifies how psychotropic medication is overvalued and overused. For some individuals, medications can significantly decrease both positive and negative psychotic symptoms and should not be overlooked, but psychotropic medications should also be considered as merely *part* of the treatment, if at all, and not the exclusive solution. Psychotropic medications are not without risks and come with numerous serious and unwanted side effects.

Psychiatrists are informally considered the top of the mental health chain of command. Because neurobiology and psychopharmacology are the primary foci of the field of psychiatry, psychiatrists and their historical overvaluation of psychotropic medication influence almost all other mental health professional disciplines. The interesting question is this: Why are the conclusions of psychiatry passively followed without question or without influence from other mental health practitioners and their professional perspectives? Upon my own reflection, I am reminded of attempts to challenge this psychotropic medication-only perspective. Some individual psychiatrists are open to other explanatory perspectives and interpretations, whereas others may respond demeaningly and dismissively. These responses may be attempts to invalidate other mental health professions as a way of protecting the status of psychiatry. Additionally, some individual psychiatrists will simply and overtly refuse to engage in conversations in which other explanatory perspectives are discussed. Since psychiatrists culturally hold the most authority in the mental health professional team approach, their opinions are often the final word and impact everyone else's perspectives, including those of patients. The following adage comes to mind. "If you cannot beat them, join them." When the authoritarian holds the belief that psychotropic medications are the only intervention to treat psychotic symptoms, this belief becomes mainstream for all others. Why is the field of psychiatry so vehemently defended? At the very least, there seems to be a fragility that must be defended.

Just as there is a pecking order in the world and every subgroup, there is one also in the field of medicine. I have personally heard conversations, on a few occasions, from medical physicians referring to psychiatrists as the lowest on this physician pecking order, saying, "Let a REAL doctor manage this medical crisis." The neurobiological theory that purports to explain the cause of mental illness, suggested David Healy in his book *The Creation of Psychopharmacology*, was embraced by psychiatrists because it "set the stage" for them "to become real doctors" (2002, p. 217). This theory allowed psychiatrists to be viewed as practicing hard science with a specialization. Prescribing psychotropic medication became what legitimized them in an extremely competitive scientific field. Robert Whitaker and Lisa Cosgrove (2015), in their book *Psychiatry Under the Influence: Institutional Corruption, Social Injury, and Prescriptions for Reform*, as well as other writers, scientifically questioned psychiatry's mantras and assumptions about the connection between mental illness causation and brain chemistry inevitably leading to the conclusion that medication is the only option. Stability and sustainability of the field of psychiatry are indeed in question, because if we take away the focus on medication, the strength of the field of psychiatry goes away.

A more patient-focused question would be, "What additional health risks (such as an increased risk for cardiac disease, stroke, and serious weight gain) could result from long-term psychotropic medication use?" This is a very serious question to ask. The Hippocratic oath that all physicians, including psychiatrists, commit to asserts that the physician will not cause harm or damage, and when unknowingly done, this practice will not be repeated. Large doses and long-term use of psychotropic medications contribute to serious medical problems, including diabetes, high blood pressure, heart disease, and kidney disease, and a large number of acute and serious side effects, such as extrapyramidal symptoms, including muscle contractions, restlessness, tremors, and systematic tics in the facial muscles, mouth, and fingers (Gardos & Cole, 1977; Whitaker, 2011).

Psychotropic medications save some people's lives. However, psychotropic medications are overvalued and overprescribed as a quick fix for the intervention and treatment of positive and negative psychotic symptoms. Additionally, many people who manifest psychotic symptoms are snowed or heavily sedated with psychotropic medications. While heavy sedation is necessary for individuals who pose an imminent threat to self and others, there is no true indication, and, in fact, much to point to the contrary in my experience, that heavy sedation helps manage loss or traumatic experiences. The overuse of these medications is very commonly reported by individuals who receive them as an additional layer of trauma (iatro-genic trauma). These psychotropic medications are often received out of one's own control or choice, have severe and altering aftereffects, render a person helpless, and are experienced as a violation of one's own dignity.

The use of psychotropic medications is not the only way to reduce psychotic symptoms. Clinicians, including psychiatrists, who apply these concepts of *Listening with Psychotic Ears* in their clinical work with individuals who experience psychosis can and do give testimony, time and again, to how closely listening to, staying committed to the well-being of, and clarifying and verifying interpretations with the person who is actively experiencing psychosis can, without medications, immedi-ately reduce both positive and negative psychotic symptoms. On multiple occasions, I have witnessed people come out of psychotic experiences with only close clinical work with a clinician without medications.

Furthermore, there is a portion of the population of people who experience pos-itive psychotic symptoms who do not respond to any type of psychotropic medica-tion. This is because the origin of psychosis lies in the meaning system, or psychology of the person's mind, and not with brain chemistry or brain tissue. Thus, we consider the following question: What effective and humane symptom-relieving options are considered for people who do not respond to medications? For this population, other methods of management and intervention are obligatory. *Listening with Psychotic Ears* is an effective and humane option for healing, understanding, and accepting psychotic experiences. Personal testimonies reflect these results. All of this discussion is not to say that psychotropic medications are not useful in some respect, and more on their usefulness in congruence with other therapeutic approaches will be discussed in later chapters.

FINAL THOUGHTS

There are several symptoms of psychosis, and these symptoms manifest in a va-riety of ways. Although many of these experiences are similar within the different conditions, the manner in which people experiencing psychosis are treated should not be standardized. Medication and the perpetuation of stigmatizing myths hinder effective and successful development of treatment options, and new ways of addressing the unique aspects of psychosis should be incorporated and respected to achieve a positive quality of life.

2

Traumatized by "Treatment"

ANTHROPOLOGICAL AND SOCIAL INTERACTIONAL

PERSPECTIVES OF THE PERSON WHO LIVES

WITH PSYCHOSIS

WHY IS IT that a person with symptoms of psychosis can often be spotted in a crowd? Why do people with symptoms of psychosis tend to severely isolate themselves from others? What environmental factors and systematic experiences have contributed to the person's decline in functioning and quality of subjective experience? Why is receiving treatment for a mental illness so very different from receiving treatment for cancer or a cardiac condition? Why do most people who have been diagnosed with a mental illness live a quality of life that is well below the poverty rate? Why can most states in America claim that their jails are the largest mental health treatment providers in their state and in the country? These provocative questions raise concern about the poor quality of life for people who live with psychosis and the social and anthropological influences that paved this unnecessarily bleak path.

Throughout history, people with mental illness have been deeply discredited and written off by society. Acknowledging these behaviors and asking these questions will cause any caring and conscientious person to take notice of the afflicted and the issues that people who live with psychosis endure. So, what is it that causes this group to be treated so differently than the rest of the human population?

Social anthropology and social interactional theory facilitate the understanding of these phenomena by use of language that underscores the perspectives of those with mental illness. From this perspective, we find the veridical truth and become aware of how interactions with others, including therapists, psychiatrists, case managers, family, and the general public, lead to the beliefs and behaviors experienced by individuals who experience symptoms of psychosis. Thus, social anthropology allows us to study mental illness from the perspective of the other side of the same coin—from the patient's perspective.

Erving Goffman, one of the most important sociologists of the 20th century, studied observable, everyday human social interactions, especially around people with mental illness. In 1961, Goffman conducted ethnographic studies of the notorious St. Elizabeth's Hospital, funded by the National Institutes on Mental Health (NIMH). This work led to the publication *Asylums: Essays on the Social Situation of Mental Patients and Other Inmates*, which has become one of the most influential texts in sociology. Goffman begins by identifying populations, including mental patients, who have been marginalized and discredited as worthless by society (1961). In the name of civilization, these individuals have been deemed to have something unremittingly wrong with them or have consciously done something extremely and unforgivably atrocious. Simply looking closer at these assumptions shows us the inherent need of society to categorize people who are different and even label those we do not understand as dangerous. Yet, for people experiencing symptoms of psychosis, unless evidence of the contrary exists, what reprehensible deed have they committed except having the misfortune of experiencing severe trauma or alternative brain functioning? Rather than pigeonhole these individuals into a *deviant* box, why not offer our humane, neighborly compassion to people who experience psychosis, as we would any other person we encounter who is suffering in some way?

Taking the suffering of another into consideration requires much compassion, and the process can be overwhelming for some. One might ask, "How do I hold compassion for a group of suffering people AND continue to check off the many task-oriented items on my never-ending to-do list?" "How do I acknowledge the extreme loneliness of those with mental illness and then go about my day as usual, picking up the children from school and getting supper together?" As a society, continuously expressing compassion for this seemingly burdensome population is difficult. The strain is often too much for the usual mind and heart to bear, and many do not have the scope to comprehend how every aspect of a person's quality of life is altered because of psychiatric symptoms that cannot be willed away.

Instead of learning about and addressing the impact that distressing events and subjective experiences have on people's lives, what most often quickly and unconsciously occurs are avoidant or self-brainwashing tactics that categorize this individual into a more digestible perspective (Goffman, 1961). Removing his or her humanity and sense of uniqueness objectifies the person. We sweepingly assign labels, categories, and identities, such as *the mentally ill* or, more commonly, *crazy person*. The act of objectifying creates interpersonal distance from others so the person's suffering does not distract us. The US military banks on this phenomenon and trains combat soldiers to view the enemy as "an evil that must be banished" to protect the country and its family values (Coll, Weiss, & Exum, 2010). A sense of *he is not like me* arises. With physical and psychological distance and less social interaction, we have fewer opportunities to check out and debunk these myths through natural interactions and connections with others who are unlike us.

What happens, instead, is that the unknown becomes synonymous with the few related stories that are heard. Overgeneralization becomes easy, and additional erroneous myths, such as *all people with mental illness are unpredictable and without boundaries, and they will hurt you if you get too close,* become standard beliefs. As people blindly believe inaccurate myths like these and others, it is easy for even deeply connected people to follow the flawed and reductionist logic that *all people who experience psychosis are incompetent, and must be completely cared for.*

When people come face to face with something or someone they do not understand, a common reaction is fear. The causes and treatments of psychosis are not well understood; thus, there is a lot of fear toward people who live with psychosis. Some people unfoundedly worry that they can *catch* symptoms of psychosis, as one might catch tuberculosis. Another misconception is that people working with clients with mental illness must be doing so because they have a personal experience with mental illness, such as themselves or a family member. The inclination is to assume that the origin of a worker's sense of compassion and commitment toward seemingly undeserving individuals with mental illness must be due to a personal plight and not simply because the individual cares about this population. Granted, a person who had a family member die of cancer is often moved to commit her career or finances to the exploration and treatment of cancer. However, few question whether scientists and researchers who are devoted to cancer discoveries have cancer or a family member with cancer. These professionals are lauded for the dedication to eradicating this devastating illness, including the development of unconventional and experimental treatments.

Naturally, workers sometimes have emotional reactions to the extreme and pervasive suffering that their clients experience. In their early training, many mental healthcare professionals report experiencing nightmares about the traumatic situations that their clients have discussed. In his or her nonworking hours, the worker may ruminate about wanting to provide a client the resources that are needed. New workers may be sensitive about destigmatizing mental illness and may perceive things more personally than is warranted. These effects may be manifestations of secondary trauma, to which all healthcare workers are quite vulnerable.

Secondary trauma for mental healthcare professionals is natural, common, and resolvable. However, the healing process requires the worker to face psychological pain, which may be an overwhelmingly difficult task for some. In these cases, it is common that the worker will create distance with the client and others that remind him of his original psychological pain, all the while continuing in the worker role. This process is unfortunate for both the worker and the client because the worker will have unresolved pain, which can lead to more interpersonal pain. Furthermore, since the relationship is the conduit for the healing process, if the relationship is strained, so is the healing process. Too often, the client has become used to people being interpersonally distant with her, so she does not protest by asking for, or demanding, the worker's full attention. People with mental illness get used to unengaged and unresponsive mental health workers, as this is all too common. Thus, the cycle continues, with the health worker not facilitating much therapeutic progress and the people with mental illness continuing to suffer.

Are these the values and principles we want driving our mainstream mental health treatment system? How well is this working? Robert Whitaker offers the following facts: "In 1955, 1 in every 468 Americans was hospitalized (usually long term) due to a mental illness. In 1987, when Prozac was made publically available, there were 1.25 million people receiving an SSI or SSDI payment because they were disabled by mental illness, or 1 in every 184 Americans" (2011, p. 6). In 2007, this population was 3.97 million (1 in 76), and in 2011, approximately 4.5 million Americans received SSI and SSDI because of mental illness disability (Whitaker, 2011). With these outcome statistics, despite the development and availability of so many new, *promising* psychotropic medications, one cannot help but acknowledge the obvious failure of mainstream public mental health treatment in the United States.

CABRINI-GREEN HOMES

Cabrini-Green Homes, a housing project operated by Chicago Housing Authority and one of the most impoverished and notoriously crime-ridden housing projects in the United States, was, at its peak, home to 15,000 residents (Saulny, 2007). This community was located near downtown Chicago, Illinois, and less than a mile from a well-known teaching hospital, where I worked for almost 12 years. These housing projects were rat and cockroach infested, and trash would sometimes back up in the garbage chutes, reaching as high as the 15th floor. The toilets would often back up, windows were broken, elevators were often not working, and both the heat and water were often out of order. The environment was so depraved that the tenants could not dial 911 and expect the Chicago Police Department to respond. Instead, they had their own police squad, which had a reputation for being corrupt and self-serving.

There are many stories of strength and hope that come out of Cabrini-Green Public Housing Homes, but even these narratives are bursting with beastly situations and dynamics that most other Americans do not ever have to endure. When these residents had medical or psychiatric crises, they would come to the medical facility where I worked for almost 12 years, and I saw these citizens on a regular basis. The stories were consistent. Almost every woman I spoke with who grew up in the Cabrini-Green Homes told a similar story of experiencing multiple sexual assaults, beginning at an early age. Almost every person was closely related to individuals who experienced severe addiction, physical abuse, unreported gang violence and murder, parental abandonment, disrupted family relationships, frequent gunshot wounds, extreme poverty, suicide, violent death, and preventable accidents and illnesses that caused severe alterations in quality of life (i.e., gunshot wounds causing paralysis; amputation of toes, feet, or legs as a result of unregulated diabetes due to poor diet and exercise practices; etc.). Any of these situations would contribute to medical and mental illness vulnerability factors. Some residents experienced only a few of these life events, whereas others' lives were riddled with these experiences.

She's Making It Up

Tara was born and raised in the Cabrini-Green Homes. She was the third child of seven. Her mother was addicted to heroin and was intermittently in and out of Tara's life. Her maternal grandmother, who also lived in Cabrini-Green, stepped in from time to time but resented having to care for the kids and ended up frequently physically abusing Tara and her siblings. Tara did not know who her father was.

Because of her mother's addiction lifestyle and impaired judgment, many predatory men were in and out of their home. Tara's older brother and sister tried to protect Tara from the sexual abuse and all the other daily harrowing occurrences, but they were not around all the time. Tara experienced sexual abuse beginning from the age of three, and as she reached adolescence, she sustained a sexually promiscuous lifestyle to support her own crack cocaine habit. Tara could not remember how many times she had been sexually assaulted in her lifetime, as these were such frequent experiences. She relied on any kind of drugs, from anyone who was offering, for any price or exchange, to block out these gruesome memories and emotions.

At the age of 10, Tara witnessed her younger brother's murder while he was caught in gang war crossfire, which was common in the housing project. The elevators were broken, and Tara had to climb 12 flights of stairs to tell her mother what had happened. When she arrived to her apartment, she could not arouse her mother, who was alone. The paramedics took two of Tara's family members to the hospital that day.

Tara stopped going to high school at the beginning of her sophomore year. She became pregnant many times, miscarrying, undergoing abortions, and carrying the babies to term twice, only to have them immediately removed because the babies were born with drugs in their tiny bodies. Tara became HIV positive and was so disorganized that she was unable to consistently connect with any medical provider and follow any prescribed treatment regime.

At the age of 19, Tara began hearing voices of men calling her name and saying the most derogatory things imaginable. This caused her to become so afraid and experience intolerable emotions that she coped the only way she knew how—using drugs to dissociate from her reality. By the time she was 20 years old, she was psychiatrically hospitalized for the first time. It was there that she was first diagnosed with schizophrenia. She was referred for supervised housing but constantly found her way back to all she had ever known and become imprinted by. She was so impaired that she was not ever able to take the prescribed psychiatric or HIV medications for very long, as she would lose the bottles or it would be stolen.

Tara's only consistent attachment figures were her drug suppliers and the general staff in the Emergency Department at the local hospital, which she frequented almost as often as her drug suppliers.

On one particular night, Tara walked in to the Emergency Department reporting that the voices were too loud and she could not quiet them. She was sobbing. Tara would often report psychiatric symptoms that were directly related to her original trauma. For example, she could not tolerate sitting alone in the interview room because she thought someone would come in and hurt her and she had no way of getting out. Tara was very verbal and would talk with great detail, as long as the clinicians would listen. Tara often seemed noticeably soothed by the simple act of telling her story to someone who was interested and who believed her. Sometimes being out there and alone would get the best of her, and she needed a break from her intense and toxic world. Approximately eight to ten times a year, she requested to be admitted to the psychiatric hospital.

The process of the psychiatric admission was long, tedious, and time consuming. After the presenting problem details were collected, the next step in the psychiatric admission process was to request that a psychiatrist interview the client and document the appropriate physician orders, including the legal papers required to hold a person in a locked facility and to dispense psychotropic medications. Time and time again, the psychiatrist would go into the interview room with the client and ask similar questions as those that I, the crisis worker, had asked. Sometimes, I would be in the room, and sometimes, I would be just a room away, listening to the client tell the same story she had previously told to me.

In the beginning of this work, when the psychiatrist would come out of the interview room, I would be eager to participate in an academic conversation about the manifestation and organization of the psychiatric symptoms that the client presented. To the psychiatrist, I would say, "So, what do you think?" The psychiatrist, who was not able to imagine that these Cabrini-Green experiences could be real would say, "She is making it up." Each time I heard these aloof and reductionist conclusions, I was emotionally alarmed, and it took my breath away. Tara's horrific story, the psychiatrist's cold, reductionist conclusions, and my reactions were no different. The accusation that Tara was fabricating these detailed stories, which basic human experience and imagination could not have independently constructed, was utterly shocking to me. What would Tara be hoping to obtain from these *malingered* stories? What did the psychiatrist have to gain by reducing Tara's story to a lie?

Another common response from the psychiatrist was, "She's just gone off her medication." Well, indeed, she may have; however, was the psychiatrist suggesting that by ingesting the prescribed antipsychotic medication, Tara would suddenly be free of the trauma-induced stress she was experiencing and avoid a psychotic relapse by simply keeping the auditory hallucinations at bay, if that was the outcome of taking the medications? There may have been some truth to a relapse; as a person goes off the antipsychotic medication, dopamine production increases. Initially, the medication dampens dopamine production. When the medication is abruptly withdrawn, dopamine production is fast and furious, causing an acute onset of psychotic and uncomfortable physical abnormalities (Chouinard & Jones, 1980). Chouinard and Jones suggest that these symptoms may be why psychiatrists suggest that a person needs to take the medications for life. However, this view of Tara's acute onset of symptoms suggests that most, if not all, of Tara's suffering is neurobiologically based.

The personal stories I consistently heard from people recalling their mental health treatment experiences were astonishingly consistent. Conclusions asserting that a patient was either making up a story or the story was invalid because "she was off her psychotropic medications" were also disconcertingly consistent. Yes, one could argue that these conclusions were the result of how these psychiatrists were trained, that is, focusing only on the origin and manifestation of neurobiological symptoms. Yet, my social work training and personal intuition prompted me to ask more questions, and ideally, a sufficiently trained mental health treatment provider should have a similar pang of curiosity that urges them to further question the person and the context of their situation. These similar harrowing stories would all too frequently result in similar reductionist conclusions of *malingering* or *off his or her medications* by the interviewing psychiatrists. How can we accurately understand this phenomenon that mental health clinicians would devalue the contextual factors that contributed to the deep suffering of another?

FRIEDA FROMM-REICHMANN

One uneventful day in the Psychiatric Crisis Center at the hospital where I worked, I was doing some reading. A psychiatrist walked into the room and engagingly said, "Hey there! What are you working on?" I explained that I was doing some reading for my PhD dissertation, which was on the topic of the causes of acute psychiatric decompensation among people who have been previously diagnosed with a severe mental illness (SMI). He enthusiastically offered, "Oh! You must be reading the work of Frieda Fromm-Reichmann." Up until that moment, surprisingly, I had never heard her name. By the next day, I was immersed in the work and publications of this German-born psychiatrist.

Fromm-Reichmann was extraordinarily focused on the therapeutic relationship with individuals who suffered from psychotic symptoms. She believed that psychotherapy was to the treatment of symptoms of psychosis what physical therapy was to the outcomes of strokes (Fromm-Reichmann, 1950). She believed that patients needed to have at least one person who never gave up on them to maintain hope for recovery from schizophrenia, and she embodied this hope for her patients. These and other treatment ideas were published in *Principles of Intensive Psychotherapy*, one of Fromm-Reichmann's most famous and classic publications (Fromm-Reichmann, 1950).

Fromm-Reichmann followed in the footsteps of many other psychiatrists who never gave up on their patients, no matter how troubled they were. These psychiatrists, their theories, and the programs where they conducted their work are explored further in Chapter 5, "Historically Ethical and Effective Mental Health Approaches for Healing the Distress of Psychotic Experiences." Mainstream historians and the contemporary mental health treatment delivery community have paid little to no attention to these revolutionists, portraying a negatively distorted image of psychiatrists and their great work with people who experience psychosis. Painting these pioneers into the mental health treatment delivery picture makes the whole field of psychiatry and mental health treatment look radically different, and more hope and direct strategies are present for healing and recovery from psychotic experiences.

In her work, Fromm-Reichmann asks the following two important questions:

1. "Can the therapeutic relationship heal even the most severe symptoms of mental illness?"
2. "Why are psychiatrists fighting the hardest against this idea?"

There is obviously a significant philosophical gap among mainstream psychiatrists and other mental health treatment delivery professionals, as the therapeutic relationship is embraced and not so rigidly fought against by the latter.

DEFENSIVE COUNTERTRANSFERENCE

One day, while poring over the works of Fromm-Reichmann, I stumbled across a phrase she coined: *defensive countertransference*. She explained this idea with the following ideas. The client tells his story. The therapist cannot tolerate the client's despair. The therapist flees from and dismisses the experiences of the client (Fromm-Reichmann, 1950). Reading those words struck a significant emotional chord in me. I felt compelled to read and reread her description, as Fromm-Reichmann had just explained the common and devastating dynamic that I had continually witnessed between many patients and psychiatrists. I was merely a witness to this behavior, so what impact must this defensive countertransference have had on the people seeking treatment who directly experienced this dynamic?

Goffman asserts that defensive countertransference shuts people down in the most essential form (Goffman, 1961). Therefore, the inclusion of defensive countertransference in the therapeutic relationship can cause those seeking treatment to buy into the mistaken belief that they are untreatable and unworthy. We now think of this as internalized shame and hatred and can identify its effects among the many populations who experience stigma, including LGBT individuals, African Americans, gang members, and women, to name just a few populations.

In the following days, as well as over the coming years, I watched for this defensive countertransference dynamic to manifest in the broader world. Defensive countertransference was everywhere and was used as a way of coping with the pervasive suffering of others. One example stands out. After Hurricane Katrina devastated the Gulf Coast Region in 2005, approximately 15,000 refugees from Louisiana and Mississippi were temporarily relocated and found shelter in the Reliant Houston Astrodome (Plyer, 2014). Former First Lady Barbara Bush made the following statement on the National Public Radio (NPR) show *Marketplace*:

> What I'm hearing, which is sort of scary, is they all want to stay in Texas. Everyone is so overwhelmed by the hospitality. And so many of the people in the arena here, you know, were underprivileged anyway, so this is working very well for them. (*New York Times*, September 7, 2005)

The White House qualified the controversial remarks as a *personal observation*. This aloof statement was in line with a privileged culture of disconnection with the Hurricane Katrina victims' catastrophic suffering, suggesting that the refugees were better off in the temporary shelter of a sports arena than in their own homes before the storm.

The normalizing culture of defensive countertransference is contagious and pervasive. If one stops and looks around with open eyes, other subgroups that have been impacted by pervasive and normalized defensive countertransference become apparent, such as people who find themselves homeless, addicted to drugs, or in domestic violence situations. Another all too common defensive countertransference reaction is that the approximately 110,000 to 120,000 Japanese who, in 1942, were forcibly relocated off the Pacific Coast and incarcerated in internment camps in the interior of the United States, losing most of their personal property, "did not have it all that bad." This same defensive countertransference occurs as individuals deny the historical Holocaust experience and the pervasive and extreme racism toward African Americans in the United States.

Many professional mental health practice textbooks will suggest that countertransference is a natural phenomenon. In clinical terms, Sigmund Freud coined the term "transference" to illustrate how his patients would relate to the clinician, as they would relate to previous important attachment figures, such as mother, sister, grandfather, in their lives. An example is when one has that intuitive sense, "We've met before. How do I know you?" and they really have not ever before met. The individual has an unconscious reminder of a previous person and interacts with the person as if he or she were the original person.

Countertransference is the clinician's emotional reactions in response to the client's situations or reactions. The clinician reacts as if the client is an important person in the clinician's life, such as other patients, family members, or work colleagues. For example, the clinician may be guarded without conscious cause because the client reminds the clinician of someone who caused the clinician harm in the past. Mental health clinicians think of countertransference reactions occurring as *when*, not *if*, as these reactions are going to happen at some point. Countertransference reactions can be positive (giving one client more time than the others) or negative (feeling bored or irritated by a particular client). Regardless of the quality of the countertransference reaction, it is all potentially destructive if not consciously reflected on and intentionally regulated by the clinician. The unique purpose of defensive countertransference is to protect the mind so that the person can go on functioning as needed. Defensive countertransference reactions are natural, common, and contagious, but they do not have to be pervasive or normalized.

Resolving defensive countertransference takes courage and commitment to the therapeutic process and the client and self-reflection. The clinician should begin by identifying and accepting this occurrence as having distracted the attention from the present. Next, the clinician reengages with the client, with presence as the guiding principle. The clinician asks, overtly or privately, "What is going on right now?"

Now, some might wonder whether this inquiry would draw critical attention to the clinician. For example, "Would this question erode the client's trust if I let it be known that I was not paying full attention to him?" There is not one general and correct answer here. Some individuals are so fragile that this attempt to reconnect will be experienced as an interpersonal loss, and the client will emotionally and interpersonally shut down. Others might be forgiving and will appreciate the attempt to be fully heard and reconnected with. Without the attempt to be present and connect with client, interpersonal distance in the therapeutic relationship causes iatrogenic trauma for the client. With persistence and commitment, good clinicians make every attempt to recognize and regulate defensive countertransference.

Unfortunately, mainstream public mental health interventions are delivered in a professional culture that systematically oppresses and further stigmatizes the clients who come to be helped. Because of the interpersonal closeness in which clients and clinicians find themselves, clinician burnout can easily occur. Moreover, as professional passion wanes, providers may, in a defensive countertransference attempt to preserve the self, automatically become negative or distant when a particular client arrives. Thoughts such as "Argh! Not her again" or "I don't want to deal with his issues" overshadow the therapeutic relationship before the session even begins. From here, the connection between defensive countertransference and social marginalization of the client starts to form. From this marginalized perspective, stigmatizing these clients becomes almost second nature. For instance, when a person seeks services, if he does not do exactly as recommended, he or she is labeled as treatment resistant, help-rejecting, noncompliant, or even untreatable. Sometimes, a person is so symptomatic that when he does not come to appointments, clinicians do not make an effort to locate him and the case is closed based on an erroneous conclusion that the person did not want mental health services. If the person is too eager and does exactly as recommended, other pejorative labels are sometimes applied, such as dependent, med-seeking, and hopeless, thereby further marginalizing the person from mainstream society.

Concurrently, negative judgment does not stop with just the clients. The clinician who becomes interpersonally close to a client is labeled mentally ill, boundariless, or sympathizer. Even today, clinicians are overly trained to be a Freudian *blank screen*, despite having so many wishes for and thoughts about the client that intersect with his or her own experiences. What is so sinful about having a therapeutically close and committed relationship with our clients who live with psychosis? Whereas the clinician needs appropriate boundaries to keep the therapeutic focus on the client, why have clinicians so harshly taken this *blank screen* stance? Clinicians have the flexibility to engage in therapeutic closeness with clients who present with symptoms of depression, anxiety, and mood disorders. Why is it so unthinkable to engage in close therapeutic inquiry with clients who experience psychosis? The following questions represent the inquiries that mental health practitioners could be asking to truly address the issue of defensive countertransference and the underlying issues of their clientele:

- Do we ever inquire about the subjective experience of the person who experiences psychosis? Why are we only focused on stopping the psychotic symptoms? How can we better understand the origin and meaning of the symptoms and embrace how these symptoms *work* for the individual?
- What is so forbidden about accurately understanding the meaning of the psychotic symptoms? What might be the meaning of hearing oncoming footsteps, the constant static on TV, constant coughing, or a fascination with Spiderman or a paranoid fixation on Steve Jobs?
- At what point does the person find these psychotic experiences distressing, even unbearable?

TOTAL INSTITUTIONS KILL THE INDIVIDUAL SPIRIT

Goffman (1961) was a noteworthy sociologist with special interests in anthropology and psychiatric patient subjective experiences. Through his writings, he examined the tone of life inside the mental hospital. His first wife, Angelica "Sky" Choate, suffered from a mental illness, possibly bipolar disorder I. She spent time in mental institutions, and on April 27, 1964, took her own life by jumping off the Richmond–San Rafael Bridge (Shalin, 2010). In *Asylum* Goffman unpacks the term "institutionalization" as it pertains to the psychiatric patient who has been living in a psychiatric institution for long periods of time, often a lifetime.

Goffman applies the term "total institution" to life in monasteries, boarding schools, prisons, concentration camps, and mental hospitals. He defines total institutions as places where people are "cut off from the wider society" and form an "enclosed, formally administered round of life" (Goffman, 1961, p. xv). He asserts that, in these institutions, the residents sleep, play, and work 100% of their time in the facility, and their behaviors are monitored, judged, and sentenced to punishment or privileges by a single authority, the staff. Goffman refers to the milieu as *batch life*, where the inmates publicly conduct their lives, and they are all interacted with in the same way and required to do the same activities together (Goffman, 1961, p. 6). These activities are prearranged on a regimented schedule, designed to meet all inmate needs, and geared toward fulfilling the mission of the institution, which, in the case of mainstream mental health treatment, is seemingly mental stabilization. However, since the mental status of the American people is becoming increasingly unstable, as evidenced by the increase in individuals receiving Social Supplemental Income (SSI) and Social Supplemental Disability Income (SSDI) for mental disabilities and skyrocketing addiction rates, whose needs are actually being attended to in contemporary mainstream mental health treatment?

Goffman also articulates that, on first glance, a separation is apparent between the inmates or mental patients (those who have restricted access to the world at large) and the supervisory personnel or staff (those who come and go). Both, he asserts, have hostile skepticism for the motives of the other. A *we/they* situation is created. Whereas both groups are socialized to be civil with one another, Goffman asserts that mental health clinicians often perceive patients as "bitter, secretive, and untrustworthy," whereas patients often perceive staff as "condescending, highhanded, and mean" (Goffman, 1961, p. 7). Although these descriptions were published in 1961, these dynamics are sadly still applicable today in some mainstream mental health treatment facilities, whether inpatient, residential, or outpatient.

Although both groups spend a significant amount of time together, there are explicit and implicit boundaries. There are designated areas where staff rest, eat, and work. Patients who attempt to cross these boundaries are summarily penalized and labeled as brown-nosers or sellouts by the other inmates. The following story exemplifies this issue.

Tuesdays at the State Hospital

Beginning in 1984, each Tuesday afternoon just before 2 pm, I went to my volunteer job at the maximum-security women's unit at the state psychiatric hospital. Beverly was a patient there. Her skull, mouth, and entire left side of her body were physically deformed because of a domestic violence assault by her husband, during which she was shoved out of a moving car. Every Tuesday, she waited by the door for me. Beverly would stay by my side until my shift was over.

On one occasion, as I approached the door, I could hear Beverly asking the staff with her warped speech, "What time is it?" Just as I opened the door, the nurse threw down her keys on the desk and screamed out, "I told you, Beverly, that if you asked me one more time, you were going into the Quiet Room. Let's go!" The nurse proceeded to enlist the help of an aide, and each hooked their arms into Beverly's arms. She was literally dragged down the hall and shoved into the Quiet Room, where, for the next 45 minutes, in a soft oppressed voice, she called for me by name and begged to be let out of the isolation room.

How is it possible to understand any part of the situation in the story as *treatment*? Was there any part of this situation that was intended to be a learning experience for Beverly? If that interaction was intended to teach Beverly something, I am certain that Beverly learned a lot that day about when, and when not, to speak, mostly never to speak about anything that makes her vulnerable. That lesson is something that many people with mental illness quickly learn: "Do not feel interpersonal attachment toward other people, especially those whose care you are under;" "Do not bother staff, and most of what you do is a bother;" and "The staff hold all authority, and you will do exactly as instructed or else you will be severely punished and socially segregated."

This nurse had a moment when she did not regulate her negative countertransference reactions and impulsively raged at Beverly. However, what exactly was the nurse raging about? Was Beverly interrupting her work? Beverly's well-being *was* the essence of the nurse's work. Possibly, the nurse wished that Beverly would wait for *her* at the door and perhaps was envious of the relationship that Beverly and I were able to enjoy. Perhaps, Beverly's plight seemed so helpless and low, because of her physical disfigurements, social isolation, and oppression, that the nurse could not tolerate Beverly's despair and fled from her own possible empathic reaction toward Beverly. The nurse could also have been exercising a coping skill called *reaction formation* and truly wished she could drag me down the hall and lock *me* up in the Quiet Room. All of these scenarios are likely, but I will never know what caused that type of reaction, because the incident was never addressed.

Beverly may have obsessively looked forward to this interaction as her only connection with the outside world, and, it may have given her something to hope for, among the monotonous and lonely days. The nurse obviously missed this opportunity to connect with Beverly, who was so desperately available. While this is just one story, the foundation of psychiatric survivor groups is constructed from thousands of people who have countless experiences of similar tonality. The history and philosophy of these groups are elaborated in Chapter 8, "Consumer/Psychiatric Survivor/Ex-Patient (C/S/X) Movement."

Goffman asserts that in total institutions, minor privileges, such as meaningful conversations, extra food, pleasant tone in conversations, and other examples of being in the right place at the right time, are extremely regulated by the authorities and become the essence around which inmates/patients build their culture. Outsiders often have great difficulty appreciating these highly desired dynamics and often disregard efforts to attain these highly infrequent rewards as patient overreactions and delusional obsessions.

Privileges can be overt or quite subtle, such as showing the patient a bit more respect and kindness, allowing a bit more privacy, or providing a better room. Patients who are familiar with total institutional dynamics can also rally other patients into desirable behaviors so they can get staff to allow forbidden privileges. An example of this type of interaction is provided in the following story.

In the Name of Football

Henry was locked up against his will in a state psychiatric hospital for 3 years. During the week, he reported that his days were spent engaging in meaningless groups, watching daytime television, milling around the day room, and standing in line for everything from taking medications three to four times a day, to meals and showering. On the weekends, Alfredo, a male staff member, would bring his own satellite dish and television to the hospital unit and, together, they would watch sports all day. Henry especially enjoyed watching football with Alfredo. Henry spoke of these weekends with Alfredo as "the most therapeutic activity during those three years." With Alfredo, there was an egalitarian and mutually respectful tone in their relationship. The interpersonal connection was authentic, generous, and kind. All of the patients had a job to do to make this privilege happen. Tedious tasks like taking medications and clearing meal trays were done with efficiency. Everyone cooperated, and a community was magically created where each person contributed, belonged, and was rewarded. On Monday morning, everyone returned to the humdrum of going through the motions, pretending to be delivering and receiving treatment.

In this story, I would speculate that this staff person enjoyed many personal privileges of his own, including, at the very least, a group of satisfied patients, which allowed for a peaceful work shift. Goffman refers to these practices as *secondary adjustments*. In a treatment facility, we would imagine that patients would be focused on healing, but in a total institution, patients are required to read the staff to learn how to gain the ability to have choices, such as a different food item, a specific television channel or program, or the ability to play a game, which make up these secondary adjustments (Goffman, 1961). The purpose of secondary adjustments is to create experiences where those who are detained can achieve a small sensation of choice, which feeds their sense of effective agency, or the subjective sense that a person has an intentional impact on his own world. In a total institution, only those with the capacity to accurately read and respond with the staff are able to experience this agency; therefore, a survival-of-the-fittest scenario is played out, as those without that capacity lose out on this sense of agency.

Economic and social responsibilities are also organizing (Goffman, 1961). So, why are we depriving people with mental illness of these responsibilities by having unrealistically low expectations of their abilities? For instance, many health practitioners assume that work is not an option for people with mental illness and that they do not have the capacity for social relationships. In fact, people with mental illness find their own methods of negotiating economic trades and relationships. Having unrealistically low expectations deprives a person of important opportunities to receive education, support, and guidance on such matters that would contribute to flourishing in these areas. The recovery model incorporates economic and social responsibilities into specific plans for personal and social recovery from mental illness.

Ironically, mental health treatment staff who cross these total institutional boundaries are often seen as unprofessional and are vulnerable to pejorative accusations that equate to professional suicide. After the first incident of this boundary crossing, the staff person is considered naïve and is counseled for his or her own good. Given the social banishment risk, most everyone who seeks a successful long-term career in mainstream mental health treatment delivery is invested in honoring these overt and subtle boundaries. New clinicians are made very aware of the culture that guides the undercurrent of expectations from their professional peers. Patients often speak of identifying with characteristics of new staff that include eagerness, empathy, flexibility, mindfulness, and egalitarianism. However, what is modeled to these new professionals and socially expected of them is to be authoritarian, rigid, judgmental, and distant.

And so it goes, the inmates/patients and the staff holding antagonistic stereotypes about each other and experiencing little spontaneous and real interactions to debunk these myths. Isolated clients use desperate measures, such as begging or finding underground methods to get their needs met, which are viewed as symptoms of mental illness, further marginalizing them due to the continued labeling as impulsive, poor at problem-solving, or manipulative, to name a few (Rosenhan, 1973).

Some clients buy into *The River* and what they are told about their mental illness, believing they will be taking medication forever, and develop low potential for their lives. At a closer glance, given these rigid and interpersonally cold boundaries, both populations fail to get all of their needs met and walk away from these experiences feeling manipulated, humiliated, frustrated, disillusioned, and devastated. Where is the *stabilization* and *rehabilitation* in this phenomenon? With the current philosophies of *rehabilitation* being delivered, this process actually leads people to experience worse outcomes in self-care, subjective experiences, and physical health.

GOFFMAN'S PHASES OF INSTITUTIONALIZATION
AND BREAKING OF THE SPIRIT

Goffman is well known for his exploration of institutionalization phenomena, which he outlines in three phases: pre-patient, in-patient, and ex-patient. Each phase will be identified, defined, and applied to the contemporary delivery of mainstream mental health treatment. It should be noted that whereas most people with symptoms of mental illness are not locked in asylums for years on end (with the exception of a forensic psychiatric hospitalization), the process of institutionalization is very much alive in acute inpatient units, residential facilities, and outpatient treatment agencies.

The first phase of the institutionalization process, the pre-patient phase, is when the person begins to experience symptoms of mental illness and has insight about what is occurring. Even young people are aware of the stigma from mental illness and do not want to be marginalized, so the symptoms are often denied until the behaviors come to the attention of those beyond the family, such as school administration or law enforcement. With family members feeling a variety of emotions, such as fear, embarrassment, and worry, the young person is often brought in coercively or forcibly for evaluation and treatment. The family, friends, teachers, coaches, or role models report the changes in the person's behaviors in an effort to give clinicians the full story. When these intimate details are revealed to the treatment providers, the young person often feels betrayed. The young person is now interacted with differently, distantly, and suspiciously. As compassion and affection are suspended and unconditional love is withdrawn, the young person experiences this as a spiritually fatal process. Fromm-Reichmann asserts that this interpersonal and spiritual shift is the most harrowing trauma of the whole experience of mental illness (Fromm-Reichmann, 1950).

The second phase, the in-patient phase, is what happens on the inside of the mental health treatment system. Here, the person experiences a death of his individualism, by which he or she is batched or pigeonholed and treated with stereotypical methods, such as being assigned a *treatment pathway* based on diagnosis. As freedoms are imposed on, by means such as physical searches, phone restrictions, food restrictions, and other indignities, the sense of *self* becomes standardized and replaceable.

In this in-patient phase, the young person with mental illness is often told, with a fair amount of certainty from clinicians, the grim prognosis of the remainder of his or her life. With attempts to lighten the blow, the conversation usually includes the following overt messages:

> You have a chronic mental illness. There is no cure, but if you take this medication for the rest of your life, the symptoms may be managed. We want to keep your stress to a minimum, so that means no post-high school education. You will be eligible for Social Security benefits (approximately $900 per month, which varies from state to state and increases slightly over time), so there is no need to work. Work is too stressful. This money will provide for all your needs to be met. There are many housing options for you; many are in single-room occupancy hotels or group-home settings with other people who have been

diagnosed with mental illnesses. We can get you connected with a resourceful case manager who can set you up for all these wonderful benefits.

The River treatment plan is swiftly delivered. While some of these benefits may sound enticing, especially when one has very few resources, quickly one sees that these are not enough resources needed for real stability. On first glance, young people usually reject most, if not all, of this script. The protest may include:

I don't have a mental illness! I am creative, and you do not understand me! I do not need medication. It makes me feel numb and interferes with my sex drive and performance. I do not need your stinking money because I will be able to work in an area in which I have talent and interest! Who could live off $900 a month, anyway? I am not going to meet with any therapist, psychiatrist, or case manager whose intention is to shut me down because I do not have these problems!

Michael White and David Epston (1990) would actually say that this protest script is healthy for the young person's sense of agency because the experience of protesting oppression fosters a sense of fortitude. Without protest, the civil rights movement and many other necessary civil rights amendments would not have occurred. Without protest, same-sex marriage would not be a reality. Protest preserves a sense of agency, dreams, hopes, values, personal principles, and drive. However, at this point, the mainstream public mental health treatment delivery system fails its young customers. The erroneous conclusion is made that the young are in denial of their illness and will have to learn on their own to follow treatment prescriptions. A better way to approach these young people experiencing symptoms of psychosis would be to engage with them and discover what dreams and goals are important in their lives, thereby constructing a plan that allows young persons to still have a sense of a meaningful future.

Yet, these mainstream mental health treatment clinicians back off and give the young person enough space to get into serious trouble, and as the statistics reflect, this is often what occurs. Compared to the general public, people who carry the diagnosis of schizophrenia are 50 times at greater risk to attempt suicide, which is 40%–60% of all people diagnosed with schizophrenia (CDC, 2012). Additionally, there are approximately 11 suicide attempts for every one successful completed suicide, and people who are diagnosed with schizophrenia are at 8 times greater risk than the general population to actually complete the act of suicide (CDC, 2012), most commonly occurring in young people who are newly diagnosed. Additionally, according to the American Foundation for Suicide Prevention (2015), in the general population, the highest rate of suicide is among people who are 45–64 years old, followed by people aged 85 and older; 15- to 24-year-olds had the lowest rate, followed by 25- to 44-year-olds. However, in the schizophrenia groups, the youngest age groups had the highest rates of suicide, explicably when an individual is painfully aware of their diagnosis and the grim prognosis of which they are repeatedly being told.

In the third phase, the ex-patient phase, the person finds that he or she has been oppressed by the authority in the hospital or outpatient mental health treatment system and lost any sense of self-identity, expression of personal style, and objective thinking. An inpatient hospital and the lack of resources in the outside world rob the patients of personal freedoms, such as wearing nail polish, choosing a clothing style, showering, eating what they want, learning self-care activities, cooking, budgeting money, and working to support themselves and buy things that reflect individuality, such as music, shoes, or leisure activities (Sommer, 1959). The person must now "wait for Godot." In the Samuel Beckett play, *Waiting for Godot*, two men patiently wait for the arrival of an unknown man named Godot. Despite promises to appear, he never shows up, leaving them unrewarded, yet they endlessly wait for unidentified rewards (Beckett, 1954). Many psychiatric patients who are caught in the strong undercurrent of *The River* helplessly wait for unknown and unfulfilled rewards.

The ex-patient phase is confounded when the patient attempts to reenter broader society after being released. Once the patient is released from mental health treatment, he or she comes back to a world where important attachment losses, such as close friends and family, occurred because of the stigma related to mental illness. This reality now leads to social isolation, unemployment, possible homelessness, and poverty. The only option for this person, at that point, is to turn to his or her case manager, who had promised the good life of affordable housing, psychotropic medications, and federal and state funding, which can be an incredibly humbling experience. Often, to receive the case management and housing services, the person must meet with a psychiatrist and take the medications as prescribed. From the client's perspective, these medications may have significant unwanted side effects that sometimes are perceived as worse than the original symptoms. These side effects can include weight gain, involuntary facial twitches, hand tremors, akathisia, numbing of emotions, decreased sex drive and sexual abilities, and many more conditions that contribute to serious medical problems. The client understandably has strong feelings about this process but has few to no alternatives. The person sometimes follows the regimen for a while, but there is not a solid commitment, and the individual finds himself in and out of social and emotional crises, sometimes landing him back into the hospital, like a revolving door.

Many people turn to recreational drugs or other behavioral addictions, such as eating disorders, gambling, or sex, to distract and numb the dysphoric feelings that haunt them every day. These behaviors become the default pattern of coping, and this coping style can result in a process of self-sabotage, magnifying the symptoms and profile of mental illness. Additionally, the social network that a person with SMI finds himself belonging to primarily consists of like-minded people who also understandably have strong feelings, few resources, and frequent crises.

Hartz et al. (2014) conducted a large case-control study with a multiethnic case sample of 9,142 individuals diagnosed with schizophrenia, bipolar disorder with psychotic features, or schizoaffective disorder and a control sample of 10,195 people without mental illness symptoms. The researchers found that, compared with the control group, people with psychotic disorders had significantly higher use of tobacco products, alcohol, marijuana, and recreational drugs. Additionally, while public health efforts have decreased smoking tobacco among the general population younger than 30, these efforts have been ineffective among individuals with severe psychotic illnesses (Hartz et al., 2014). Furthermore, heavy use of tobacco, alcohol, and other drugs are strongly correlated with cancer, heart disease, and other serious medical problems, contributing to the 25-year premature death rate for people with SMI (Hartz et al., 2014).

Individuals who turn to a drug lifestyle to cope often find themselves caught up in the criminal justice system. This statement is also true for people who have SMIs and fall into a distinctive category termed *co-occurring disordered*, referring to individuals with both an SMI and drug misuse. These people often find themselves in crises and participate in criminal behaviors that either (1) help them get their immediate needs met or (2) involve them in serious threats to the safety of others. This population of individuals has high rates of violence, is highly represented in media, and contributes to the myth that people with SMIs are dangerous. These individuals are involuntarily detained under the forensic penal code in jails or other correctional facilities with the sparsest of mental health treatment. People who experience co-occurring disorders are the most marginalized and the most difficult to reach. These individuals are highly institutionalized and experience the lowest quality of life.

At some point, the overburdened, tired, and oppressed person no longer has the resources to fight the mental health treatment system and *The River* treatment plan that is constantly, persistently, and rigidly shoved at them. With dignity, he suspends, maybe even surrenders, his sense of agency to the benefits of the mainstream mental health system, quieting his uniqueness to obtain the needed resources, such as housing. He compromises his beliefs to his new personal narrative script: "My name is John, and I am a schizophrenic. I cannot go to school or work because I have schizophrenia. I will meet with my case manager to get Social Security benefits and housing." When the person experiences big feelings that are disorganizing, he or she learns to get himself to the most convenient person who can prescribe psychotropic medications, most commonly the psychiatrist, and reports the most dysphoric and disorganizing symptoms. By this point, the person has usually tried several different kinds of psychotropic medications, both in treatment and found on the streets, and can ask for the preferred medication by name. Conversely, he or she can assert which medication not to prescribe because of the well-known acute side effects, such as extrapyramidal symptoms or general malaise, unless those are the results he or she is seeking to numb the senses.

In an enormously deprived environment and in an attempt to experience a whiff of effective agency, the person begins to sneak unhealthy behaviors and think and behave in a guarded manner. Quietly and purposefully, many individuals who are prescribed high doses of psychotropic medication begin to constantly smoke cigarettes and drink caffeinated and/or sugary drinks to experience any push of dopamine, the neurotransmitter that allows for the experience of pleasure, which the overuse of antipsychotic medications prevents. Extreme behaviors emerge that further marginalize the individual. Some individuals may cope with deprivation by stealing things from others, manipulating those who may be vulnerable, or remaining passive and vulnerable themselves. These behaviors are, thus, categorized as additional symptoms of mental illness (i.e., antisocial personality disorder; narcissistic personality disorder; borderline personality disorder; dependent personality disorder, etc.), causing further marginalization, stigmatization, and oppression. Then, the soul comes to a grinding halt. Describing these shifts in thinking and actions is not an attempt to categorize afflicted individuals as *bad people* but to illustrate how desperate one becomes in getting his or her needs met in a relentlessly destitute environment in which he finds himself. Given this, it is no wonder that the rates of suicide attempts are so high among people with psychotic symptoms. Quality of life in the mainstream mental health treatment delivery system can be disconnected and grim.

As the person with symptoms of mental illness surrenders to *The River*, a big portion of her identity attaches to the label "mentally ill" for years to come, and pervasive low expectations of the self and world ensue. The person can now *talk the talk* and *walk the walk* of a person with mental illness and has lost connection to the veridical *self* with dreams and goals for personal and worldly potential. This fatal *River* is where we find a large portion of people in the public mental health treatment delivery system: disconnected from self and others and scratching for extremely scarce resources and ways of coping. When a person *does* have a sense of individualism, it sometimes manifests as histrionic, underdeveloped, childlike behavior, such as wearing a chaotic mix of bright colors or riding a bike decked out with monkey bars, propaganda signage, and flags. While each individual has a right to be unique, these behaviors do not originate from the veridical self, and these unauthentic expressions can be understood as taking on society's stereotypical characteristics, further marginalizing the individual from needed resources that enhance the quality of one's life. Freedom is not authentic when expressions are in response to oppression.

Almost all SMIs (excepting diagnoses in the autism spectrum) first manifest in late adolescence or early adulthood. During this time, developmental stages of self-determination, autonomy, and freedom are felt and developed. Efforts during these important developmental stages, such as education, establishment of lifelong intimate relationships, and employment career, exponentially establish and advance one's standing in life. Because these developmental activities are disrupted and oppressed through years of mental health treatment, when he or she does return to mainstream life, many of these developmental efforts are thought of as irrevocable losses. The person with SMI is forever socially and financially marginalized.

Today, only a small fraction of people who experience psychosis are hospitalized for long periods, except for those in the forensic system. Still, Goffman's ex-patient scenario is very alive in the contemporary version of institutionalization, only without the walls and locked doors. People who are recipients of mainstream and public mental health treatment services are subject to *The River*, or iatrogenic trauma, and experience Goffman's social *total institutionalization*. At the slightest suggestion that a person may be experiencing psychotic symptoms, or even big feelings, people distance themselves and become suspicious of the person as an act of self-protection. The cycle of cultural stigma toward people with symptoms of SMI continues, resulting in the severe self-protective behavior, psychosis, addiction, psychogenic death, and suicide. Is it any wonder that young people who begin to experience symptoms of mental illness maintain such fierce denial and avoid mental health treatment when it may be so necessary? No one wants to be a mental patient and be subjected to all the social and existential marginalization and iatrogenic trauma that this role brings.

LOOKING AHEAD

The intention for this chapter and the entire book is to tell the truth about the subjective experiences of individuals who live with psychosis and offer effective and humanistic solutions to these unspoken realities. This noble endeavor of assisting a person with mental illness and healing psychosis by leading into the experience of authentic subjective experience may be overwhelming. Clinicians might find that they need to occasionally retreat and preserve their own spirits from time to time because of this enormously challenging work. People who live with symptoms of psychosis *need* clinicians and loved ones to step away and rejuvenate when it becomes too much for their minds to bear. Then, when they are ready, and sometimes when they are not ready, they are tasked with coming back to the therapeutic relationship to keep on supporting those who cannot walk away from their overwhelming experiences each day. There is hope, and continuing to learn what we can from this book and other places will help us be effective at healing the distress of psychosis.

FINAL THOUGHTS

For many people, especially clinicians, the subjective world of people who experience psychosis has not been accessible because Western society has historically discarded these people in institutions, and they have been forgotten. Goffman, Sullivan, Fromm-Reichmann, Winnicott, and other psychological theorists and anthropological pioneers have given us the vocabulary and context by which to explore the common and subjective experiences of people who experience psychosis and other symptoms of SMIs. People with mental illnesses have experienced a history of mistreatment and invalidation in the name of experimentation and treatment for the well-being of the patient. Many, including psychiatric survivors, family members, and clinicians are fed up with *The River*. Now, it is up to enlightened clinicians, family members, loved ones, and individuals with lived experience to use this information with the best intentions toward the healing of psychotic experiences and improved quality of life.

3

Brief History of Iatrogenic Trauma from the Mainstream Mental Health Treatment System

---

MANY INTERVENTION METHODS have been used in the United States and around the world to manage symptoms of psychosis and the people experiencing them. Sometimes, these methods have included humane values and efficient methods, but sometimes abuse, torture, and severe neglect have all been delivered in the name of *treatment*.

VARIOUS APPROACHES TO REDUCE PSYCHOTIC SYMPTOMS

As Europeans established themselves in the United States, people who had mental illnesses were not deemed a major social problem, because families were self-sufficient and were expected to provide for their members who were sick, aged, or disabled. As the population grew, people with mental illnesses became more visible and irksome to others, as these people were interruptions to pleasant family life and work productivity. As resources became limited, families with a person with mental illness became overburdened and were unable to provide necessary care. As a result, these people were institutionalized for very long periods of time, often their whole lives, in self-governing local community facilities that assumed responsibility for the problems presented by their most vulnerable members. Some say that these asylums were a rationalized method to purge the most inconvenient population.

At this time, mental health professionals had no formal theories to understand mental illness and no formal treatment theories. Their understanding and treatment became based on fear. The 1684 text written by Thomas Willis, *The Practice of Physick: Two Discourses Concerning the Soul of Brutes*, on the subject of insanity set the tone for the many medical guides that would be written over the next 100 years.

Willis's theory was that people with mental illness were animal-like and, in kind, needed to be kept down like animals. "Discipline, threats and blows are needed as much as medical treatment. Truly nothing is more necessary and more effective for the recovery of these people than forcing them to respect and fear intimidation" (Willis, 1684; Gregory Zilboorg, 1941).

During this time, they used water as an intervention, often for a calming effect to cool and soothe the scalp, yet other times, water was used in bursts, like that of a fire hose, to regulate and punish people. Another method used was the physical and emotional experience of shock with *The Surprise Bath*. The *lunatic* was blindfolded, led across a room, and suddenly dropped through a trapdoor into a tub of cold water. The intention was that the unexpected plunge would be so physiologically and psychologically shocking that life-threatening terror would be induced and the person's rationality would be instantly and dramatically restored (Whitaker, 2010).

Joseph Guislain built an elaborate mechanism that he called *The Chinese Temple*. The *maniac* would be locked into an iron cage that would be mechanically lowered into a body of frigid water. Again, as the individual experienced life-threatening shock, the cage would be raised out of the water. It was thought that with the life-threatening shock, often needing resuscitation, the person would take a fresh perspective on life, breaking dysphoric associations and leaving the mental illness behind. However, because the person in the cage had no power to raise the cage above the water, many likely drowned during these experiments (Whitaker, 2010).

Mercury and other chemical agents were used to induce nausea so fierce that the patient would not have the mental strength to rant and rave. Near starvation was another recommendation to rob a person of his strength. Mustard powders could be rubbed on a shaved scalp, and painful and open blisters formed. Caustic substances were then rubbed into the blisters to further irritate and infect the scalp. The belief was that the blistering *treatment* caused considerable pain, and the person's mind would become focused on the pain, rather than on his or her *usual* raving thoughts.

Bloodletting and purging were also used because the theory was that excess blood in the brain led to psychosis. These treatments caused people to become so weak, they were unable to behave frantically. Yet, like many previously believed truths about people who were different, just because an idea or behavior was popular does not mean it was humane or effective.

Another theory about the cause of mental illness was that evil spirits possessed these individuals. Exorcisms were performed to dispel these evil spirits. Individuals were coerced to carry religious devotional items, such as rosaries and holy water, to keep evil spirits at a distance. Furthermore, individuals were stigmatized and socially isolated for fear of contagion.

In 1751, Pennsylvania Hospital was the first institution that had a unit designed especially to care for the sick and mentally ill. The conditions were immoral, to say the least. Patients were locked up, beaten, and kept in an unhealthy basement with no separate location for human waste. All patients were kept together, regardless of their symptoms, including psychosis, severe depression, and intellectual impairment. The people in the town would come to the hospital to peer into the basement windows, as if the hospital were a zoo. In 1760, the hospital's managers built a fence to prevent the disturbances, but even this fence could not keep curious peepers away. In 1762, when the hospital fell on financial hard times, the hospital staff began charging a visitor's fee to let people in to observe the patients. A young physician named Benjamin Rush joined the staff at Pennsylvania Hospital and campaigned for a separate ward out of the basement for people with mental illness.

Many individuals with severe mental illness (SMI) were similarly warehoused in comparable deplorable facilities for long periods of time or whole lifetimes. Through the efforts of activists, such as Quakers and their associates, quality of life improved for individuals who lived with SMI. The efforts of Rush, the Quakers, and others to improve the quality of life of individuals experiencing symptoms of psychosis are further explored in Chapter 5, "Historically Ethical and Effective Mental Health Approaches for Healing the Distress of Psychotic Experiences."

Along the lines of these humane and effective practices, mainstream physicians organized themselves, lobbied, and gained the finances to build asylums that they could administer. By 1844, 13 asylums had formed the Association of Medical Superintendents of American Institutions for the Insane to promote their interests. The nature of their first agenda item was as follows: If an institution was to call itself a treatment facility, it should always have a physician as its administrator or superintendent. Saving time and money were the association's top priorities. Drugs, such as morphine and opium, were generously administered to sedate patients to the point that they were not able to function. Today, this practice is referred to as *chemical restraint*. As the practice of chemically restraining people became more common, so did the use of physical restraints and straightjackets, which were more digestible to practitioners. Without effective humane practices, individuals in mental hospitals did not get better. As patients were retained, the population in these hospitals increased, and quality of life and care in the hospitals drastically declined.

In 1946, *Life Magazine* published an exposé of the state of mental hospitals and treatment in the United States. This article, "Bedlam," by Albert Q. Maisel, included many photos. To read the entire article and see images, go to the website listed in Appendix B.

ELECTROCONVULSIVE TREATMENT

Agents to induce seizures for therapeutic results date back to the 16th century. The use of electricity to induce therapeutic seizures was first used on animals, specifically dogs and pigs. In 1938, two Italian neuropsychiatrists, Ugo Cerletti and Lucio Bini, used electricity to induce seizures in humans. By the 1940s, electroconvulsive treatment (ECT) was widely conducted on people with all different categories of psychiatric symptoms, especially severe depression.

The mode of action of ECT is to induce a seizure on an anesthetized person by firing electronic signals into the brain's synapses, much as a car battery would be jumped. Over the years, the procedure has been fine-tuned, targeting specifically impaired parts of the brain. Furthermore, medications are administered to circumvent adverse side effects, such as broken and dislocated bones, the feeling of being smothered, and impaired memory. One popular movie, *One Flew over the Cuckoo's Nest*, portrayed its main character, Randie Patrick Murphy, as incapacitated and a shell of his former self after receiving ECT, which made such an impact on mainstream society that the administration of ECT drastically declined (Case et al., 2013).

Today, generally speaking, a prime candidate for ECT would be someone whose brain synapses were ineffectively firing or not firing at all. These populations include the elderly and adults who experience intractable depression, meaning every available intervention and medication has been tried with little to no positive results. Electroconvulsive treatment is still widely used today, with varying results. (Kellner, 2015; McKnight, 2015).

In an unpublished study, Dr. Charles Kellner, professor of psychiatry at the Icahn School of Medicine at Mount Sinai, New York, reports high success rates using ultra-brief-pulse ECT and a low dose of the antidepressant venlafaxine (brand name—Effexor) on elderly patients. Kellner's report shows an 85% reduction of suicidality and a 50% increase in mood. Additionally, nearly 18% of these patients displayed rapid and significant improvement (reduction in depressive symptoms) in just 1 week. For some, ultra-brief-pulse ECT may be a viable consideration to achieve a significantly better quality of life when depressive symptoms have been disabling (Kellner, 2015).

TRANSORBITAL LOBOTOMY

Transorbital lobotomy was brought to the United States by the American neurologist and psychiatrist Walter Jackson Freeman II and neurologist James Watts in 1936. They performed the first surgery at George Washington Hospital in Washington, DC. Freeman wanted to bring this surgery to the people he thought needed it the most—patients in state psychiatric hospitals. There, they had no surgeons, operating rooms, or anesthesia. Freeman and Watts refined the psychosurgery so that it could be more easily conducted outside of sterile operating rooms and in outpatient settings by accessing the frontal lobes through the eye socket. Freeman frequently practiced in his own kitchen with an ice pick from the drawer and carloads of grapefruits. Freeman performed the first refined surgery on a live person in 1946. In 1947, Watts ended the relationship with Freeman because he was repulsed by Freeman's minimization and fervent promotion of the procedure and himself. By 1951, over 18,608 people had been lobotomized (Shorter, 1998; Rogers, 2011).

There are a number of highly publicized narratives of individuals who were lobotomized. At the age of 23, Rosemary Kennedy, John F. Kennedy's sister, was lobotomized and physically paralyzed, requiring institutional care for the remainder of her life (Kessler, 1996). Howard Dully was one of the youngest to be lobotomized at the age of 12 (Dully & Fleming, 2007; NPR, 2005). To hear Howard Dully's story, go to the website listed in Appendix B.

Freeman performed over 3,400 lobotomies, mostly on women, in 23 states. He sometimes performed several at one time, boasting his skill and power. In February 1967, Freeman conducted his final lobotomy on Helena Mortensen, who was one of many who died of cerebral hemorrhage. Following this, Freeman was banned from performing any additional lobotomies (NPR, 2005).

PHYSICAL RESTRAINTS

Physical restraints have been used throughout history to detain individuals who experience psychosis and other symptoms of mental illness who are deemed out of control and display unsafe behaviors. There have been a variety of materials used to construct physical restraints, including metal shackles, wood, leather wrist and ankle cuffs, and canvas straightjackets. Most people who have been psychiatrically hospitalized will be able to give reports of involuntarily being physically restrained or witnessing others who were involuntarily kept in physical restraints. While mental health professionals have historically used physical restraints in situations where they simply do not know what else to do to keep an individual and the surrounding community safe, many use physical restraints as an to control a person, instead of dealing with the situation in a more effective manner, or to simply exert power of the individual. Let's consider the following examples taken from real inpatient scenarios.

Step Behind the Line

Tina was psychiatrically hospitalized for the first time for treatment of severe depression. She witnessed another patient being wrestled by staff into the isolation room. A nurse yelled for Tina to step behind the painted line in the floor so as to keep others away and safe from the incident. Tina, having never seen this kind of *treatment* before, stood frozen and asked what was going on. Half of her foot was across the painted line on the floor. Again, the nurse yelled at Tina to step behind the line. When Tina did not follow this nurse's demands, Tina was swiftly also wrestled into restraints.

Get Out of Bed or Else You Will Be Put in Physical Restraints

Kane was in a state psychiatric hospital for the treatment of severe and paralyzing depression. When Kane was unable to follow staff's demands to get out of bed, he was placed in restraints, lying down in his bed. While staff was connecting and locking the restraints, Kane was told, "You wanted this. You like this, huh?" Believing that patients like and want restraints is a common rationalization for the emotional trauma of implementing physical restraints. This behavior is another manifestation of defensive countertransference, by overpowering someone who is so frail. The staff could not bear to empathize with Kane (Cohen, 1975).

No Hitting for Four Days

Jimmy was admitted to an acute inpatient psychiatric hospital for institutional care and the management of severely impaired impulse control. No residential treatment facility would take him in his current impaired state. The one appropriate residential facility that would consider accepting Jimmy made the stipulation that he had to "refrain from hitting another person for the magic four days." You can take a wild guess how many days Jimmy was kept in solitary confinement and five-point physical restraints so that the medical chart would reflect that he had not hit another person for four days. If you guessed four days, you are correct.

In the attempt to change the culture of implementing physical restraints, the overuse of tranquilizing medications (serial and as needed—PRN) may become the only method of managing unsafe behaviors. However, a different, more humane and effective method of dealing with unsafe behaviors is needed beyond these two options. Furthermore, colleagues at two separate state psychiatric hospitals have told me that on any given day, one-third of all payroll staff are out on medical leave as a result of being physically assaulted by patients. Therefore, when a hospital or other treatment provider uses more effective methods of dealing with escalating behaviors, the use of physical restraints, tranquilizing medication, and client and staff injuries goes down. When the risk and reality of experienced and witnessed physical and emotional injuries go down and authentic therapeutic connection occurs, we can imagine that patient and staff reward goes up. The clinical skills of *Listening with Psychotic Ears* will give clinicians an alternative tool to use and change the treatment culture.

Psychiatric survivors have come forward and told their stories to legislative bodies that have instilled laws that limit the implementation and length of time that physical restraints can be used. Because of these actions, the overuse of physical restraints has fallen from favor, law, and practice in the United States; however, some acute and long-term residential mental health treatment facilities still rely on physical restraints and tranquilizing medications. Additionally, recipients of mental health treatment have heard these stories through the movies, the news, and informal social storytelling. The most terrorized were the individuals on whom these *treatment methods* were performed or who witnessed fellow mental health patients forced into physical restraints. As the person is now in need of mental health treatment, he or she rightly feels skeptical of its well-touted *benefits*. Therein lies the veil of threat to one's physical safety and integrity as one considers mental health treatment. Here is the very definition of the term "iatrogenic trauma."

PSYCHOTROPIC MEDICATIONS

This section discusses the unethical overuse and iatrogenic effects of psychotropic medications. In the interest of space and focus, this section specifically highlights antipsychotic medications and not the wide range of other psychopharmaceuticals, such as antidepressants and antianxiety medications.

The use of psychotropic medications was introduced in the early 1950s when the tranquilizing effects of reserpine, a medication used to treat high blood pressure, were observed when given to patients in long-term psychiatric hospitals (Lopez-Munoz et al., 2004). Chlorpromazine (brand name Thorazine) was introduced during this time, as well. These medications did not treat the positive (hallucinations and delusions) and negative (cognitive disorganization) symptoms of psychosis, but had a sedating effect, which reduced the perceived need to physically restrain and isolate individuals. Over the years, other psychotropic medications, including haloperidol (brand name Haldol) and fluphenazine (brand name Prolixin) were developed that actively treated positive psychotic symptoms by working on specific dopamine receptors. Over the years, many new antipsychotic medications have been developed, tested, and marketed, each working on different neurotransmitters and synapses, carrying hope of improving mood and decreasing positive and negative psychotic symptoms, resulting in the improvement of executive functioning and quality of life.

Today, largely as a result of the partnership between the colossally wealthy pharmaceutical companies (their lobbying efforts to secure their astronomical profits) and 1980s managed-care insurance reimbursement protocols, mainstream mental health treatment for symptoms of psychosis consists of first-line use of psychotropic medications. Most commercial health insurance companies are reluctant and even refuse to reimburse for mental health treatment unless the patient is compliant with prescribed psychotropic medication. Other treatment approaches, including individual therapy, are considered helpful but secondary to the use of psychotropic medications.

Psychotropic medications come with passionate discussions about efficacy and secondary harm, and these discussions contribute to the vulnerability of integrity and efficacy in the field of psychiatry. Robert Whitaker, in his 2011 book *Anatomy of an Epidemic: Magic Bullets, Psychiatric Drugs, and the Astonishing Rise of Mental Illness in America*, summarized a large quantity of empirical studies with large sample sizes. These studies compared samples of individuals with psychotic symptoms to those who do not receive psychotropic medications. Whitaker's book (2011) is chocked full of studies with findings that show long-term use of psychotropic medications result in *more* severe impairment in cognition, mood, and physical health.

People who take psychotropic medications have mixed reviews of them. Some people say that taking the medications was a miracle, and every aspect of life is improved as a result. Others, many others, report serious temporary (i.e., extrapyramidal symptoms [EPS]) and, more often, permanent side effects (i.e., tardive dyskinesia [TD]), which most often includes emotional numbness, dry mouth, involuntary movements including tics and tremors, psychomotor energy lethargy, severe weight gain that instigates serious and life-altering medical conditions, and sexual dysfunction, to name a few.

Many individuals who are prescribed these medications report the overvaluation of neurotransmitters, or attributing dysphoric emotions, trauma ruminations, and impaired social functioning to brain chemistry. When neurotransmitters and brain tissue are reductionistically concluded to be the cause of these impairments, then, logically, psychotropic medications are equally reductionistically concluded to be the only intervention. This perspective excludes trauma and serious attachment loss as explanations for these impairments, and this denial results in not appropriately attending to the identification and necessary grieving process that can and does result in healing. Individuals with lived experience report a range of overwhelming emotional reactions to invalidation of their emotional and spiritual life and the overvaluation of psychotropic medications that may or may not provide relief of psychotic symptoms and mood impairment and may cause serious and even fatal reactions. One can easily find these psychiatric-survivor narratives on the Internet and at conferences that are organized by and for people with lived experiences of mental illness, such as Mind Freedom and The Center for Dignity, Recovery, & Empowerment. The International Society for Psychological and Social Approaches to Psychosis (ISPS) distributes the "Bibliography of First Person Narratives of Madness," which provides narratives told by individuals and families with lived experiences about the process of SMI and the results of iatrogenic trauma from mental health professionals and their interventions in the mental health treatment system (see Appendix B). Many of these narratives include the unethical administration and iatrogenic effects of psychotropic medications.

An antipsychiatry or antimedication perspective will not characterize or benefit this discussion of *Listening with Psychotic Ears*. On the contrary, the author fully acknowledges that these interventions, especially psychotropic medications, when used thoughtfully and at appropriate dosages, can save lives and dramatically improve quality of life. However, certain frequently prescribed medications can cause severe, sometimes permanent, physical side effects and impairment. Further, some medications have a history of being dispensed for punitive reasons or for the convenience of mental health care workers. In addition, the most marginalized people, including people of color, the poor, the socially isolated, illicit drug users, and those with a history of violence, will be prescribed the cheapest medications available, causing the most rapid and severe side effects, including physical impairments.

Consider the following example from the observational documentary *Hurry Tomorrow* (Richard Cohen Films, 1975), in which a typical day at Metropolitan State Hospital in Norwalk, California, is video recorded. In this hospital, a male patient was so overly tranquilized by psychotropic medication that he could not even follow verbal directions that were given by hospital staff. The nurse responded, "You are not listening to me. Do you want a shot?" Although he was already so cognitively impaired by the usual dose of psychotropic medications, she proceeded to give him an intramuscular shot of Thorazine (chlorpromazine). He was unable to either protest or cooperate. The video later documented that this patient was so lethargic from the medication that he was laying on the floor in a common day room. Another patient of the ward carried the man to a couch and stayed with him, talking with him in a gentle and encouraging tone. There was no staff in sight.

People who are physically large or from historically underrepresented racial groups (excluding Asians, who are stereotypically viewed as compliant and emotionally withholding, thus not threatening) will frequently be overmedicated with high doses of the least costly psychotropic medications. The intention is to quickly and effectively calm the individual to prevent any unsafe actions. Notice that the underlying assumption is that there will be unsafe actions. These high doses of medications are rationalized with comments such as "What if this person became emotionally disregulated? We are just looking out for everyone's safety." What narrative does this practice of overmedicating a selected few create in the recipient and others who stand witness? It is important to consider these issues when exploring the spectrum of mental health interventions, especially because medication remains the priority of public mainstream interventions for many mental healthcare providers treating people who experience psychotic symptoms.

Taking a much closer look at these oppressive and torturous practices, whether directly done to a person, witnessed by someone, or heard through the grapevine by people with symptoms of mental illness, this culture of practice deeply, deeply alters a person's belief system and behavior, and these people begin to develop their own standards of behavior. Today, the older a person is, the more intense is the impact of these practices on the person's beliefs about themselves and the world. Whereas many of these medical procedures are only done under special circumstances and are highly monitored, some, including the overuse of psychotropic medication, are not quite as restricted. Furthermore, physical integrity is often not secure, especially in mainstream treatment settings. When physical integrity is insecure, mental integrity is also insecure, causing an exacerbation of psychotic symptoms. This scenario is a perfect example of iatrogenic trauma.

Currently, when a person enters into the mental health treatment delivery system, the person is quickly labeled with some kind of DSM diagnosis for reasons of funding and treatment pathways. If the person is experiencing symptoms of psychosis, the diagnosis will most likely include schizophrenia. Because of the pressure to diagnose within the first session and the fact that diagnosis is often performed in isolation (meaning there is only one clinician interviewing the client), the working diagnosis often does not accurately reflect the manifested symptoms. When the individual returns to the treatment agency or office, subsequent clinicians are expected to follow the initial diagnosis (especially if given by a psychiatrist) and implement a treatment pathway with the purpose of packaging the person with all the resources needed to live in the community. For a person with symptoms of psychosis, this treatment pathway frequently means securing his or her buy-in to *The River*.

Whereas many of the Victorian mental asylums have now been replaced with modern, smaller institutions and the most egregious torturous practices are no longer in use, the interplay between the culture of mental health treatment delivery and the culture of *mental patient* is ever present. Subtle beliefs about the intentions, prognoses, and capacities of people who experience psychosis still oppress nearly all individuals who experience symptoms of psychosis. While we have moved away from the practice of hospitalizing individuals for long periods, there still is an attitude that these individuals matter less; do not have legitimate feelings, concerns, or reactions; and should compliantly take their neuroleptic medications and wait quietly until the symptoms pass. The culture of we/they still exists, has impact, and results in deep and pervasive oppression on individuals who experience psychosis. Once a person enters the mental health treatment delivery system and receives a DSM diagnosis, membership in this *total institution* culture is forced, and the natural progression of his or her natural roles (such as long-term friendships and career milestones) will automatically be enormously and irretrievably disrupted or eliminated, and this person will now fall victim to assumptions based on stigma. In the mental health treatment delivery system, every action receives the same reaction regardless of severity, every minute is scripted, and every response is judged.

Every once in a while, and by a miracle, a person who has been caught in *The River* is released by the strong current. He pops out of the gripping current saying things like, "I want off this medication! I want to go back to school! I want a job! I want a life partner! I want to belong somewhere meaningful! I want to feel something!" Whereas all these statements are intended to create a self-determined life worth living, he will not likely realize these dreams while in the mainstream mental health treatment delivery system; yet, this system is all he has known. The more enlightened human recovery guide will simultaneously nurture and facilitate the realization of these dreams and assist with mourning the loss of time gone by, a result of iatrogenic trauma. If a person with psychotic experiences wants to get training to be employed as a violin player for example, then that and all the steps in between will be the therapeutic goals. Having these meaningful goals will help a person to be realistic about challenges and develop coping skills and safety net problem-solving.

Now, this journey through the *Listening with Psychotic Ears* philosophy, which you are allowing me to guide you through, will have its challenges. Some of the information will be unfamiliar and radical, thus requiring the reader to stop, consider, exercise skepticism and hope, and reflect. I invite you to read at your own pace. Take your questions to people in your world who inspire you and believe in your greater well-being.

Today, people who receive mental health treatment consistently report serious omissions by their treatment providers. Their reports indicate that clinicians do not have enough time; patients are herded into various mental health treatment facilities; and psychotropic medications are given with force and overabundance. People with symptoms of mental illness want relief, acceptance, choices, and a voice. These complaints are far too common.

Mainstream mental health treatment has come a long way since the days of transorbital lobotomies, ECT, and the like. Evidence-based interventions being mandated in mental health treatment facilities across the United States are a movement toward more effective and humane interventions. Still, many mental health consumers still report significant gaps in treatment.

For many people, especially clinicians, the subjective world of people who experience psychosis has not been accessible because Western society has historically discarded these people in institutions, and they have been forgotten. Goffman, Sullivan, Fromm-Reichmann, Winnicott, and other psychological theorists and anthropological pioneers have given us the vocabulary and context by which to explore the common and subjective experiences of people who experience psychosis and other symptoms of SMIs. Many, including psychiatric survivors, family members, and clinicians, are fed up with this reductionist and literally disabling treatment perspective. Now, it is up to enlightened clinicians, family members, loved ones, and individuals with lived experience to use this information with the best intentions toward the healing of psychotic experiences and improved quality of life.

FINAL THOUGHTS

Coming to this information in a capacity to create a shift in how mental health treatment is approached relies on the willingness of the reader to accept the information. The contemporary neurophysiologist Daniel Siegel (2010a) asserts that we have a range of openness to integrate new information, dictated by subjective experience. In *reactions of certainty*, Siegel (2010a) states that we experience certainty and are not open to any additional information or options. Some readers of this book, in reaction to these fresh clinical and philosophical ideas, say, "I am comfortable with my belief in the current mental health treatment delivery paradigm. I am not taking in any new information." Of these readers, I ask that they question their dogged refusal to acknowledge new ways of working with people who live with symptoms of psychosis and try to understand what holds them back from being open to change.

Another place on the range of subjective experience is *skepticism and the openness to probability* (Siegel, 2010a). The skeptical reader might react with the following thoughts: "Hmm, I *doubt* that a person who is experiencing psychosis can be accurately understood, be communicated with, and have increased reward in his or her subjective experience and quality of life, but with additional information, there may be some possibility. Tell me more." To this reader, I acknowledge and respect the need for safety and stability. I provide practice- and evidence-based principles and narratives that illustrate these more buoyant and hopeful outcomes.

Finally, Siegel (2010a) asserts that in the *open plane of possibilities*, a person takes into consideration new information and allows for new beliefs to surface. This reader will take the abundant information being offered toward healing the distress of psychosis and leap over the constraints of history to visualize a paradigm bursting with enlightened possibilities, growth, and progressive outcomes.

The spirit of Siegel's discussion is not intended to be reductionist. There is the hope of enlightenment to the workings of one's mind and an offering of choices about how we experience and integrate new information. The reader is invited to be grounded in the open plane of possibilities. The philosophy of *Listening with Psychotic Ears* has the ability to make even the most seasoned professional a believer or, at the very least, a more effective practitioner.

4

Evidence of Unethical and Ineffective Mainstream

Mental Health Treatment

THE MAINSTREAM MENTAL health treatment delivery system is filled with self-serving and coercive ineffective practices. Both long-term scientific studies and the majority of individuals who receive mainstream public mental health treatment have discouraging stories to tell about their treatment experiences. Let's face it, mainstream public mental health treatment and services have limitations in showing improvement in quality of life and continue to cause iatrogenic trauma, for many individuals who live with symptoms of severe mental illness (SMI), especially psychosis. While there are pockets of effective and humane avenues of mental health treatment, much of mainstream public mental health treatment focuses on psychotropic medications and is both ineffective and inhumane. Research and narrative findings of these ideas are explored in this chapter. Moreover, we explore how the mainstream mental health treatment system got to be so unethical and misguided.

PHARMACEUTICAL COMPANIES ARE UNETHICAL DICTATORS OF MENTAL HEALTH PRACTICE GUIDELINES

Much of the information in this section is drawn from the investigative and detailed work of Robert Whitaker and Lisa Cosgrove, *Psychiatry Under the Influence: Institutional Corruption, Social Injury, and Prescriptions for Reform* (2015). We are grateful for their expertise, time, and efficient efforts to identify and summarize these pivotal details from original documents that shed light on where the mental health treatment system and its customers exist today.

Currently, when talking to anyone about mental illness or mental health treatment, the topic of psychotropic medications always comes up in the conversation, usually within the first few minutes. Taking a step back, we ask, "Why has the public mainstream mental health treatment system decided that the administration of psychotropic medication should be the focus of mental health practice guidelines?" Healy, in his book, *The Creation of Psychopharmacology* (2002), shares his insights on the answer to this question.

In 1980, the APA published the DSM-III, which "marked the moment that the APA moved away from psychoanalytic explanations for mental disorders and adopted what it considered to be a more scientific way to think about psychiatric difficulties" (Whitaker & Cosgrove, 2015, p. 9), essentially tossing out subjective experiences and associations in favor of neurobiological factors. Additionally, in the United States, in 1985, around $800 million were spent on psychiatric drugs. This number increased to more than $40 billion in 2011 (Wilker, 2009). One cannot deny the correlation between a shift in cause toward biology and the skyrocketing numbers in dollars spent on psychotropic medications. But how, exactly, did this happen?

In 1976, the APA received a mere $294,842 in pharmaceutical company grants, which were used for training its psychiatrists. Just prior to this, in 1974, the APA board worried that "APA's relationships with pharmaceutical companies were going beyond the bounds of professionalism [and] were compromising our principles" (Pollock, 1981, pp. 1415–1417). In response to this concern, the APA formed a task group to explore the suggested potential dependency of APA on pharmaceutical companies and the impact on APA operations, just in case this money were ever to dry up. The APA task force concluded that without this money, many local APA organizations and training programs could no longer survive. The APA then established that their principles were *not* compromised and that obtaining these and more pharmaceutical grant and contract dollars would be "top priority" (Pollack, 1981). In 1980, the APA received an additional $1.36 million in pharmaceutical company grants.

In 1980, the APA adopted the disease model of mental illness, which asserts that all symptoms of psychosis and some of mental illness are caused solely by altered brain tissue or functioning and are best treated with psychotropic medications that normalize brain functioning. Through the DSM task forces, this terminology saturated the DSM-III. The pharmaceutical companies could not have been more tickled, as this gave legitimate reasons for them to interchangeably work with the APA, marketing and providing treatments for mental illnesses. The APA began allowing pharmaceutical companies to sponsor scientific papers and presentations, which were delivered by medical school faculty at formal and social meetings at the APA annual meeting (Whitaker & Cosgrove, 2015).

Additionally, on December 12,1980, the Bayh-Doyle Act was passed that now allowed individual persons to license their discoveries to pharmaceutical companies and then receive royalties from their federally funded (i.e., National Institutes of Health [NIH]) research studies and discoveries. Pharmaceutical companies jumped on this and courted individual psychiatrists. The year 1980 was pivotal for economic partnership between pharmaceutical companies and individual psychiatrists, as the Bayh-Dole Act was passed the same year APA decided it was legitimate for pharmaceutical companies to sponsor scientific symposiums at their annual meeting. The APA annual meeting had become the most profitable fundraising event for pharmaceutical companies to lavishly stroke the senses of psychiatrists, including symposiums, meals, giveaways, massages, social activities, and "even sitting to have their portraits painted" (Whitaker & Cosgrove, 2015, p. 34). In 1980, meeting revenues were a mere $1 million. In 2004, the APA's annual meeting revenue rose to $16.9 million, enjoying a profit of $9.8 million for that year alone (APA Annual Reports 1980–2011).

These profit dollars are funneled back into the companies for many things including research, marketing, advertising, and training. As any experienced researcher knows, massage the data enough and research can tell you anything you want. This self-serving skewed research goes into medical school textbooks and professional journals, influencing mental health practitioner decision-making. Consider the following example:

Pharmaceutical companies fund short-term research that shows how psychotropic medications are, indeed, effective by quickly reducing psychotic symptoms and quieting bothersome behaviors. Antipsychotic medications do reduce the amount of dopamine in the synapses, resulting in temporarily more clear thinking. Some of the antipsychotic medications are also considered major tranquilizers, and, upon ingestion, they significantly reduce energy levels. However, Steve Hyman, former director of the NIMH, showed that the brains of people with symptoms of schizophrenia were not *born* with too much dopamine or an overabundance of dopamine receptors, stating, "There is no compelling evidence that a lesion in the dopamine system is a primary cause of schizophrenia" (Nesler & Hyman, 2002, p. 392). Upon the administration of antipsychotic medication, as the brain seeks equilibrium, additional dopamine receptors grow, which causes the brain to be more sensitive to dopamine, causing substantial and long-lasting alterations in neural functions, including both positive and negative psychotic symptoms (Hyman, 1996).

Yet, this study and others like it end up on the cutting room floor, and the short-term findings alone are going into medical books, with which medical students are educated, trained, and socialized. Thus, the continual flow of new physicians entering the field come to believe that the disease model is the ultimate word on how to treat symptoms of mental illness. Pharmaceutical companies also have departments of staff devoted to marketing these findings to insurance companies and other administrative groups with the intention for these groups to conduct their business policies in a way that ultimately benefits the pharmaceutical companies. As a result, most insurance companies have limits on coverage, including refusal of reimbursement for mental health treatment services unless the patient is taking psychotropic medications as prescribed.

People who experience symptoms of SMI actually get better with time and accurate supports. Why are the psychotropic medications pushed so very aggressively? In the year 2007 alone, $25 billion was spent on antidepressants and antipsychotic medication (Whitaker, 2011). Health insurance companies, including commercial companies (i.e., Blue Cross Blue Shield, Aetna, etc.), federal insurance (Medicare), and state insurance (Medicaid) fund most of these prescriptions. Most individuals and families could not afford an ongoing supply of these medications, as pharmaceutical companies have marked up the cost so much. As a result of pharmaceutical companies marketing to health insurance companies, insurance companies have bought into the pharmaceutical company's propaganda that psychoactive medication administration is the quickest, most efficient, and humane way to interrupt symptoms of mental illness.

Furthermore, pharmaceutical companies fund some of the work of psychiatrists. Through psychiatrist's public speaking, advocacy, and media campaigns, this financial sponsorship influences their decision-making and, thus, the public's perspective on the causes and treatments of mental illness. Some examples of how psychiatrists are influenced include workshops on how to interact with the media, public affairs campaigns, subscriptions to APA publications, an increasing number of leadership fellowships for psychiatry students, APA job searches and salaries for those positions, and documentaries about mental illness, such as *Healthy Minds*, a television program that airs on national PBS television stations. These funding efforts were characterized by then-APA-medical-director Melvin Sabshin as a way to help them grow from a "Mom and Pop" organization into a "business-like mammoth organization" (Sabshin, 2008, p. 62). Annual revenues for APA increased from $10.5 million in 1980 to $65.3 million in 2008 (APA Annual Reports, 1980–2011).

Many prominent individuals began to aggressively question and expose the influential economic partnership between the APA and pharmaceutical companies. In December 1998, after a 35-year APA membership, the psychiatrist Loren Mosher wrote a provocative resignation letter to the APA, which he condemningly renamed the "American Pharmacological Association." He asserted, "psychiatry has been almost completely bought out by the drug companies" and calls psychiatrists "drug company pats[ies]," as their primary focus is now "prescription writing" (Mosher, 1998). He criticizes the efforts of the APA to align with the National Alliance on Mental Illness (NAMI), which aims to enhance the pharmaceutical companies' fraudulent practices of posing as healers for their true purpose of making money. The letter can be viewed in its entirety at the website listed in Appendix B.

Uncovering industry funding, Iowa Senator Charles Grassley asked the APA for a "complete accounting of APA revenues, except those from advertising in our journals, from pharmaceutical companies, starting in 2003" (Silverman, 2008, para. 6). Senator Grassley asserted the obvious influence on nonprofit organizations that claim to be independent in philosophy and practices. The APA decided to form a task group, the Work Group on Future Relationships with Industry, to address the future of this financial partnership (Yan, 2010). Policies that had been in place and resulted in mammoth profits were now revised. The APA meeting revenues plummeted from $65.3 million in 2008 to $42.6 million in 2012 (APA, 2011).

FOR WHAT WAS/IS THIS APA/PHARMACEUTICAL COMPANY PARTNERSHIP MONEY USED?

Pharmaceutical companies hire academic psychiatrists to be spokespersons, advisors, and consultants for their products (i.e., tests, monitoring devices, and medications) (Carey, 2008).

> They could be involved in every aspect of the drug-development process; providing advice on how to design the trials; serving as investigators in media after those results were published; and then, following the FDA's [Food and Drug Administration] approval of the drug, speaking about it and the related disorder at CME [Continuing Medical Education] conferences and dinners organized by the pharmaceutical company. (Whitaker & Cosgrove, 2015, p. 40)

The exact details of these partnerships are available through the disclosure reports submitted by the 273 speakers at the 2008 APA annual meeting, in which the following contracts were revealed: 888 consulting contracts and 483 speakers' bureau contracts (APA Annual Meeting Program, 2008). Additionally, pharmaceutical companies fund many prominent persons of psychiatric professional literature and standards, including professional journal editors, editors of psychiatric medical school textbooks and clinical practice guidelines, developers of diagnostic criteria, and chairs of psychiatric departments at medical schools (Whitaker & Cosgrove, 2015). Because of the definitive status of psychiatrists in the mental health chain of command, the opinions of psychiatrists are pervasively influential over all mental health professionals and treatment services.

The DSM has been heavily influenced by the financial interests of pharmaceutical companies through academic psychiatrists who influentially speak with an industry-skewed agenda. In the 1990s, 57% of DSM-IV-TR task force members (writers) reported contracts with pharmaceutical companies; all of the groups that worked on mood disorders and schizophrenia had such financial contracts, which undoubtedly influenced their DSM disease model contributions (Cosgrove, 2006). For the DSM-5, 69% of task force members reported receiving money from the pharmaceutical industry (Cosgrove 2012). In an effort to practice more ethically and accurately, the NIMH, the United States' largest federal mental health research organization, asserted that any grant proposal that uses the DSM as mental illness nosology (categorization) would be rejected, favoring a more accurate, updated, and independent Research Domain Criteria (RDoC), "a research framework for new ways of studying mental illness" (Insel, 2013; NIMH, n.d., para. 1).

Additionally, these academic psychiatrists are being contracted with by pharmaceutical companies to serve as key opinion leaders (KOLs), whose positions hold a great deal of desired rewards, including money, power, and professional and social opportunities beyond imagination. To resist these insidious and seductive remunerations goes against survival instincts but must be considered for ethical practice to occur. Ethical and legal writers assert that the occurrence of this economy of influence was not intentional, but allowing its pervasiveness to continue is unethical and suggestive of corruption (Fava, 2008; Lessig, 2014; Whitaker & Cosgrove, 2015).

FINDINGS OF LONG-TERM STUDIES OF CHRONIC PSYCHOTROPIC MEDICATION USE

These pharmaceutical companies have conveniently omitted from their educational documents the long-term studies on people who have been taking these psychotropic medications for many years. The results of these long-term studies on chronic administration of antipsychotic medications are quite grim.

The outcomes in schizophrenic samples that have taken antipsychotic medications for many years and those who have not (or who have taken placebo medications) greatly differ. Among those who have continually taken the psychotropic medications, the following outcomes are repeatedly observed (DeSisto,

Harding, McCormick, Ashikaga, & Brooks, 1995): Individuals are more likely to have more relapses with greater severity. They are more frequently hospitalized, which is not only a disruption in the individual's life process and identity but also quite financially burdensome to the individual, their families, and taxpayers. These individuals experience psychotic symptoms that are more persistent and intensifying, emotional numbness, decreased motivation, and social disengagement. These individuals experience more physical symptoms including nausea, vomiting, diarrhea, agitation, insomnia, headaches, unusual motor tics (including tardive dyskinesia), and lethargy. These individuals are more likely to be dependent on the finances of social service benefits, including Social Security, Medicare, and Medicaid (Bockoven, 1975; Gardos & Cole, 1977). Additionally, the higher the medication dose, the greater the severity of these symptoms and probability of relapse (Prein, 1971). Finally, people who are chronically administered antipsychotic medications experience early death, dying 15 to 25 years earlier compared to a general population sample (Morgan, 2003; Tiihonen, 2006). The seriously mentally ill are dying of cardiovascular ailments, respiratory problems, metabolic illness, diabetes, and kidney failure (Whitaker, 2011).

Many studies exist that compare outcomes of medicated people with schizophrenia to those with schizophrenia who did not take antipsychotic medications (or placebo) (Bola, 2005; Bola & Mosher, 2003; Carpenter, 1977; Carpenter & McGlashan, 1977; Perry, 1998; Rappaport, 1978). These studies found that the unmedicated populations were discharged from mental hospitals sooner, had lower rates of symptom relapse, experienced reduced rates and severity of depression, displayed less blunted emotions, and suffered less lethargy. In several studies, the subjects who experienced psychotic episodes and did not take antipsychotic medications reported their emotions as gratified and informed (Carpenter & McGlashan, 1977; Harding et al., 1987; Harding & Zahniser, 1994; Rappaport, 1978).

David Helfgott, a renowned pianist whose life is depicted in the Academy Award–winning movie *Shine*, was diagnosed with schizophrenia (Scott & Hicks, 1996). In a documentary about his life, Helfgott asserted that he does take psychotropic medications, but he takes less than his psychiatrist prescribes so he can experience his feelings, as the prescribed dose left him emotionally numb. Many individuals who have been diagnosed with a psychotic disorder report in social conversations that they can think more clearly on the medications, but that a lower dose of the antipsychotic medications offers more optimal thinking and functioning without so many side effects. Some individuals who live with psychotic symptoms report that the right combination and dosages of medications has saved their lives. Again, these studies are not commonly found in mainstream education that focuses on shaping the mental health profession's and practitioners' treatment philosophies.

INCREASED MENTAL DISABILITY ENROLLMENT IN SSI AND SSDI

We would expect, since 1955, when psychotropic medications were first made publically available and their use pronounced, that rates of enrollment in Social Supplemental Income (SSI) and Social Supplemental Disability Income (SSDI) for mental disability would decrease, since the medications are so *promisingly effective*. In fact, these rates (i.e., mental disability rates) are skyrocketing. In 1987, 1.25 million (one in 184) Americans received SSI or SSDI as a result of a mental illness. In 2007, there were 3.97 million (one in 76), and in 2011, there were approximately 4.5 million individuals who received SSI or SSDI as a result of a mental illness (Whitaker, 2010, p. 6). These results show a sixfold increase in the mental disability rate since 1955. So, at the very least, with this focus on psychotropic medications, we can confidently say that psychotropic medications are not effective in decreasing mental disability. Other humane and effective interventions to SMI are urgently needed.

INCREASED SPENDING ON PSYCHOTROPIC MEDICATIONS AND LESS ON HOUSING

The Substance Abuse and Mental Health Services Administration (SAMHSA) Spending Estimate Project (2010) compared national spending for mental health prescription drugs and levels of treatment (residential, outpatient, and inpatient). In 1986, approximately $6 million or 7% of $32 billion was spent on prescription drugs. In 2005, this figure increased to $141 billion or 27% of $113 billion. Comparatively, in 1986, money spent on residential treatment facilities accounted for 22% of $32 billion earmarked for national mental health. This figure declined to 22% of $113 billion in 2005. While national mental health dollars are increasingly being spent on psychotropic medications, fewer dollars are spent on housing. This discrepancy in the allocation of funds is detrimental to progress for those living with mental illness because the longer a person is in the mental health treatment system, the more they will be marginalized from society, including work. Thus, their poverty level will become more certain, and more people with mental illness will join the many who are already homeless, in transitional housing, or in very low-income neighborhoods with high crime rates because that is all they can afford. What would be more beneficial is to put money into making affordable and safe housing available to people living with mental illness.

INCREASED ILLICIT DRUG USE

To cope with a severe lack of hope and helplessness, individuals who find themselves living with paralyzing symptoms of SMI often turn to recreational drugs.

In a large sample size of 9,142 individuals diagnosed with schizophrenia, bipolar disorder with psychotic features, or schizophrenia, Hartz et al. (2014) conducted a large case-control study. The researchers found that, compared with the control group (n = 10,195), people with psychotic disorders had significantly higher use of tobacco products, alcohol, marijuana, and recreational drugs. Additionally, while public health efforts have decreased smoking tobacco among the general population younger than 30, these efforts have been ineffective among individuals with severe psychotic illnesses (Hartz et al., 2014).

As we are painfully aware, heavy use of tobacco, alcohol, and other drugs is strongly correlated with life-altering results. These results include medical problems such as cancer, heart disease, and other serious medical problems contributing to the 25-year premature death rate for people with SMI (Hartz et al., 2014). A drug-influenced lifestyle inevitably leads to dealings with the criminal justice system or medical problems, which can continue to severely alter an individual's life course. Individuals who live with drug addiction and SMI find themselves faced with a multitude of negative consequences, including more frequent crises, longer and more severe episodes of decompensation, lower rates of education, unemployment, poverty, few reliable social supports, more frequent and more severe medical problems, homelessness, social isolation, significantly higher stress rates, and physical and sexual assault.

INCREASED SUICIDE RATES

To reiterate what was discussed in Chapter 1, "Types of Psychosis and General Intervention Approaches," the suicide rates for people living with schizophrenia differ in severity and age range from the rates for the general population. Despite the assertions of successful treatment outcomes using psychotropic medications, mental health treatment has seemingly been so ineffective that social marginalization becomes inevitable. At that point, when a person realizes that living with mental illness is all the future holds for him or her, the option is often so grim that, for some, suicide is considered a "better" option (Palmer, Pankratz, & Bostwick, 2005).

VERMONT STUDIES LONG-TERM OUTCOMES

The classic Vermont and Maine studies compared long-term outcomes in samples of individuals who received psychosocial rehabilitation (Vermont) and traditional treatment that focused on psychotropic medications (Maine). Sample subjects were matched by age, sex, diagnosis, and chronicity. Results revealed more positive outcomes in the Vermont sample that had more live individuals, more productivity, fewer symptoms, better community adjustment and higher global functioning (DeSisto et al., 1995; Harding et al., 1987). Both samples consisted of individuals who met the schizophrenia criteria from the DSM-II (later and retrospectively rediagnosed with DSM-III), excluding those who were elderly, criminally mandated (forensic population), diagnosed with organic brain disorder, and had alcohol- or drug-induced diagnoses. Every attempt was made to exactly match the Vermont and Maine samples, including age, gender, diagnosis, and length of hospital stay (DeSisto et al., 1995; Harding et al., 1987). While there was a large sample to draw from, after exact matching occurred, the final sample size was 296.

Treatment principles in the Vermont State Hospital were more congruent with a psychosocial rehabilitation model. The Vermont State Hospital and the Vermont Vocational Rehabilitation Division paired to provide a comprehensive program that drew from the fields of medicine, vocation, and sociology. The following principles were emphasized: self-sufficiency, blurring of staff/patient roles, meaning more authenticity and egalitarian power structure, intensified relationships, higher expectations for both patients and staff, community residences, employment placement, and linkage to natural supports in the community.

The Maine treatment principles included that of traditional care, meaning public mainstream mental health treatment. The following principles were emphasized: psychotropic medications (considering this treatment was delivered in the mid-1950s, this included early tranquilizing medications, including reserpine and chlorpromazine (brand name Thorazine) and outpatient care from hospital workers and then community mental health centers. There were little to no vocational efforts, and halfway houses were not yet available to the Maine resident sample.

According to Harding and colleagues, the findings in the Vermont sample were surprisingly optimistic, contrary to common thought about individuals who were considered severely mentally ill (Harding et al., 1987). Following a 3-hour interview, 68% (82 people) who previously met DSM-III criteria for schizophrenia no longer had any signs or symptoms of schizophrenia. Forty-five percent showed no mental health symptoms at all. Twenty-three percent shifted symptoms and diagnosis to affective or organic disorders.

While 82% of these Vermont sample individuals had been prescribed psychotropic medications (75% low to medium dose range), patients reported variation in how these medications were actually ingested. During official interviews, 75% reported compliance with medication prescription. In additional interviews, about 25% reported always taking medication; 25% took medication when symptoms were present; and 34% did not take their medications. Add the 34% who did not comply with the 16% who were not prescribed medications, and this leaves a total of 50% who did not take psychotropic medications.

The long-term follow up outcomes (5, 10, 20, 25, and 32 years) were surprising, despite the low function assumption of the Vermont sample, who were chosen because of their assumed chronicity of illness, evidenced by long-term stays on the maximum security hospital wards. The findings showed few to no mental symptoms, classifying these individuals as recovered or significantly improved, as evidenced by the following. The Vermont sample had little to no need for any inpatient or outpatient supportive services, had frequent meetings with friends, with at least one close friend, had employment or school enrollment, and were able to adequately meet their own basic needs. These findings are contradictory to many myths, including that individuals who are diagnosed with schizophrenia are disabled and need to be completely cared for. These myths and the methods by which these individuals are approached and worked with are in need of serious reconsideration, favoring recovery efforts that allow for the individual to be supported in creating a rewarding life and simply being humanely treated as a person.

The Maine sample, who had traditional mental health treatment that involved long-term hospitalization, psychotropic medications, and little or no involvement in vocational services, had very different outcomes at follow-up. First, the Maine sample had more attrition as a result of death (180 Vermont vs. 119 Maine). The Maine sample was kept in the hospital longer and had less education. The Maine sample were found to be working less (26%) than the Vermont sample (47%). The Maine sample displayed more limiting symptoms of mental illness (emotional withdrawal, conceptual disorganization, guilt feelings, mannerisms/posturing, depressed mood, hostility, hallucinatory behavior, unusual thought content, blunted affect, disorientation, auditory hallucinations) and had less community adjustment. The functioning rating of at least "pretty well" was Maine at 49% and Vermont at 68%, showing that the Maine sample had an overall lowering functioning rating (DeSisto et al., 1995).

FINAL THOUGHTS

In this chapter, the massive wealth and power of the pharmaceutical companies has been exposed. Pharmaceutical companies have been insidious in their influence over what phenomena are researched, the outcomes are skewed, and these massaged outcomes go into medical textbooks and the eager minds of medical students. Because of historical trends, these medical students, then, are blindly escorted in as leaders in the mental health field, thus influencing the practice of other mental health professions. With pharmaceutical companies leading the mental health treatment delivery system, with health insurance companies in tow, we are seeing layers of severe iatrogenic trauma, including physical health decompensation, overall low quality of life, and premature death. Unethical and ineffective mental health treatment is alive and well in the mainstream and public mental health system. An urgent paradigm shift in how psychotic symptoms are understood and addressed is needed.

5

Historically Ethical and Effective Mental Health Approaches

for Healing the Distress of Psychotic Experiences

HISTORICAL CONTRIBUTORS TO HEALING PSYCHOSIS

To truly understand the details and depths of any current situation and accurately assess feasible and effective future potentials, an exhaustive identification and exploration of past theorists, clinicians, and communities who have enjoyed successful outcomes must ensue. This chapter provides detailed information about the important historical work of individual people, programs, and communities—some that have been already briefly discussed in previous chapters—who believe in the work of healing by hearing, communicating, and holding real recovery hope with people who actively experience symptoms of psychosis. While the clinical techniques of *Listening with Psychotic Ears* have not yet gone through the rigorous investigation to be categorized as evidence-based practices, many clinicians, family members, friends, and people who experience symptoms of psychosis hold these techniques in esteemed regard and refer to them as *practice-informed* interventions.

This group of people is in desperate desire for effective and humane tools for healing the distress of psychotic experiences. Anyone, including clinicians, whose scope of practice does and does not include prescribing neuroleptic medications can be inspired by a number of principles and techniques from these giants who have walked before us.

Quakers—The Religious Society of Friends

Quakers, or the Religious Society of Friends, have had a long and significant impact on the historical and contemporary delivery of mental health services. In 1790, a young widowed Quaker woman, Hannah Mills, was hospitalized for the treatment of "melancholy" at the York Asylum (now Bootham Park Hospital) in the Bootham District of York, England. Her family made attempts to visit her and were refused, with the reasoning that she was in private treatment. After being there for 45 days, Mills died in the institution. The Quaker community was outraged and shocked by the horrid squalor living conditions that were discovered upon investigation.

William Tuke

In response to these unthinkable living conditions, the Quakers enlisted William Tuke (1732–1822), of York, to construct the kind of treatment facility where Quakers with mental illness could be cared for by Quakers and symptoms of mental illness could be healed. Tuke enlisted funds and knowledge from friends, other Quakers, and physicians. In 1796, the York Retreat was opened in Lamel Hill in the countryside of York, England (website listed in Appendix B). Treatment was based on individualized attention, kindness, benevolence, and restoration of self-esteem and functioning. Unlike other asylums of the time, all forms of punishment were banned. Quaker philosophy was embedded in all levels of facility construction. The buildings were small, homelike environments with comfortable furniture, paintings on the walls, and curtains on the windows. The buildings were housed on a large and serene piece of land, where patients were encouraged to explore. There was a low staff-to-patient ratio, and staff saw themselves as subservient to the patients.

Patients were fed nutritious and delicious foods that were thought to naturally stabilize the body's functioning. There were daily activities, such as tea parties and puppet shows, scheduled to encourage patients to get formally dressed and socialize. Patients were encouraged to engage in productive work, such as vegetable gardening, tending to farm animals, laundry, and cleaning, which made the campus self-sustainable. Physicians were intentionally excluded because of the Quaker disbelief in Western medicine. With extended stays, egalitarian values, restorative nutrition, and a predictable daily structure, people got better and were discharged from the hospital to live, once again, in the community, often after 18 months of treatment.

Samuel Tuke

Samuel Tuke (1784–1857), also of York and the grandson of William Tuke, carried on these traditions of mental health treatment reform with his commitment to the York Retreat. Samuel wrote about the treatment philosophy and practices in his book

Descriptions of the Retreat near York (1813). With the wide distribution of his book, Samuel Tuke made famous the concept of *moral treatment*. Many audiences are initially put off by the term "moral treatment," with its implied derogatory judgment of behaviors and, especially, the character of individuals. However, borrowing from the work of Jean-Baptiste Pussin and Philippe Pinel, Tuke explains the true French origin of the term—*traitment moral*—suggests the essence of the meaning is more closely to *morale*, meaning feelings, subjective experience, and the way one feels about himself. With this historical explanation, a more accurate definition of moral treatment refers to the treatment and recovery of self-esteem.

The York Retreat and moral treatment inspired many other similar treatment facilities, including American Brattleboro Retreat, Hartford Retreat, and Friends Hospital. Again, these care centers had positive treatment outcomes, and individuals were able to be discharged and live in the communities from which they came.

A Radically Benevolent Pair: Phillipe Pinel and Jean-Baptiste Pussin

Phillipe Pinel (1745–1826) was born in Jonquières, in the countryside of France, to a lineage of physicians. Despite holding his physician's degree, he didn't practice medicine in his early career, partly because of a lack of medical knowledge and partly because of dissatisfaction with being ostracized by the elitist, traditional realm of the *old school* closed system/regime because of his more moderate perspective.

In concordance with many who devote their lives to the exploration and reform of mental health treatment, Pinel had a personally moving experience. He had a close friend who developed debilitating symptoms of depression and mania who ultimately took his own life. Considering this to be an avoidable tragedy as a result of poor mental health treatment and care, Pinel was motivated to seek employment at the most prestigious asylum in Paris, where he remained for 5 years. Here, Pinel observed, explored, and discovered the foundational ideas that he carried throughout his career.

During 1793–1795, Pinel served as *physician of the infirmaries* of Bicêtre Hospital, which housed approximately 4,000 mandated male prisoners, 200 of whom were categorized as mental patients, in whom Pinel showed enthusiastic interest. There, Pinel banned torturous treatments, including blistering, purging, and bleeding, preferring observation and individualized and relational methods with his patients (Weiner, 1992). In 1794, Pinel published *Memoir on Madness* as an appeal to the French Revolutionary government to use more decent methods of working with the mentally ill (Weiner, 1992).

Jean-Baptiste Pussin (1745–1811) had been successfully treated for scrofula (tuberculosis of the neck/lymph nodes) at Bicêtre Hospital. Later, both Pussin and his persistent and empathic wife, Marguette Jubiline, were recruited as live-in custodians (not medically trained) of the mental ward of Bicêtre Hospital. There, both were observant, patient, empathic, and respectful of the patients. In 1797, Pussin banned the use of chains and iron shackles with these patients, preferring a more benevolent psychological approach.

In 1795, Pinel left Bicêtre Hospital for the Hospice de la Salpêtrière, an enormous and bureaucratically entangled hospice village for approximately 7,000 frail and indigent women. In 1802, Pinel arranged for the transfer of Pussin to Hospice de la Salpêtrière. Upon Pussin's arrival, chains and iron shackles were banned there also (Weiner, 1992).

Pinel's most important contributions revolved around the then radical ideal that mental patients needed individualized care and understanding, which was based on observations and benevolent and exploratory conversations. Additionally, Pinel was convinced that under even the most bizarre and incomprehensible manifestations of mental illness, there could be rationality. He asserted that symptoms of mental illness often originate from surrounding events, especially heartbreak or disillusionment in relationships. Pinel asserted that insanity is almost always intermittent and not a complete abandonment of reason. Pinel successfully made efforts to understand and communicate with even the most disturbed patients.

These ideas have remained true among prominent psychological healing communities throughout history and are viewed as accurate to this day. Pinel remained at Hospice de la Salpêtrière and continued his nonmedical and benevolent psychological work, also known as moral treatment, with these women until his death in 1826.

Benjamin Rush

Benjamin Rush (1746–1813) was born in the countryside of Philadelphia, Pennsylvania, to a family of seven children. When he was 5 years old, his father died, leaving his mother to care for a large family. At the age of 8, Benjamin was sent to Maryland to live with an aunt and uncle. Benjamin Rush had the finest education that was available, attending a very prestigious boarding school, now called West Nottingham Academy, Princeton University (Bachelor of Arts), and University of Edinburgh in Scotland, where he received his medical degree. At age 24, he returned to the United States, opened his own medical practice in Philadelphia, and taught chemistry at the now University of Pennsylvania. Rush was fluent in French, Italian, and Spanish and wrote the first textbook on chemistry.

Rush opposed slavery and capital punishment, and advocated for public education and public healthcare. Because his views were congruent with those of the Quakers, he has often been mislabeled as a Quaker. In fact, he was Presbyterian and very active in his religious beliefs. He was quite active and outspoken in the political arena, as well, ultimately being an original signer of the United States Declaration of Independence.

In a time when addiction and mental illness were thought to originate from weak moral character (indulgence) and willfulness, thus resulting in maltreatment and extremely marginalizing stigma, Rush asserted that the brain played a significant role in these mental illnesses. Because of this, he was named the father of American psychiatry. He advocated for the humane treatment of people with mental illness. In 1812, Rush published *Medical Inquiries and Observations upon the Diseases of the Mind*, in which he categorized symptoms. Rush said the causes of these mental disorders included blood circulation and sensory overload. His cures included bloodletting, purging, and the tranquilizing chair.

In 1783, Benjamin Rush joined the staff at Pennsylvania Hospital, where he remained until his death. As previously stated, seeing the appalling living conditions of people with mental illness, including being restrained and confined in the cold basement and sleeping on piles of hay, Rush campaigned for a more respectable and humane unit all to themselves. Pennsylvania Hospital was the first hospital in the United States to have a separate ward, out of the basement, for people with mental illness. Rush suggested placing a high stone wall around the hospital to protect the patients from the onlookers who had been allowed to peer through the windows at the mentally ill patients. He also suggested that manual labor, reminiscent of moral treatment, would prove to benefit both men and women in their recovery.

One of Rush's sons returned from his tour of duty in the US Navy with severe depression and was unable to care for himself. Rush admitted him to this mental health treatment ward of Pennsylvania Hospital, where he remained for 30 years and until his own death. Benjamin Rush died at the age of 68 of typhus fever in 1813 and was buried in Philadelphia (Landsman, 2001).

Dorothea Dix

Dorothea Dix (1802–1887) was born in Hampden, Maine. She was the eldest of three, with two younger brothers for whom she cared. Until she was 12, they lived in Worcester, Massachusetts. Then, fleeing her alcoholic and abusive father and intellectually delayed mother, who suffered from severe and frequent headaches, she ran away to her wealthy grandmother's home in Boston. At age 14, Dix was severely punished for not conforming to the wealthy lifestyle and giving away her new clothes to the poor. As a result, she was sent to live with her aunt.

Having had only sporadic education herself, Dix opened up her own school, where she taught the daughters of wealthy families. Later, she taught the children of poor families in her own home.

Dix had episodes of illness that included a cough and fatigue, especially during the winter months. During the years of 1824 to 1830, her health was so fragile, she removed herself from teaching and committed herself to writing. Her most famous manuscript, *Conversations on Common Things* (1824), was written in the style of a conversation between a mother and her child about things that a successful schoolteacher should know. Believing that women should be educated equally as men, and encouraged by her second cousin Edward Bangs, between 1831 and 1836 she established another school, a secondary school for girls in Boston. Again, Dix became very ill. At this time, Dix was encouraged to go to England for an extended respite period. The family of the social reformer Rathbone, a Quaker family, took her in. She was also introduced to the prison reformer Elizabeth Fry and to Samuel Tuke. Her own episodes of depression afforded Dix an affinity for determination for advocacy work for humane care for the mentally ill.

She was briefly engaged to marry her second cousin Edward Bangs but broke off the engagement and never married. After the death of her grandmother, in 1837, Dix returned to the United States. Her grandmother left her a significant financial inheritance, which allowed her the freedom to continue her charitable reform work.

In 1841, Dix began teaching Sunday school to women at East Cambridge Jail. During these visits, Dix noticed women with mental illness were horribly mistreated. Additionally, Dix documented the mistreatment of poor mentally ill individuals who were cared for in private homes contracted by the state. She documented the details of these situations and took the documents to be read, by a male, to the Massachusetts state legislature. (At this given time, women were not allowed to have a presence in the court.) In one inflammatory report, *Memorial*, Dix wrote, "I proceed, Gentlemen, briefly to call your attention to the present state of Insane Persons confined within this Commonwealth, in cages, stalls, pens! Chained, naked, beaten with rods, and lashed into obedience" (Dix, 1843, para. 5). Dix is noted for the reform and addition of many asylums and the building of 32 new asylums in the United States, Canada, Japan, and Scotland (Dix, 2006).

In her elder years, overcome with tuberculosis and unable to care for herself, Dix took up residence at the Greystone Park Psychiatric Hospital, a hospital she helped to reform from crowdedness and other horrid conditions. The administration gave Dix a private suite for as long as she lived. Despite her courageous and tireless advocacy for better living conditions for mentally ill in every state east of the Mississippi River and in many other countries including Japan, Scotland, Italy, England, France, Austria, Greece, Turkey, Russia, Sweden, Holland, Denmark, and Belgium, Dix refused to have any hospital named in her honor and rarely spoke about her accomplishments, as this would have produced tremendous embarrassment for her. She died on July 17, 1887, and was buried in Mount Auburn Cemetery in Cambridge, Massachusetts.

Clifford Beers

Clifford Beers (1876–1943) was a psychiatric survivor, turned activist, whose work had great impact on national and international mental health policies. When Beers was a child, he witnessed his younger brother's death—a result of having a seizure and drowning in a tub of water. Beers complained of many obsessional worries and paranoia and made several suicide attempts. As a result, he was hospitalized several times.

At one point, Beers was held against his will for 3 years. He snuck out letters begging for his release. Upon his release, Beers wrote an autobiography, *A Mind That Found Itself,* documenting the human rights violations and many abuses he and his peers suffered while under mental healthcare in the hospital. He wrote of individuals who were so far out of their minds that they were unable to follow staff directions, and for this they were beaten and forced in isolation. He spoke of being held, only in his underwear, in a straightjacket that was so tight that the circulation in his fingers was compromised (Beers, 1903).

Beer's book had a major impact on changing stigma about mental illness and improving both the quality and quantity of mental health services. The book was given an enthusiastic review by the psychiatrist Adolf Meyer, who joined Beers in his mental healthcare reform efforts. Additionally, others, including the physician William H. Welch and philosopher William James, collaborated and constructed the Connecticut Society for Mental Hygiene, whose mission was to help improve attitudes toward individuals with mental illness, develop better standards of mental healthcare, prevent mental illness, and promote thriving mental health. These efforts were adopted by other states that established their own work groups. In 1909, Beers founded the National Committee for Mental Hygiene, whose efforts reformed mental health law reform, developed grants for the purpose of researching the causes of mental disorders, and trained medical students (Manon, 2010).

Although Beers married, he and his wife decided not to have children to avoid any biological intergenerational mental illness risks. Beers's two other siblings also had a severe mental illness (SMI), were psychiatrically hospitalized, and ultimately died in the institutions by suicide.

In 1930, Beers organized the International Congress for Mental Hygiene, which was attended by representatives from 53 countries. The gathering initiated international mental healthcare reform efforts and led to the development of the International Committee for Mental Hygiene. Beers became overwhelmed by all the stress and admitted himself to Butler Hospital in Providence, Rhode Island, where he died 4 years later.

Carl Jung

Carl Jung (1875–1961) was born in Kesswil, Thurgau, Switzerland. He was the fourth and only surviving child in his family. His father was a poor rural pastor in the Swiss Reformed Church, and his mother was part of a wealthy family. His mother experienced depressive moods and most nights she retreated to her separate bedroom, enthusiastically communicating with spirits (Jung 1995). Jung's mother was occasionally physically absent as a result of hospitalizations and interpersonally absent as a result of depression and other symptoms of mental illness. At one point, Jung's father took young Carl to live with and be cared for by the father's unmarried sister. Jung acknowledges the impact that his mother's emotional distance had on him.

Young Carl was a quiet and introspective boy. At age 12, in a tussle with a classmate, Jung was pushed to the ground with such force that he became unconscious. For the next 6 months, each time he went to school or began his homework, he experienced a fainting episode. At one point, he overheard his father speaking with concern about his condition and the limitations of his future learning and career potentials. Alarmed, Jung reconsidered his ability to upgrade the family's financial resources and immediately began applying himself to his studies. He fainted only three more times and was able to more adaptively manage his fears (Jung, 1963/1989/1995).

Jung unintentionally discovered his own branch of the field of psychiatry and was captivated by the inclusion of both biology and spirituality. He obtained his medical degree in 1900. In 1906, at age 30, he published *Studies in Word Association* and sent a copy to then-50-year-old Sigmund Freud, which led to an intense friendship and correspondence that lasted 6 years. Freud viewed and endorsed Jung as his successor. Together, they traveled, delivering speeches that would forever impact the world of psychoanalysis. During these travels, Jung became acquainted with the indigenous people of Alesheim, or the *tjurungas* of Australia. In their ritualistic practices, he saw great similarities to his own early experiences of isolative and ritualistic behavior, which he felt brought him in touch with his true essence. His assertions on psychological archetypes and the collective unconscious were greatly inspired by these early important insights. However, in 1912, a theoretical difference over the nature of libido and religion ruptured Jung and Freud's friendship, which would never recover. Jung steered away from Freud's sexual developmental assertions, preferring his ideas of collective unconscious.

In 1903, Jung and Emma Rauschenbach married, and eventually had five children: one son and four daughters. They remained married until Emma's death, but the union was stormy, involving Jung's openly exhibited relationships with other women (Hayman, 1999).

At age 38, Jung began experiencing psychotic symptoms (auditory and visual hallucinations) and called these experiences "a horrible confrontation with the unconscious" (Jung, 2009). Valuing these experiences, he recorded everything he felt and kept small journals about his personal insights, revelations, and experiences. He then began to transcribe his notes and illustrations into a red leather bound book, which Jung called *The Red Book* and which can be viewed at the website listed in Appendix B. Jung left no posthumous instructions about his *Red Book*. Until its publication in 2009, only about 12 people had ever seen the document.

Jung was a devout believer in depth psychology, which is the exploration of the conscious, unconscious, and semiconscious mind. He also was strongly influenced by the collective unconscious, a collection of past ancestral experiences and wisdom that is available to any individual or group open to spiritual incoming intuitive energy.

Jung categorized individuals by their unique method of energetic rejuvenation. The *introvert* is preoccupied with his or her own mental life. Energy and reflection dwindle during social interactions. The introvert prefers solitary activities such as reading, computer work, artistry, and invention (Jung, 1995).

The *extrovert* receives gratification or energy from that which is outside the self. This person tends toward social situations, rather than isolative activities, and is talkative, energetic, and enthusiastic. Most personalities are some mixture of both introverted and extroverted but side with one.

Jung thought of individuals in terms of archetypes, the collection of past ancestral experiences, the unconscious, life milestone events, and current cultural manifestations. All this is then formulated into a stereotypical archetype such as mother, wise old man, trickster, hero, maiden, child, and many others.

Currently, Jung's work is thriving and is pervasive in many arenas that exclusively uphold the details of his philosophy. The C. G. Jung Institute was founded in 1948 in Zurich, Switzerland. Other organizations with the same name exist in the United States, including Boston, Chicago, Los Angeles, New York, San Francisco, Santa Fe, and Washington, DC (see Appendix B for websites).

Frieda Fromm-Reichmann

Frieda Fromm-Reichmann (1889–1957) was born in Karlsruhe, Germany, to an Orthodox Jewish German middle-class family. She was the eldest in a sibship of three girls. Her mother was educated, clever, confident, and enthusiastic. Her father, an iron merchant, was warm and sensitive and had a love for music and literature. Her father and mother were entirely devoted to their children, at the risk of their own relationship, for which Fromm-Reichmann often was the mediator. These experiences groomed Fromm-Reichmann to be a discerning listener—patient and personally generous. An exemplary student and privileged eldest daughter, she went to medical school and earned her medical degree in 1908. In 1911, she completed her psychiatric residency. Fromm-Reichmann directed a clinic for brain-injured German soldiers. She studied neurology with Kurt Goldstein (Bruch, 1982; Cohen, 1982).

Fromm-Reichmann became fascinated with the work of Freud and received psychoanalytic training in Berlin. In 1926, she married Eric Fromm, the renowned sociologist, psychoanalyst, and philosopher. They began a psychoanalytic training institute, and in 1930, they opened a residential sanitarium for the healing of psychosis. It abruptly closed in 1933, when Hitler came to power. That same year, the couple separated. The marriage is said to have not been a mutually rewarding relationship from the beginning, as Fromm burdened Fromm-Reichmann with his desires for a motherly figure. Fleeing the persecution of Hitler's regime, she made her way to France, Palestine, and then to the United States, where she lived for the remainder of her life. She conducted her most important and famous work at the private mental hospital Chestnut Lodge Sanitarium in Rockville, Maryland, where she remained until her last days (Hoff, 1982; Gunst, 1982; Cohen, 1982).

At Chestnut Lodge Sanitarium, in her work with her patients she had a unique reputation for radical commitment and respect toward them. She prioritized the therapeutic relationship, which included listening until she accurately understood their communications. Through this, she conducted psychotherapy with individuals who were diagnosed with schizophrenia, radically differing from Freud's followers. She was fiercely protective of the most vulnerable individuals.

Following the era of Freud's psychoanalytic theory and its rigidly conformist and closed community, Fromm-Reichmann's focus on the subjective experience and belief in recovery from mental illness was unorthodox and radical. Along with her mentor from Chestnut Lodge Sanitarium, Harry Stack Sullivan, she developed *interpersonal theory*. Chestnut Lodge was well known for its innovative healing work with the most severely disturbed patients through the modality of listening, interpreting, and communicating with their expressions. Other noteworthy Chestnut Lodge Sanitarium clinicians included Kurt Goldstein and Harold Searles (Stanton, 1982; Stevens & Gardner, 1982).

Unlike others who believed that people with schizophrenia could not develop meaningful interpersonal relationships with others and develop transference reactions, Fromm-Reichmann believed that an intense personal relationship was quite possible. She recognized that a potential distorted transference was common, and it was her task to reflect this distortion to the patient and prove that she was not this person that was imagined. She valued a continuous and persistent effort to nurture a ripe environment in which a person could come out of hibernation and be involved in a mutually warm, authentic, interpersonal relationship.

Fromm-Reichmann often mimicked her patient's behavior so they could experience the seemingly invisible obstacles that impeded their own progress and instinctively make necessary changes. At Chestnut Lodge, one of Fromm-Reichmann's patients was a despondent man whom no one could reach. As many hospital staff did, Fromm-Reichmann lived on the grounds of Chestnut Lodge. She instructed the staff to call her at any hour if this patient were to make any attempts at all to communicate. Once, at two o'clock in the morning, Fromm-Reichmann got a call. Her patient was in a day room, jumping from chair to chair. She came running, still wearing her nightgown. Fromm-Reichmann made every attempt to talk with him, but her efforts were unsatisfied. In an effort to join him and to mimic his behavior for him to see, Fromm-Reichmann began jumping from chair to chair like him. These radical and committed efforts reached this patient, and from there, he was able to open up and communicate with her (Hornstein, 2005).

Fromm-Reichmann made many important and unique assertions about the subjective experiences and intrapsychic motivations of people who experience psychosis. Most importantly, she asserted that this person, being exquisitely sensitive to interpersonal relationships, had had abject experiences of social rejection and continued marginalization, leaving him exceptionally guarded to new social opportunities. This type of isolation results in high levels of frustration, aggression, anxiety, depression, and other symptom formation. Fromm-Reichmann believed in the importance of working closely and frequently with clients so they could identify, discuss, and accurately understand any nonverbal communications and not again have them be misunderstood as rejecting (Weigert, 1959; Fromm-Reichmann, 1954).

Fromm-Reichmann believed in listening closely and understanding accurately and completely that which her patients were attempting to verbally and nonverbally communicate. She recognized that some of the communications were mysterious and bizarre and that, with patient waiting and attuned connection, even the most bizarre communications had the potential to be understood. "This might take months, even years, but if the doctor could stand the uncertainty, the pattern would emerge. Frieda's main technique was waiting, a method she deployed so skillfully it looked like magic" (Hornstein, 2005, p. xv). Her patients rewarded her by opening up and sharing with her, which was their healing modality, thus creating a very mutually rewarding relationship.

Fromm-Reichmann, along with Eric Fromm, Clara Thompson, Harry Stack Sullivan, David Rioch, and Janet Rioch, founded the William Alanson White Institute, a world-renowned psychoanalytic institute in New York City. This institute is thriving still today (see Appendix B for website information).

Donald Woods Winnicott

Donald Woods Winnicott (1896–1971), or D.W., was born in Plymouth, Devon, England. His family enjoyed financial wealth and social status. He was the youngest in a sibship of three, having two older sisters. His mother experienced strong depressive moods, and the young Donald believed that his own livelihood depended on his keeping her in cheerful spirits. Yet, Winnicott derived a good deal of tender loving care from his nanny and was very close to her. His early sufferings and anxiety were the underpinnings of his curiosity and devotion to working with the development and stability of young children.

Winnicott spent his whole life working with troubled children as a pediatrician and psychoanalyst in institutions (Paddington Green Children's Hospital, London, England), camps for evacuated children and their families during World War II, and in private practice. He was twice psychoanalyzed, by the famous analysts James Strachey and Joan Riviere. While trained by Melanie Klein, Winnicott ultimately belonged to a branch of the Object Relations School, called the Independent School, contributing many important and unique ideas that are still used today (Rodman, 2004).

The following paragraphs describe some of Winnicott's most noteworthy contributions, which are still widely used to this day.

The *holding environment* is the context in which the person is physically and psychologically maintained (Winnicott, 1964). This context includes physical items, such as furniture, computers, colors, people, and space. The holding environment also refers to the quality of these items, such as their working condition and comfortable/soothing tone. For example, an elementary school classroom can be chaotic, with too much furniture, flamboyant colors, overwhelming smells, and loud noises, causing an overstimulating atmosphere. Alternatively, a classroom can have just enough furniture in working order, complementary colors, and minimal smells and noises, creating a more soothing holding environment that allows the brain to focus on learning rather than defensively coping. Most importantly, the qualities of interactions that occur in the holding environment are the focus. For example, when administering activity directions, a teacher's style can be joyful and encouraging or callous and discouraging. Winnicott thought of the mother–child relationship as the first and most important holding environment, as this is where security and expectations for the future are established. Additionally, he saw the client–therapist relationship as equally essential.

Winnicott did not believe in the concept of a *perfect* mother or her idealized impact. Instead, he believed an empathic and pervasively generous standard of care kept the infant from extreme physical or emotional discomfort or distress; he called this "good enough mothering/parenting" (Winnicott, 1971). This quality of care resulted in optimal security and psychological development. It depended on a sincere and accurately attuned caregiver, whose responses to the child were timely and correct (Winnicott, 1965a, 1971).

Winnicott believed the *true self* is rooted in a pervasive sense of security that allows one to feel connected to one's own authentic feelings, to be connected to others, to be creative, and to not have to invest in an excessive amount of defensive energy (Winnicott, 1965a). He asserted that this authenticity originates from good enough parenting, consisting of the caregiver's accurate attunement, accepting all emotions, timely responding, and embracing his or her own true self.

Winnicott asserted that when a child's needs and emotional life are not attended to, causing experiences of extreme physical or emotional discomfort, he or she contorts his or her own needs and emotional reactions to meet the caregiver's needs. This defensive mask, the *false self*, is developed to keep the caregiver afloat so that he or she can continue to provide the best possible care (Winnicott, 1965a). As one can imagine, this process leaves the child's physical and emotional needs unmet, which alters his sense of security and leaves him with overwhelming emotional states. As the child takes on this false self identity and seemingly gets his needs met, he may come to confuse these efforts as his true self, yet feeling empty, unsatisfied, obsessively rigid, or even dead (Winnicott, 1971).

Winnicott's idea of the *transitional object* comes from within the holding environment, specifically that which soothes. The child will choose his first transitional object around age 3, when he becomes aware of his separateness from the world and others. The transitional object is the first manifestation of the child's imagination or play with symbolism. The child chooses an object that represents a similar quality of soothing that he received from his caregiver. This transitional object allows the child to feel soothed without the presence of the caregiver, genuine in relationships, and creative (Winnicott, 1964). Adults, as well as children and adolescents, have transitional objects in the form of physical things (mobile phone, clothes, coffee, alcohol), people (best friends, admired celebrities), places (home, vacation spots, stores), and activities (sports, pornography, dancing, and music).

Initially, Winnicott asserted that psychosis was the result of caregiving failure in infancy or very early childhood. Given this, his *prescription* for recovery was to intentionally manage a family's environment and, through the interpersonal actions and tone of the familial relationships, *nurse* the personality development back to a healthy track. In several case reports, Winnicott instructed the family to arrange the family home as a hospital (Kanter, 1990; Winnicott, 1955). They had brief consultations for intentional guidance throughout the week, but Winnicott stressed that the therapeutic work occurred in the quality of the caring environment, which could be internalized by the person seeking comfort. Later, as the promotion of a neurobiological etiology for schizophrenia became mainstream, the willingness to acknowledge or examine the idea that the family could have caused the illness (i.e., schizophrenogenic mother) became a highly sensitive topic.

Here, Winnicott lists some guiding principles in successful work with people who experience psychotic symptoms:

> You apply yourself to the case. You get to know what it feels like to be your client. You become reliable for the limited field of your professional responsibility. You behave yourself professionally. You concern yourself with your client's problems. You accept being in the position of a subjective object in the client's life, while at the same time you keep both feet on the ground. You accept love, and even the in-love state, without flinching and without acting-out your response. You accept hate and meet it with strength, rather than with revenge. You tolerate your client's illogicality, unreliability, suspicion, muddle, fecklessness, meanness, etc. etc., and recognize all these unpleasantness as symptoms of distress. (In private life these same things would make you keep at a distance.) You are not frightened, nor do you become overcome with guilt-feelings when your client goes mad, disintegrates, runs out in the street in a nightdress, attempts suicide and perhaps succeeds. If murder threatens you, call in the police to help not only yourself, but also your client. In all these emergencies, you recognize the client's call for help, or a cry of despair because of loss of hope of help. In all these respects you are, in your professional area, a person deeply involved in feeling, yet at the same time detached in that you know that you have no responsibility for the fact of your client's illness, and you know the limits of your powers to alter a crisis situation. If you can hold the situation together the possibility is that the crisis will resolve itself. (Winnicott, 1963, p. 229)

Winnicott asserted that the psychotic episode was the most authentic expression that a person could have. His reasoning was this. In a psychotic and highly emotional episode, the repression barrier between conscious and unconscious are so thin that, for better or worse, the individual becomes incapacitated from holding back his true feelings, which true self expressions thrust beyond the false self (Winnicott, 1964; 1965).

In Winnicott's time (mid-1950s–mid-1970s), many extreme behaviors were categorized as psychotic, including diagnoses such as major depression, borderline personality disorder, and conduct disorder. However, Winnicott did work with people who experienced classic symptoms of psychosis, including the famous

Dr. Margaret Little, who wrote about her own psychoanalysis under Winnicott's care: *Psychotic Anxieties and Containment: A Personal Record of an Analysis with Winnicott* (Little, 1985).

Winnicott had two marriages: one to Alice Taylor for 28 years and the second to the famous psychiatric social worker Clare Britton for 20 years until his death 1971. Britton worked primarily with children, and Winnicott often referred readers to her work for further elaboration, as he considered her more articulate than himself. Winnicott thought that the holding environment management principles, developed in work with children, could be generalized to adults with psychotic disorders (Winnicott, 1963). Winnicott died in his sleep after a series of heart attacks.

Ronald David Laing

Ronald David Laing (1927–1989), an only child, was born in Glasgow, Scotland, to a middle-class Presbyterian family. The members, especially his mother, were materially privileged but emotionally bleak. His father experienced some symptoms of mental illness and was fully incapacitated for a period of 3 months while young Laing was a teenager. Young Laing was forbidden to play with other children until middle school; the reason given to him was that "he was evil" (Miller, 2004).

While he displayed a consistent and persistent interest in existential philosophy, Laing received his medical degree from the University of Glasgow, especially choosing this university for the opportunities to study birth and death, which were of particular interest to Laing. Laing had a history of heavy alcohol and drug use, preferring the hallucinogen LSD. These substances served to both numb dysphoric emotions and expand his emotional and cognitive abilities.

Laing spent several years in the British Army working as a psychiatrist attending to people who were severally mentally distressed. Before and after Laing's military service, he worked with patients with SMI in psychiatric hospitals. Between 1956 and 1964, Laing trained at the Tavistock Clinic in London, with now-legendary colleagues John Bowlby and Winnicott. In 1965, Laing wrote his first book, *The Divided Self: An Existential Study in Sanity and Madness*, making the subjective experience of madness accessible to all through existential principles influenced by Jean-Paul Sartre and Georg Wilhelm Friedrich Hegel (Laing, 1965).

From 1965 to 1970, Laing conducted his most famous and radical antipsychiatry experiment at Kingsley Hall, London, England. Here, people with mental illness were invited to live in a communal therapeutic safe-haven environment with psychiatrists who did not push psychiatric medications. Residents were encouraged to play, regress into childhood for the chances of release and a corrective experience, and participate in Eastern practices, especially meditation.

The activities at Kingsley Hall were quite controversial. The program was developed in an enthusiastic time in which everything in society was being questioned, including authority, family, roles, social rules, illness, and sexuality. The most famous resident, Mary Barnes, regressed into childhood, was fed with a bottle, and would frequently smear feces as painting. Belongings were thrown out of windows and the facility was constantly in disrepair. Residents were given LSD (legal at the time) for the purpose of allowing the repressed material that haunted the unconscious to be released and healed. At least two residents jumped off the roof, and at least once, the home was raided by the drug squad.

Dominic Harris tracked down 13 of 130 who passed through Kingsley Hall, including Laing's colleagues and residents. He collected profound individual anecdotal stories and photographs documented in a self-published book called *The Residents*, which can be viewed at the website listed in Appendix B (2012). Harris's purpose was to give the participants a legitimate voice as a survivor of a social experiment, among all the derogatory stories and judgments that were being said. These stories disclose intense experiences during which residents ingested LSD under Laing's direction, the delusional and regressed behaviors of residents, conversations with Laing and his friend Sean Connery, and the squalorous conditions in which they lived. A nonnarrative documentary called *Asylum* also recorded the daily happenings of Kingsley Hall (Robinson, 1972).

Laing was married twice. He fathered six sons and four daughters by four women. By his children's reports, Laing seemed physically and emotionally unavailable to his first set of children and more comforting and available to his later-born children.

In 1987, Laing was forced to resign from the medical register of the General Medical Council as a result of his questionable behavior, including heavy alcohol use and extreme divergence from mainstream psychiatry. Laing died in August 1989 of a heart attack while playing tennis in St. Tropez, South of France. To read the story of his death, see the website listed in Appendix B.

John Weir Perry

John Weir Perry (1914–1998) was born in Rhode Island, United States of America. He attended Harvard Medical School. As a young medical student, in Switzerland, Perry met Carl Jung, who forever impacted Perry's personal perspectives and style. Perry served in the US Army and, during World War II, worked as a medic in China. There, Perry was especially taken by the ancient philosophy of Taoism. Perry particularly noticed the similarities between the Tao principle that the universe is a *self-organizing system* and Jung's idea that the symptoms of schizophrenia should not be stopped, but that a *spontaneous healing process* would occur with the facilitation of a trained psychological escort. He incorporated this idea into his work by allowing for things to naturally happen, rather than focusing on interventions. Following the war, Perry, a medical doctor, psychiatrist, and psychotherapist, moved to the San Francisco area, where he lived and worked for the remainder of his life.

In 1952, Perry published his first book, *The Self in Psychotic Process: Its Symbolization in Schizophrenia*, for which Carl Jung wrote the introduction. Based on his work in mainstream mental health treatment delivery settings, Perry believed the current mental health treatment delivery system was, at the very least, not working and, more commonly, traumatizing people, especially with the forced use of neuroleptic medications, electroshock therapy, and locked facilities. He asserted that people who experience psychosis were rarely, if ever, listened to or met at their visionary or altered state of consciousness. "Instead, every imaginable way to silence the patients—to ignore and to disapprove of their non-rational language and experience—was called into play, thereby increasing their sense of isolation, alienation, and so-called madness" (Perry, 1974).

During the 1970s, Perry founded an alternative residential treatment facility, called Diabasis, in San Francisco. It was designed to be a sensory-appealing homelike environment where young adults who were experiencing their first psychotic episodes could be empowered through the episode and emerge "weller than well" (Menniger, 1963, p. 406). The treatment included experiential opportunities such as painting, dance, massage, sand tray, meditation, martial arts, and conversation. Activities were not mandatory. There were no locked doors, and no violence to person or property was allowed by anyone. A rage room was used, where a person could express his anger, often with a primary therapist also in the room. There were conversations with the primary therapist three to four appointed times a week.

The workforce was small, consisting of both paid and volunteer staff. Workers were chosen based on the capacities of empathy and hearing depth-oriented (involving the unconscious) conversations. It was believed that everything else could be communicated through on-the-job training. Diabasis operated on a model of expressing, releasing, and discovering thoughts and self rather than suppressing these personal aspects. Individuals lived in the supported home environment for about 3 months and then were moved to a lesser-supervised residential treatment home for another 3 months. Usually, within a few days of admission to the supervised home, patients experienced significant stabilization.

While mainstream mental health treatment would expect that these individuals would be dependent, take medications for the remainder of their lives, and be in and out of acute and long-term locked psychiatric facilities, these individuals had few, if any, relapses. The program enjoyed an extremely high success rate, asserting that 85%–90% of patients were able to return to living in the community without relapse

(Perry, 1974). In 1974, Perry published *The Far Side of Madness*, a book that offered the workings and results of Diabasis.

Below are some additional and essential tenets that guided the work of Perry:

People with big ideas keep so much of their thoughts, ideas, and beliefs inaccessible in the unconscious in attempts to fit in to mainstream society. When the person is stressed or tired, the repression barrier thins and the unconscious reveals itself. Psychosis is an altered state of consciousness in which a person has a capacity of a spiritual awakening to both what is and is not working for him. Addressing these thoughts offers spiritual and intellectual openness and stronger life perspective. Also, the subjective experience carries hope of being more meaningful than ever before. The psychotic vulnerability or visionary state can now be included in the person's narrative to create an accurate and comprehensive story and explore the meaning and strength of now having a mental illness. (Perry, 1998)

When we focus on the inner life or subjective experience of the person who experiences psychosis, this is when and how clinicians can be truly helpful (Perry, 1998, p. xii). In the medical model, there is no room for mystical material (Perry, 1998, p. xii).

Perry followed Jung's assertion that myth, symbol, and ritual are the common manifestations of psychosis. He asserted that the ideas of myth, symbol, and ritual are often misunderstood and misdiagnosed as *religious preoccupation* and left out of contemporary understanding and knowledge of psychosis. Perry asserts that "if we want to deeply understand people who experience psychosis, go back to learn myth and ritual forms of antiquity" (Perry, 1998, p. xi). In attending to unconscious material and viewing this through myth and ritual, the clinician may "be diverted into many mysterious areas. As a result, the person with these kinds of episodes is allowed to reach their fruitful outcome" (Perry, 1998, p. xiv).

Perry was skeptical about the belief that psychosis is caused only by faulty brain structure or neurotransmitters. He noted that the symptoms of psychosis can be relieved without medication and even during a single conversation in which favorable rapport and open connection can be reached in the relationship, and this coherency could last a few hours, a few days, or forever. Additionally, with unfavorable conditions, a person who has been taking prescribed neuroleptic medication can immediately experience psychosis. Any clinician who values the therapeutic relationship and allows for the expression and accurate understanding of unconscious material has seen these amazing and immediate results (Perry, 1998).

The unconscious mind knows best how to heal itself. Clinicians must trust that. This means that clinicians and family members must be patient and tolerant of not knowing and not being in control.

Perry revered individuals with psychotic experiences, terming them *visionaries*. At the website listed in Appendix B, you can view an interview of Perry by Jeff Mishlove, in which they discuss how visionaries are viewed and treated in the mental health treatment system.

On October 29, 1998, Perry died from cancer at the age of 84 in his Larkspur, California, home. His tombstone reads, "Some individuals are by their innate endowment called upon to escape the bounds of the average and to venture free" (Perry, 1998, Preface).

Loren Mosher

The maverick psychiatrist Loren Mosher (1933–2004) was born in Monterey, California. Not much is publically known about his early life. He attended medical school at Stanford University and did his psychiatric residency at Harvard University, where he graduated with honors. Mosher was the inaugural chief for the Center for Studies of Schizophrenia at the NIMH from 1968 to 1980. He was the founder and first editor in chief of the prominent academic journal *Schizophrenia Bulletin*. He coauthored the book *Community Mental Health: Principles and Practice* (1989) with Italian colleague Lorenze Burti.

Mosher devoted his entire life to humane and effective treatment for people who have been diagnosed with schizophrenia, and his assertions were often incongruent with mainstream mental health treatment delivery in the United States. His work was congruent with the principles of moral treatment, which emphasized equality between patients and workers. In 1966, Mosher was strongly influenced by his training at the Tavistock Institute and his visit with Laing there (Mosher & Burti, 1989).

From 1970 to 1992, Mosher was an investigator for Soteria Community Services Alternatives, where alternative treatments for people with first episodes of schizophrenia were found to be humane, effective, and at least 40% cheaper than mainstream mental health treatment. During 1971–1983, Mosher founded and investigated the experimental Soteria Project, based in Palo Alto, California, and with facilities in San Jose, California, San Mateo, California, and Bern, Switzerland. In Greek, *soteria* means relaxation and protection. Here, young people who were newly diagnosed with schizophrenia could receive treatment in a home-like environment.

Mosher had unique beliefs about the use of psychotropic drugs. He made them available to those who were violent and severely suicidal but did not push or force them. Neuroleptic medications were given at a far lower dose than usual treatments and were not the focus of treatment. The staff were mostly nonprofessional peers supervised by professionals. The Soteria Project patients were compared to usual mental health treatment patients and found to be dramatically more functional than those who received neuroleptic medications. Further details of Soteria House can be found at the website listed in Appendix B and in Mosher's written publications (Matthews et al., 1979; Mosher, 1999; Mosher et al., 1975, 1990; Mosher & Menn, 1978; Wilson, 1982). Mosher authored *Soteria: Through Madness to Deliverance* (2004), to describe the tone and effective practices of Soteria House. This book was published just 5 months after he perished. In 1983, Soteria House closed its doors, primarily because of the fatal lack of supportive funding, which Mosher believed to be the result of powerful pharmaceutical industry influences because the use of psychotropic medicines were incongruent with the Soteria philosophy.

Because he largely avoided the use of pharmaceuticals in his work, Mosher was severely marginalized by the APA, and later in his career, he was not invited to present to American audiences. His work, however, is well known and prominent in many other European countries, especially Switzerland, where a Soteria House is still in operation.

After Mosher criticized the APA for taking money from pharmaceutical companies and resigned (see Chapter 4 for discussion and Appendix B for a website with the resignation letter), he worked closely with individuals and groups of psychiatric survivors, especially one called Mind Freedom International, whose tag line is "Win human rights in the mental health system!" (See the website listed in Appendix B.) Mind Freedom International's goals, as listed on its website, are as follows:

- Win human rights campaigns in mental health, such as opposing coerced, forced, and fraudulent mental health procedures.
- Challenge abuse by the psychiatric drug industry.
- Support the self-determination and voice of psychiatric survivors and mental health consumers.
- Promote safe, humane, and effective options in mental health.

In Mosher's obituary, David W. Oaks, Mind Freedom International's director, referred to Mosher as "a hero for fighting the good fight," the fight against his own profession, and the abuses of psychiatry (http://www.moshersoteria.com/tributes/david-oaks-tribute/).

Mosher's work is archived at Stanford University. Soteria House, in Bern, Switzerland, is still in strong operation. To view its website, see Appendix B. This type of small milieu and supportive therapeutic work is widespread in European countries.

On July 10, 2004, Mosher died of liver cancer in Berlin, Germany. His last residence was in San Diego, CA.

Murray Jackson

Murray Jackson (1922–2011) was born in Sydney, Australia. His father was a soldier who became securely established in the Department of External Affairs and United Nations Temporary Commission on Korea. His mother was also quite accomplished in her professional career at the *Australian Women's Weekly*, becoming the second editor in its history. Murray Jackson both began, through an internship, and ended his long psychiatric career at Maudsley Hospital in South London.

Jackson's philosophy and style were strongly impacted by psychoanalytic principles of the day (Melanie Klein, Herbert Rosenfeld, and Henri Rey), as was reflected in his style of work with people who experienced symptoms of psychosis. He both directed and treated patients with the psychoanalytic modality on Maudsley Hospital's Ward 6, a 10-bed inpatient psychiatric unit. His unique approach to finding meaning in even the most bizarre psychotic communications was recorded in his two most famous books, *Unimaginable Storms: A Search for Meaning in Psychosis* (1994) and *Weathering the Storm: Psychotherapy for Psychosis* (2001). These books contain edited transcripts from actual treatment conversations between patients and Dr. Jackson. Ward 6 of Maudsley Hospital closed with Murray Jackson's retirement in 1987.

Grof and Grof: Christina Grof and Stanislav Grof

Stanislav Grof (b. 1931) was born and educated in Prague, Czechoslovakia. He received his medical degree at Charles University in Prague in 1957, where he specialized in psychiatry. He received his PhD at the Czechoslovak Academy of Sciences in 1965. Grof was one of the founders of transpersonal psychology and an innovative researcher and explorer into the use of nonordinary states of consciousness. Grof is well known for his work with psychedelic medications that induce an altered state of consciousness for the purpose of exploring and healing the unconscious depths at which a person makes all decisions.

Christina Grof (1941–2014), raised in Honolulu, Hawaii, first met Stanislav Grof when her professor suggested that she seek help for her own powerful spiritual experiences. From these experiences, her deep interest in nonordinary states of consciousness grew. Christina Grof was an avid student and teacher of hatha and Kundalini yoga (to view her biography, see the website listed in Appendix B).

In 1989, Stanislav Grof and his wife, Christina Grof, edited and published *Spiritual Emergency: When Personal Transformation Becomes a Crisis*. There are many chapter contributors to this book, including Laing and Perry. The book explores episodes of spiritual growth that may seem overwhelming and that in mainstream mental health treatment would be diagnosed and treated with locked acute psychiatric hospitalization and neuroleptic medications, which he refers to as *traditional suppressive therapies*. The contributors to the book identify, explore, and normalize these experiences. Grof asserts that confronting and processing "the emerging unconscious material helps to clear the rest of the day from unwelcome intrusions of its disturbing elements" (Grof & Grof, 1989, p. 196). He identifies ways in which healers, friends, and family members can accurately assist people with these experiences, including trusting relationships that are open to spirituality with trained or untrained people, around the clock support if necessary, flexibility, creativity, support groups, and testimony from those who have successfully gone through a spiritual emergency and other nonordinary states.

> The most important task is to give the people in crisis a positive context for their experiences and sufficient information about the process they are going through. It is essential that they move away from the concept of disease and recognize the healing nature of their crisis. (Grof & Grof, 1989, p. 192)

Other specific techniques that are used to facilitate and accelerate the transformational process are meditation, acupuncture, movement including shaking and dancing, group chanting, going within oneself with music, emotional expression including crying and screaming, journaling, drawing, painting, and intense physical activities, including manual work, swimming, or jogging. If experiences or emotions become overwhelming or dysphoric, one can stop these experiences, change nutritional diet, and be soothed by humming sounds.

Heavily influenced by Kundalini yoga, gestalt therapy, and Reichian body work, Grof and Grof developed *holotropic breathwork*, which is specialized and controlled breathing conducted in a supportive environment, often with evocative music and sound, to naturally induce an altered meditative and mystical state of transpersonal consciousness. To see a video of Stanislav Grof describing holotropic breathwork, see the website listed in Appendix B. The details of holotropic breathing can be found in Grof's book *The Adventure of Self-Discovery: Dimensions of Consciousness and New Perspectives in Psychotherapy and Inner Exploration* (1988).

Grof was greatly impacted by Carl Jung and the ideas of collective consciousness and cultural mythology. "When we are working at the deepest levels of the mind, we can have access to a synchronous connection to all other happenings of the

Universe." This quote and many other details about Stanislav Grof and his work can be found at the website listed in Appendix B.

In 1980, together, Stanislav and Christina Grof founded the Spiritual Emergence Network (SEN). Its purpose is to facilitate human development and meaning and connection beyond personal identity, which leads to a greater capacity for wisdom, compassion, respect for all life, and a deeper sense of personal security and inner peace. (Find the Spiritual Emergence website listed in Appendix B. Here, one can find information, support, and referrals to specially trained counselors.)

Stanislav Grof is now a notable adjunct faculty member at the California Institute of Integral Studies in the Department of Philosophy, Cosmology, and Consciousness, in San Francisco, California. He has published over 150 articles and 20 books that discuss theoretical and clinical implications of nonordinary states of consciousness for the purposes of exploration and healing.

Oliver Sacks

Oliver Sacks (1933–2015) was born in 1933 in London, England. He was the youngest of four boys. Both his Orthodox Jewish parents, themselves children of poor Jewish immigrants, were thriving physicians. His father, a general practitioner who gave up his dream to be a neurologist, made house calls to the poor communities of the East End. His mother, the 16th of 18 children, became one of the first female surgeons in England and eventually specialized in obstetrics and gynecology. She enthusiastically worked closely with Oliver at home, dissecting the brains of malformed fetuses from her work. Both parents were hard working and committed to their patients, which pulled them from emotional intimacy with their children. Sacks was raised by a nanny—his first words were her full name, "Marion Jackson" (Brown, 2005).

Having a near *perfect life*, when Oliver was just 6 years old, he and his brother were sent to a country boarding school to avoid The Blitz, systematic and frequent bombings by Nazi Germany. The boarding school headmaster was extremely sadistic, conducted severe beatings, and allowed the children only very little to eat (Epstein, 2008). They remained there for 4 years. His brother eventually experienced symptoms of psychosis. Upon Sacks's own reflection and diagnoses, these experiences undoubtedly impacted his pervasive and pathological shyness, capacity for bonding, social awkwardness, and tendency toward isolation (Epstein, 2008).

Oliver Sacks had a winding career trajectory, making his way from failing at conducting research on human nutrition at Oxford, to working as a neurologist at UCLA, to researching neuropathy and neurochemistry at Yeshiva University's Albert Einstein College of Medicine in New York City, to working in a migraine clinic. Here, he wrote his first book, *Migraine*, in 1970 about the peculiar life stories of his patients and himself. Later, he worked at Beth Abraham Hospital in the Bronx, with patients who had survived the 1917–1928 encephalitis lethargic epidemic that left them catatonic for approximately 10–12 years and who were considered hopeless. After much research, Sacks administered a new drug called L-Dopa, which awakened these patients back to consciousness and into their own life in a different time, after having lost so many years. Sacks wrote the book *Awakenings* about these experiences (Sacks, 1973). This book was later made into a 1990 American motion picture by the same name, starring Robin Williams, who portrayed Oliver Sacks (Marshall, 1990). Between 2007 and 2012, Sacks held the position of Professor of neurology and psychiatry at Columbia University.

In 2013, Sacks published *Hallucinations.* Borrowing the narratives from the lives of his own patients, and using his neurological expertise, Sacks makes every attempt to normalize and humanize a variety of common sensory hallucinogenic experiences that impact cultural storytelling and art (Saks, 2013). To watch an Oliver Sacks Ted Talk: *What Hallunication Reveals About Our Minds,* Ted Talk of Dr. Oliver Sacks discussing his perspective of how common sensory hallucinations are (10% of population), yet very few (only 1%) report for fear of the stigma of being considered insane, see the website listed in Appendix B (Sacks, 2009). We were fortunate to live in contemporary times with such a genius. Sacks gave many public presentations and interviews, and we have numerous opportunities to be a member of his live or digital audience by doing a quick Internet search.

For most of his life, Sacks claimed to be celibate and to have given up on romantic relationships. In his obituary, condolences were offered to his partner, Dr. Billy Hayes. Sacks was a professor of neurology at the New York University School of Medicine and the author of many additional fascinating renowned books and articles, even up to the week before his passing. Sacks died at age 82 on August 30, 2015, of cancer in his New York City home.

CONTEMPORARY CONTRIBUTORS TO THE RECOVERY OF PSYCHOSIS

The following individuals have made significant contributions to the world of recovery from psychosis. These individuals pride themselves on listening to clients for accurate understanding and wellness among people who experience SMI, especially symptoms of psychosis.

Patricia Deegan

Dr. Deegan was diagnosed with schizophrenia during her adolescence. Because of her lived experiences with psychosis and mainstream mental health treatment,

Deegan now is devoted to the recovery and wellness of individuals who experience SMI and psychosis. Deegan developed the *Hearing Distressing Voices Toolkit*. The professionally guided experience allows individuals to have a virtual psychotic experience by listening to a prerecorded audio track and conducting instructed tasks. This experience allows others to have an understanding both of what psychosis feels like and of the social stigma faced by those with these lived experiences. The toolkit can be accessed at the website listed in Appendix B.

Mary Ellen Copeland

Mary Ellen Copeland is an author, mental health advocate, and a psychiatric survivor. As a child, Copeland's mother spent 8 years in a mental institution. Mary Ellen, herself, was diagnosed with bipolar disorder I (aka, manic-depression). Drawing from these personal lived experiences, Copeland has published articles, books, and a prevalent toolkit for the recovery and wellness of individuals with SMI. Her toolkit, *Wellness Recovery Action Plan* (WRAP), an evidence-based practice, gives step-by-step instructions for creating a mental health treatment advanced directive document, based on recovery model principles of hope, respect, accountability, connections, and self-advocacy (Copeland, 2012). Copeland is the founder of the Copeland Center for Wellness and Recovery, which provides trainings, retreats, and a recovery community. More information can be found at the website listed in Appendix B.

Robert Whitaker

Robert Whitaker is a medical journalist and world-renowned author. Whitaker has taken a special interest in investigating and exposing the self-serving and infamous historical and contemporary practices of neuroleptic pharmaceutical companies and the field of psychiatry. Whitaker has written several books that many mental health alternative treatment groups have embraced and the field of psychiatry has unscientifically criticized.

- *Mad in America: Bad Science, Bad Medicine, and the Enduring Mistreatment of the Mentally Ill* (Whitaker, 2010)
- *Anatomy of an Epidemic: Magic Bullets, Psychiatric Drugs, and the Astonishing Rise of Mental Illness in America* (Whitaker, 2011)
- *Psychiatry Under the Influence: Institutional Corruption, Social Injury, and Prescriptions for Reform* (Whitaker, 2015)

Whitaker was afforded a research department and years to explore the explicit details of research studies, court proceedings, and other paramount documents on which he based his provocative assertions. He documented the winding and scandalous history of neuroleptic medication promotion by pharmaceutical companies and psychiatrists. Mainstream media and the general population do not have access to these resources because of the time and money required to find and promote them. The opinions of the general population are then vulnerable to what is heard through news and movies, in which the details are quite thin and even questionable. Whitaker makes the results of these studies available to everyone. Alternative (to neuroleptic medication) mental health treatment groups and individuals have embraced Whitaker's work and used his research findings to base their arguments for a desperately needed effective mental health treatment alternative.

RECOVERY COMMUNITIES

There are several therapeutic communities whose efforts are designed to assist in the process of healing from SMIs and improve quality of life. While there are a few pockets of these recovery-oriented communities in the United States, most of the long-term recovery-oriented research and sustainable care comes out of Sweden, Finland, Norway, Belgium, and Australia.

Gould Farm

Founded in 1913 by William Gould, Gould Farm was the first and is now the oldest therapeutic farm. It was built on the principles of "respectful discipline, wholesome work, and unstinting kindness" (website listed in Appendix B). The farm has room for about 100 people, 40 adult guests and about 60 staff members and their families. There are clinical staff onsite, including social workers, psychiatrists, nurses, and nurses' assistants. Guests are assigned to a sustainable work program including Forest and Grounds Team, Farm Team, Garden Team, Harvest Barn Team, Kitchen Team, Maintenance Team, or Roadside Store and Café Team. Gould Farm works with adults, volunteers, and staff and their families.

Geel, Belgium

Geel, Belgium, with a population of approximately 35,000, has a history rooted in the principles of community recovery and a foster family model of care for people who live with mental illness (Goldstein, 2009). Beginning in the Middle Ages, people came to the church of Geel, Belgium, specifically to Saint Dymphna, to be treated for symptoms of mental distress. In 1296, it is said that Saint Dymphna achieved sainthood because of her miraculous works and by choosing martyrdom over her insane father's incestuous demands. As more and more people sought healing in Geel, there was no more room in the church. The church canons trained families who took in the suffering visitors.

This centuries-old foster care family model is still in operation today and is considered an important element that fits into the Openbaar Psychiatrisch Zorgcentrum (OPZ), the mental health treatment system. The OPZ serves adults, children, adolescents, and older adults with any type of symptom of mental illness. They offer a comprehensive range of professional services via group and individual therapeutic modalities. More information can be found on the OPZ website, listed in Appendix B. Geel, Belgium, considers itself a successful community recovery model. This family-assisted-care living model has been adopted by Germany, Italy, Austria, and Switzerland. A comprehensive explanation of how this psychiatric foster care system works within the larger community mental health system is available in a book with DVD, *Geel Revisited After Centuries of Mental Rehabilitation* by Eugeen Roosens and Lieve Van de Walle (2007), with a foreword by Oliver Sacks.

Open Dialogue Treatment

Open dialogue treatment (ODT) is a client-centered mental health treatment modality that has its original roots in Western Lapland, Finland. It was developed between the 1980s and 1998 by Jaakko Seikkula, PhD; Markku Sutela; and their multidisciplinary team at Keropudas Hospital in Tornio, Finland (Seikkula, Alakare, & Aaltonen, 2000).

The main principles of ODT are as follows:

- An immediate response to the crisis during the first 24 hours.
- Avoiding inpatient treatment by organizing home visits as often as needed in an attempt to avoid hospitalization.
- Open dialogue *with* the client, not *about* the client, at treatment meetings about all the issues concerned.
- Flexibility and mobility is guaranteed by means of adapting the treatment response to the specific and changing needs of each case using the therapeutic methods that best fit each patient and his or her family. The first meeting is usually at the patient's home.
- Responsibility. Whoever contacted is responsible to organize the first meeting, in which the decision of treatment is made and the case-specific team takes charge of the entire treatment.
- Psychological continuity. The team takes responsibility for the treatment for as long as needed both in outpatient and inpatient settings.
- Tolerance of uncertainty in behavior and speech from the patient by family members is managed by building up a safe enough home environment.

During a psychotic crisis, this level of enough safety is provided by daily visits from the clinician to the home for at least the first 10–12 days. Immature conclusions and treatment decisions are avoided. For instance, neuroleptic medication is not started in the first meeting, but instead is discussed in at least three meetings before starting it.

Because it considers effective psychotic treatment alternatives to neuroleptic medications, some people erroneously conclude that ODT is based on antipsychiatry principles. In fact, neuroleptic medications are made available after considering potential risks, are given at the lowest possible dose, and are discontinued at the earliest possible time.

Open dialogue treatment assumes there is meaning in the manifestation of psychotic symptoms and includes the person in their own treatment process. One major difference in ODT is helping the social network understand and appropriately respond to the person, rather than holding the attitude that the person has a problem in his or her head. Open dialogue treatment recognizes that some people who experience symptoms of psychosis come from abusive families. It asserts that there is some benefit to staying engaged with the family so that the perpetrator can be confronted and the survivor can express his emotions. However, ODT respects that in some cases, the survivor may not want to be involved or that the family dynamics are too volatile.

Compared to mainstream mental health treatment, where nearly 100% of individuals receive neuroleptic medications, ODT outcomes are quite favorable. Two important follow-up outcome studies, one at 2 years and one at 5 years, report the following outcomes:

Individuals who receive ODT have fewer psychiatric hospitalizations; use less neuroleptic medications; have less crisis occurrences; and show increased rates of returning to work. At the 5-year follow-up, 83% of ODT recipients returned to their jobs or school or were job seeking and not on government disability benefits (i.e., Social Security Disability or Public Aid, etc.) Moreover, these outcome studies reflect a significant reduction in psychotic symptoms over the years (Seikkula, Alakare, & Aaltonen 2000; Seikkula et al., 2003; Seikkula et al., 2006).

Daniel Mackler produced several video documentaries on the topic of recovery from schizophrenia using ODT: *Open Dialogue* (2000a); *Healing Homes* (2000b); and *Take These Broken Wings* (2000c). These documentaries can be viewed on YouTube or purchased from Daniel Mackler's website listed in Appendix B.

Currently, ODT is in use in Finland and now in the United States, at the University of Massachusetts Medical School, by Mary Olsen, PhD; Douglas Ziedonis, MD; and Jaakko Seikkula, PhD. Of course, such an innovative treatment method that is contrary to the myopic view of neuroleptic medication intervention will bring criticism. Marvin Ross (2013) wrote an affect-laden article, *Don't Be Too Quick to Praise This New Treatment*, in the *Huffington Post* that dismissed the positive ODT outcomes. Without accessing the actual numbers, he suggested that the ODT outcomes may not be any better than the *Merck Manual,* a pharmaceutically based medical textbook that has been used in medical education for many years. Olsen, in an ODT blog retorted, "Don't Be Too Quick to Disparage and Dismiss the New Treatment Either, thus quashing further scientific inquiry and reinforcing the status quo" (Olsen, 2014, para. 20).

FINAL THOUGHTS

This chapter has taken us through a historical journey of the theorists, practitioners, groups, and places where individuals with mental illness have received iatrogenic trauma and ultimately respect and healing. No matter our position (clinician, family member, person with lived experience), we all might challenge the mainstream mental health status quo that continues to cause iatrogenic trauma, consider what *has* been effective, and further these interventions and the philosophy of addressing individuals with mental illness and psychosis.

I caution you about speaking completely freely about and insisting on these treatment methods among mainstream mental health treatment providers, as this conversation will surely bring some surprising consequences. Hopefully, these treatment philosophies will be heard and respected. However, mainstream mental health treatment providers will often respond with benign dismissiveness, such as, "Isn't that nice," or "It is anecdotal," and even harshly criticize them as ridiculous or wacky. For support and further exploration of this effective and humanistic healing work, identify and associate yourself with like-minded people. This work can be practiced within most therapeutic relationships, regardless of time frame and theoretical orientation, with the exception of modalities that do not embrace speaking about hallucinatory and delusional content.

While some of these programs mentioned in this chapter still exist, the current status of most will read "CLOSED." The gargantuan financial weight of Big Pharma has equally colossal political influence and lobbies for insurance companies to only reimburse for treatment that includes neuroleptic medications because neuroleptic medications are thought to more rapidly stop psychotic symptoms. Many of the programs described here used, but did not push for, neuroleptic medication. Government funding and insurance reimbursement was not feasibly granted, thus, they could not meet expenses on their own and, sadly, had to close their doors, severely limiting these treatment options for people who struggle with psychotic experiences and cannot afford the expense of private treatment in the United States. We look to these incapacitated programs so that we might identify some of the effective and humane treatment aspects to be incorporated into contemporary mental health treatment modalities and programs.

For a list of like-minded organizations that provide treatment and/or empowerment for individuals, families, and groups who live with mental illness, please see Appendix B. Please consider this list a living document, keeping in mind that creating a comprehensive and contemporary list is impossible, as facilities and organizations are forever coming and going.

Summary of Unit I

THIS UNIT ADDRESSED the types of mental illness pervasive among people experiencing symptoms of psychosis and the manner in which societal beliefs and marginalizing behaviors have contributed to further decompensation and diminished self-worth for people living with mental illness. By acknowledging the misguided and dishonorable treatment practices used throughout history to condemn this population and the work of those who took a different, less offensive approach to engaging with and managing symptoms of psychosis, we begin to sort out the puzzle of what works, what is acceptable, and what is needed to help bring about a better quality of life and the development of an empowered spirit for individuals living with psychosis. *Listening with Psychotic Ears* carries forward the admirable work of the pioneers of ethical treatment and provides a legitimate option for those willing to accept this open and holistic perspective of mental illness.

UNIT II

New Discoveries About the Causes and Healing Approaches of Psychosis

6

The Relationship Between Early and Severe Trauma and Psychosis

---

A poised poet and motivational worker, Sheila, a 51-year-old woman, reads her personal story from a well-worn notebook. She is dressed in a business suit with native mother of pearl hoop earrings, wooden beads, and a scarfed headband. The cadence of her sermon-like rhythmic speech is confident, humble, and mesmerizing. The following story is Sheila's lived experience with the mental health treatment system. It is an eye-opening vicarious look at what reality is like for those immersed in it.

Sheila begins by existentially questioning who she is, given her history of cultural and personal trauma. Her biological mother came from a family that was impoverished of secure attachment and resources, and she continued this *mothering* with Sheila.

Sheila was adopted into another family, where she was severely neglected and, between the ages of 2 and 16, sexually abused by the foster father. The foster family requested to adopt Sheila. At a family interview, Sheila revealed the abuse. Sheila was immediately removed from the family, and they never spoke again.

Sheila says this severe detachment from her family and the severe neglect and sexual abuse that occurred in the foster family had great impact. She was given many erroneous diagnoses, including retardation, attention deficit disorder, bipolar disorder, and schizophrenia. She joined a street gang and was revered for her ruthless acts. As she removed herself from gang life, she began doing drugs to soothe her deep depression.

Sheila reports that from a very young age, she lost time. Later, others told her stories about her behavior in these moments. It took many years for Sheila to stumble across a clinician who accurately heard her story and connected the horrifying details to her historically violent behaviors and dissociative emotional reactions. Ignoring the details of a person's past can lead to inaccurate diagnosis and treatment, which occurs all too often among people who experience psychotic symptoms. Now, Sheila has received a diagnosis that more accurately captures her symptoms and lived experiences, and, as a result, is receiving more accurate treatment to resolve her most distressing symptoms.

TYPES OF TRAUMA AND MENTAL ILLNESS VULNERABILITY

When asked, a large percentage of people, but certainly not all, who experience positive symptoms of psychosis say they experienced significant trauma in early life. These experiences include any number of the following: parent abandonment; witnessing parents and other adored family members in the process of domestic violence or substance addiction; enduring physical and emotional beatings; experiencing punitive neglect; being sexually assaulted, often at the hands of a trusted family member; caring for and protecting younger siblings from abuse; fearing for life and loss of integrity from walking to and from school in violent neighborhoods; and living in extreme poverty. Furthermore, if the trauma occurred prelanguage, at times before the brain could understand, organize, put words to, and make meaning of the events, then the traumatic experiences result in altered brain tissue and impaired brain functioning. Read, Perry, Moskowitz, and Connolly (2001) noted the correlations between traumatic life events and brain structural and chemical differences found in people who have been diagnosed with schizophrenia.

As previously stated, a large population exists in which psychotropic medications do not have a diminishing effect on positive psychotic symptoms. How do we explain this phenomenon? How do we begin to help this person? What roles do brain structure and neurotransmitters play in resolving such phenomena? Is there more information that we can work with to help connect these events? One idea is the following:

The word "vulnerability" comes from the Latin word *vulnerare*, which means *to wound*. Vulnerability suggests a greater capacity to be wounded in the future. As a result of being wounded, one's capacity to be wounded again is exponentially greater. Some people use drugs or engage in activities such as casual sex with strangers, shopping, Internet play, social media and gaming, or work to buffer these ever-present deeply painful feelings of vulnerability. Some people consciously or unconsciously prefer even the most egregious negative consequences of addiction (homelessness, shattered family, social relationships, and intimate relationships, un-employment, and serious health problems, to name a few) to the devastating pain of past traumas. However, there are others who do not use substances or distracting behaviors in excess to dull the pain of these horrendous traumatic experiences. For this population, positive psychotic symptoms can serve as a defense or buffer against the effects of the horrific experiences and emotions stemming from the memory of more trauma than the mind can bear.

When a person experiences deep loss or trauma, he or she can experience *the un-bearable emotion*, where a person is left feeling alone, abandoned, immobile, reduced to a nonhuman, and unsoothed. People with psychotic vulnerabilities have layers of early life traumatic experiences, many of which include severe trauma. When an-other experience has a whiff of an unbearable emotion relating to a previous ex-perience, the person, in an attempt to not experience the emotional distress, flees into defenses, including disorganization, delusions, and auditory hallucinations, as Sheila experienced during adulthood, which contributed to her varied mental illness diagnoses. Left untreated, these defenses and coping styles can develop into lifelong patterns that include the continued themes of persecution, grandiosity, or the feeling that one is dead or will imminently die, just to name a few common psy-chotic themes (Allen & Coyne, 1995; Allen, Coyne, & Console, 1996; Allen, Coyne, & Console, 1997; Honig et al., 1998; Romme & Escher, 1989).

Because of high rates of premorbid traumatic experiences, including childhood sex abuse, physical abuse, and interpersonal violence (Davidson & Smith, 1990; Goff et al., 1991; Jacobson & Richardson, 1987; Masters, 1995; Mueser et al., 1998; Read, 1997; Ross & Joshi, 1992), studies suggest that psychotic symptoms emerge as a reac-tion *to* these traumatic experiences (Ellason & Ross, 1997; Read, 1997). In a sample of 275 people who carried a diagnosis of severe mental illness (SMI), Mueser et al. (1998) found that 98% had experienced at least one traumatic event in their lifetime. Additionally, 68.5% of 426 individuals who were living with psychotic disorders and were experiencing their first time in psychiatric hospitalization reported traumatic experiences (Neria, Bromet, Sievers, Lavelle, & Fochtmann, 2002). Concurrently, studies have found that approximately 70% of people who experience auditory hallucinations developed this symptom *after* a traumatic experience or an event that recalled the memory of an earlier traumatic event, suggesting that the positive psy-chotic symptom of auditory hallucinations may be part of a coping style (Honig et al., 1998; Romme & Escher, 1989).

Sexual Abuse and Psychosis

Sexual abuse is one of the most frequently reported, deeply traumatic experiences that can occur. An overwhelming number of studies suggest a strong correlation between childhood sexual abuse and the experience of positive psychotic symptoms (Morrison, 2001; Morrison, Frame, & Larkin, 2003; Larkin & Morrison, 2015; Read, 1997). Several surveys have indicated that between 34% and 77% of patients with general SMI, specifically schizophrenia, reported childhood sexual abuse or physical abuse (Darvez-Bamez, Lemperiere, Degiovanni, & Gaillard, 1995; Goff et al., 1991; Livingston, 1987; Ross, Anderson, & Clark, 1994), and 56% of patients admitted to a psychiatric hospital for first-episode psychosis reported childhood sexual abuse (Greenfield, Stratowski, Tohen, Batson, & Kolbrener, 1994). Beck and van der Kolk (1987) found that 46% of 26 chronic, hospitalized patients with a psychotic disorder reported a history of childhood sexual abuse. Friedman and Harrison (1984) found that 60% of 20 patients with a diagnosis of schizophrenia had experienced childhood sexual abuse. Read, Agar, Argyle, and Aderhold (2003) reviewed the case notes of 200 mental health treatment consumers and found that those who had experienced sexual abuse (in childhood or as an adult) were significantly more likely to endorse two or more of the characteristic symptoms of schizophrenia (as defined in the DSM). Such findings suggest that many people with psychotic symptoms may have endured specific, or cumulative, experiences of trauma *before* the onset of their psychosis (Honing, 1988), and people who report childhood abuse are more likely to experience positive psychotic symptoms (Ross et al., 1994).

Dirty Magazine Cover

Gloria walked into the store hunched over, urgent in pace, with one arm covering her face and the other held close to her chest. She had a suspecting look in her eyes, yet she appeared to see no one. The clerk had seen her in the bookstore a few times before and nothing much ever seemed to happen. She was just one of the characters who wandered the streets of this small town. Every town had a few. They were usually pleasant or at least unassuming. Yet, the clerk never tried to engage with Gloria, mostly due to the enveloped nature of Gloria's physical demeanor. She held herself wrapped tightly, like a safe wrapped in chains. Gloria seemed closed off from the world, as she plunged deeper into whatever hole she had intrapsychically crawled into. It was clear that Gloria did not want to be approached, and the clerk felt no need to force her.

On this particular day, Gloria was milling about by the magazine rack when she started to make loud hissing noises and lunging motions at the cover of the current issue of *Rolling Stone*. This particular issue showed the celebrities of the hit show

True Blood, posed nude and covered with blood. The other customers who were standing near the rack backed off as Gloria continued to mutter angry statements under her breath, finally reaching out and turning the magazine around. The clerk could make out the word "DIRTY," as Gloria reacted to the magazine.

Gloria left shortly after she had turned the magazine around, only to return the next day to reenact the scene. Again, the hissing and muttering persisted, and the magazine was eventually flipped backward. The clerk was aware Gloria was likely experiencing some sort of reaction to the cover, maybe religious or maternal, but she gave it little thought.

A few weeks later, the clerk was walking down a side street with a friend when they saw Gloria walking with the same harried pace and protective hunched posture, one arm hiding her face. Gloria made haste in the opposite direction across the street. The clerk could see she was saying something, but she was too far away to hear. When the clerk told her friend the story about Gloria and the magazine, her friend said that Gloria had been in town for a long time, and "she has never been normal." The friend had worked with a newspaper journalist and learned that, as a child, Gloria's stepfather had sexually assaulted her for many years.

As it turns out, Gloria's husband and some of his friends also viciously attacked her. After the attack, she ran away so he would not find her. With nowhere to go, she found herself on buses, in random woman's shelters, and on the streets. These experiences were just too much for Gloria's mind and brain to bear. Yet, without the proper help, Gloria relived these sexual assaults every day.

When an individual has a history of childhood sexual or physical abuse and then experiences psychotic symptoms as a defensive reaction, the person is vulnerable to experience additional traumatic experiences, creating layers of trauma and loss. This was very true for Gloria and many others like her. Being violated in such a severe way by a trusted person shattered Gloria's idea of trust in others. She then chose a life partner who was familiar to her. This man violated Gloria in similar ways as had her stepfather. Gloria did the best she could to protect herself from her husband and found herself homeless on the street and in temporary homeless shelters, where all women are vulnerable to unwanted sexual advances, sometimes violence.

The Government *Made Me Do It*

Max was a 48-year-old male. At age 17, Max enlisted with the US Air Force. By the time Max was 20, he had been given a psychiatric medical discharge. Max believed that the government was forcing him to look at young boys and become sexually aroused, which was happening with more and more frequency. Max responded with rage toward the government and began sending them threatening letters through the mail. Max also developed a fear of being in public areas, known as agoraphobia. Max's father had abandoned the family when Max was just 2 years old. His mother remarried when Max was 4 years old. Max's stepfather sexually molested Max from the age of 5 until he was 9 years old.

Hopefully, by this point in the discussion, the understanding of how the qualitative imprint of Max's trauma manifested into psychotic delusions is apparent. Because of the almost certain physical response of sexual contact, Max likely became sexually aroused despite the abuse. The neurobiology field has an explanatory mantra: "What fires together, wires together." Because Max was sexually abused by his stepfather, he, too, became entrenched in a twisted mental environment where young boys were sexually arousing. Max associated the authority figure of his stepfather with the government, who was making him look at and become sexually aroused by young boys. Subsequently, the development of agoraphobia occurred as Max's way to control these unwanted sexual impulses.

We can clearly see the connection between the early and cruel sexual abuse that Max endured and his current delusion about the government forcing him to look at and become sexually aroused by young boys. A common defense mechanism is to project one's own unwanted thoughts onto another who is safe to rage at without experiencing consequences in return. Max attributed his current unwanted sexual arousal toward young boys to another authority figure, the government. Max externalized these imprinted impulses because of his well-developed set of moral values.

Max currently experiences many layers of loss, or consecutive losses, as a result of the early trauma he experienced at the hands of his stepfather. He developed a disabling psychiatric disorder at the age of 20, a time during which Max should have been focusing on his lifelong employment career. Instead of a military career with all the social and financial benefits, Max now has a mental health treatment career that is loaded with iatrogenic trauma because the treatment is focused only on psychotropic medications and not on the impact and meaning of the severe trauma he endured. Max is unable to work, and his fixed Social Supplemental Income (SSI) does not allow for much in the way of safe and affordable housing. Max rents an apartment in the Skid Row area of downtown Los Angeles, known for housing the largest homeless population in the United States. His psychiatric symptoms, including paranoia, shame, and extreme social isolation, cause him to be unable to make sustainable social connections, which, in turn, increases his symptoms of mental illness and social marginalization.

I Own Skid Row

Along this same Row is Alicia, a 37-year-old woman who believes she owns all of Skid Row. She collects clothes and blankets and donates them to the people of Skid Row.

Although Alicia could live in more comfortable housing because of her SSI income, she prefers to live in an apartment in Skid Row "to watch over the people there." In fact, she believes her SSI checks "originate from the CIA, which is supporting her protective efforts." Alicia brings her psychiatrist and case manager brand new clothes because she believes they are her parents.

Alicia grew up in a household where her alcoholic mother was not able to protect her and her younger siblings from the predatory men with whom she associated. Alicia and her younger siblings were alternatively sexually assaulted and physically abused by most of the adults in her home environment. When she was 12 years old, she was able to report the abuse. She and her siblings were removed from her mother's custody and lost contact from one another. Today, Alicia has no family to call her own. Alicia's perceived protection of the people of Skid Row allows her to experience her vital need for belonging, connection, and mastery in the form of protection from predatory abusive people. Alicia overtly attaches to her psychiatrist and case manager as her loving and protective parents and she their beloved daughter.

Alicia was homeless and lived on the streets of Skid Row for many years. Housing was finally arranged for her in independent and minimally supervised housing in Skid Row. Alicia requested a room change because she reported that every night, people were breaking into her room and raping her. Alicia frequently washed her vaginal and rectal areas with bleach water. When her room change was granted, she believed this criminal behavior stopped. She was so grateful for her room change that she took it upon herself to tidy up the main lobby of the apartment building on a daily basis.

Like Max, the early and severe abuse that Alicia sustained was the foundation for a lifetime of subsequent losses. Alicia was most comfortable in the Skid Row area, where there is an abundance of mental illness, drug trafficking, violence, and prostitution. Because she had no family to call her own, she attached to her mental health treatment providers as primary family members. There were limits on the availability and intimacy of these relationships. Additionally, because of her delusional attachments to her psychiatrist and case manager and the obligation she feels to buy new clothing for them, her income, which should be available for her own well-being, is significantly reduced. Yet, some might argue that these attachments and spending her limited money on them, while delusional, made up her spiritual sustenance. Nevertheless, Alicia experienced layers of continued losses that originated from the early and severe abuse that imprinted her attachment and belief systems.

Psychosis and PTSD: No Longer Ignoring the Facts

Psychotic symptoms have long been observed and documented in the aftermath of a broad range of traumatic events across the lifetime. Grimby (1993) found that in a sample of older adults, 82% experienced either hallucinations or sensory *illusions* 1 month after losing a loved one. Among the Latino culture, auditory, visual, tactile, and olfactory hallucinations of deceased loved ones are so common that the DSM-5 specifies this symptom as a culture-bound syndrome and discourages the diagnosis of a psychotic disorder (American Psychiatric Association, 2013; Anglin & Malaspina, 2008; Blow et al., 2004; Strakowski et al., 1996). Furthermore, in 1944, Lindemann documented reactions from survivors of the Cocoanut Grove Nightclub fire in Boston, Massachusetts, in which 492 people were killed and many others severely injured. Auditory and visual hallucinatory experiences were among the common reactions of survivors of the fire and their loved ones (Lindemann, 1944).

Lifetime exposure to interpersonal violence experienced by people with SMIs varies between 48% and 81% (Hutchings & Dutton, 1993; Jacobson & Richardson, 1987). In a sample of 458 undergraduates, Berenbaum (1999) found that reported childhood maltreatment was associated with higher levels of unusual perceptions and beliefs. Several studies document the emergence of psychotic symptoms and meeting criteria for the diagnosis of schizophrenia following the most severe political trauma, including concentration camp survivors (Eitenger & Grunfeld 1966; Klein, Zellermayer, & Shanan 1963; von Baeyer, 1977), Pacific Theater prisoners of World War II (Beebe, 1975), and Cambodian refugees during the Pol Pot regime (Kinzie & Boehnlein, 1989). Most recently, more studies than can be listed here that include severe PTSD reactions, including auditory and visual hallucinations among veterans of the Iraq and Afghanistan wars. Given these strong findings across multiple studies and among large samples, it seems undeniable that there is a strong correlation between traumatic experiences and the reactionary development of psychotic symptoms (Shaner & Eth, 1989).

Study after study asserts the correlation between the nature of the traumatic experiences (especially childhood sexual and physical abuse) and the content and quality of the psychotic symptoms that individuals experience, especially the command auditory hallucinations, paranoid delusions, thought insertions, flashbacks, intrusive images, and reading others' minds, often for many years after the events (Goff et al., 1991; Heins, Gray, & Tennant, 1990; Read & Argyle, 1999; Read et al., 2003; Ross, Anderson, & Clark1994; Sansonnet-Hayden, Haley, Marriage, & Fine, 1987).

Read and Argyle (1999) examined the relationship between three positive symptoms of schizophrenia (hallucinations, delusions, and thought disorder) and childhood physical and sexual abuse among psychiatric inpatients. They found that 17 of 22 patients with an abuse history exhibited one or more of these three symptoms, and half of the symptoms for which content was recorded appeared to be related to the abuse. However, this study had a small sample size and obtained its data from analysis of clinician case notes, which may bring into question the reliability and validity of these reports of symptoms and abuse. More recently, Read et al. (2001) found, in a sample of 200 community patients, that hallucinations were significantly related to sexual abuse and childhood physical abuse. This relationship was particularly the case for commenting voices and command hallucinations. Goff et al. (1991) have also suggested that such a history of childhood sexual abuse may contribute to the symptomology and course of a psychotic illness. It is common for victims of sexual abuse to experience general flashbacks, intrusive images, and bodily flashbacks associated with the abuse years after the event (Heins, Gray, & Tennant, 1990; Sansonnet-Hayden et al., 1987). Somatic delusions, such as delusional parasitosis (the belief that one is infested with parasites such as mites, lice, insects, or bacteria) are also documented following traumatic life events such as rape and sexual assault (Oruc & Bell, 1995). Furthermore, in Beck and van der Kolk's (1987) study of chronically hospitalized psychotic women, it was found that patients reporting histories of childhood incest were more likely to have sexual delusions. This congruence between the concrete details and nature of traumatic experiences and the form and content of psychotic symptoms suggests there may be a causal link. However, an alternative view would be that psychotic symptoms are always related to persons' developmental histories, and if these histories contain traumas, these events will be used in their development of explanations for anomalous experiences.

This striking congruence between a patient's life events, early experiences, and the content of his or her symptomology is often observed. In one study, empirical support for this congruence was found by Raune, Kuipers, and Bebbington (1999), who reported some association between themes expressed in delusions and auditory hallucinations and the characteristics of stressful events *before* symptom onset. In addition, Fowler (2000) reported that 14 of 26 patients in a treatment trial of cognitive-behavioral therapy for psychosis had a trauma history, but the presence of a trauma history can often be masked by the psychotic presentation. He also reports that careful assessment can reveal syntonic links between the nature of trauma and the content of hallucinations and delusions and suggests that a trauma history may make patients more likely to develop a chronic illness or have drug-resistant symptomology.

This connection between early and severe trauma and the similar-natured manifestation of psychotic symptoms is vital to the treatment of individuals who experience psychotic symptoms. The wide range in study time frames (dated and contemporary) illustrates the sustainability of this information. All of this information suggests a strong positive correlation between early and severe traumatic experiences among people who later develop psychotic symptoms, especially positive symptoms (Butler et al, 1996; Janet, 1893).

What's interesting is that during the coursework for my bachelor's degree in psychology, master's degree in social work, and PhD in clinical social work, which emphasized the study of mental illness, this relationship between psychosis and early and severe trauma was not presented. There are many possible reasons for this omission. There is a significant amount of information on the topic of traumagenic neurodevelopment (TN), or the nature in which early traumatic experiences change brain matter and functioning, as an explanatory model (Read, Perry, Moskowitz, & Connloy, 2001), specifically for schizophrenia. Yet, translational science suggests that the use of knowledge-based research in the applied world involves a 20-year gap between when the knowledge is gained and when it is used in practice (Brekke, Ell, & Palinkas, 2007). Therefore, because most of these TN studies were published in the late 1990s, these accurate understandings and effective interventions are only now available for clinical practice. Much of the intention of the publication of this book is to speed up the time frame in which this knowledge is administered into clinical and administrative mental health treatment settings.

A significant portion of this TN model research and knowledge is conducted and published in British, Norwegian, Australian, and New Zealander professional journals that are independent of the influence of pharmaceutical companies. If this information is available in the United States, it is produced in an alternative or protesting venue. These researchers and authors are not readily available at professional mainstream conferences, and thus are not *spreading the word* in the United States.

Another speculation about the reason for the absence of this TN knowledge in mainstream professional education is this: We reflect back on the discussion of defensive countertransference and consider that this information is just too difficult for professionals to hear and then be productive all day long. If mental health professionals are not trained to even discover this material, then most will not, and few will know what to do with this revealed traumatic material. Moreover, the pharmaceutical industry has attempted to brainwash us all in believing that the origin of all emotional states is neurobiological and can be solved by the administration of the right combination of psychotropic medications. This significant evidence of early and severe traumatic experiences among those who have psychotic experiences places room for doubt on the truth of this statement.

SEVERAL NEW DIAGNOSTIC CATEGORIES AND CLINICAL SKILLS THAT INCLUDE TRAUMA AND PSYCHOSIS

Kingdon and Turkington (1999) have suggested a new psychiatric diagnosis, *obsessional psychosis*, which includes repetitive and distressing auditory hallucinations of the perpetrators associated with traumatic experiences, especially sexual abuse. For instance, Alicia's belief that intruders were sexually assaulting her nightly in her apartment actually represented repetitive delusions focused on similar sexual assaults from her childhood. The nature of the early abuse has strong correlation with the quality of symptom manifestation.

Because of the bizarre nature of psychotic symptom manifestations, the trauma of an individual's history may be overlooked. The phrase "Don't poke a sleeping bear" comes to mind. Mental health clinicians often do not know what to say or do in response to these seemingly bizarre expressions, they think it is best to avoid examining them for fear of further decompensation. Furthermore, mental health professionals worry what this person may experience as provocation and how he or she will react to it.

Fly Like a Butterfly

When Jackie was a child, her mother's brother emotionally and sexually abused her for a significant period. Already socially marginalized and alone often due to her mother's lack of attention and affection, Jackie was vulnerable to her abuser. When she finally came forward to her mother about the abuse, her mother's reaction was to blame Jackie and restrict all social activities, including afterschool sports or events and friends.

As an adult, with her mother no longer able to threaten her, Jackie took to traveling to countries ruled by abusive dictators and protesting while dressed like a butterfly. Engaging in such bizarre and provocative behaviors in places where she had no legal status was all but asking for severe trouble, with results that could be a tremendous threat to her life. Yet, she felt the safety of being able to protest because the original object of Jackie's protesting, her deceased mother, was unable to respond. She was compelled to pursue these protests because of her emotional history.

As a result of her bizarre and disorganized expressions, Jackie was alternatively ignored, not taken seriously, or overpathologized, causing an infinite amount of social marginalization and personal, social, and financial losses. She was compulsively recreating her early life, using all her income to travel to these countries where the main figure served as a representation of her cold and critical dictating mother. So, how is the butterfly costume explained? Possibly, Jackie had a wish to flee from her abusers and transform her life into a meaningful one worth living. Are Jackie's symptoms more accurately categorized as schizophrenia, PTSD, or obsessive-compulsive disorder?

The individuals whose stories resemble Jackie's may be overdiagnosed with schizophrenia or other SMIs that include symptoms of psychosis. We are reminded of Sheila's story. Sheila had experienced every kind of abuse, and it was always severe.

As she grew into adolescence and adulthood, Sheila was diagnosed with every possible SMI listed in the DSM, including schizophrenia. In fact, according to Fowler (2000), a more accurate diagnosis may have been an extreme form of PTSD. Fowler and others also emphasize that because there is such a strong correlation between traumatic experiences and the manifestation and nature of hallucinations and delusions, clinicians must take a careful trauma history and be alert for ongoing psychotic symptoms, especially those that are not affected by psychotropic medications (Ellason & Ross, 1997).

The origin of most psychiatric diagnoses in children is trauma, whether *Big T* or *Little t* trauma. Big T trauma refers to serious traumatic experiences, such as childhood sexual abuse, physical abuse, and natural disasters. Little t trauma refers to subtle but equally serious themes that occur over time, such as ongoing interpersonal and emotional neglect, bullying, experiences of being shamed or humiliated, and other experiences that diminish self-esteem and dignity. Little t traumatic experiences can be just as serious, if not more serious, because these experiences go ignored or are normalized, and the child has no external means to validate or put words to his or her intrapsychically distressing experiences. When a child is traumatized, he or she may not have the cognition and language to metabolize and express the feelings that he or she is experiencing. A child's big emotions are often expressed so bizarrely that, without knowing the content of their traumatic experiences, the manifestation of symptoms sometimes appears as psychosis. With this manifestation, the child is often diagnosed with a psychotic disorder, such as schizophrenia.

In the advanced mental health professional practice courses that I instruct, students report their internship experiences where they are working children who have been diagnosed with psychiatric disorders. The following similar story is often told. The child has been diagnosed with a psychotic disorder, such as schizophrenia, and is taking several different psychotropic medications with little to no effect on hallucinations and delusions. In 9.9 out of 10 of these stories, there is almost always one or a series of huge, identifiable, severe traumatic experiences that this young child has endured. The experiences are just too much for this young mind to bear, and the delusions are the only way to make sense of the unthinkable traumatic turn of events.

We often hear case after case like this in which the child's expressions of his emotional reactions to the traumatic experiences are so extreme that he is misdiagnosed with schizophrenia and medicated with psychotropic medications, often causing serious side effects, such as tics, weight gain, or emotional numbing. What is equally alarming is that the child's emotional reactions to the trauma, including the new diagnosis and medications are not talked about. Especially now, with this diagnosis of schizophrenia, the child will not have help with his traumatic experiences, as many mental health clinicians believe that this depth of conversation would overstimulate the child, causing him to experience an acute psychotic decompensation. The child with the diagnosis of schizophrenia is now thrown into the grips of *The River*. Again, would a more accurate diagnosis of this child's psychiatric symptoms be a severe form of PTSD? Further and comprehensive assessment would be necessary for an accurate categorization of the symptoms. When any mammal, or attachment-driven animal, is scared or hurt by another, one natural reaction is to retreat into physical and interpersonal safety. When strong emotional reactions are not attended to, an individual will find creative means to express him/herself.

When Bizarre Is Normal: Understanding Symptoms and Finding the Best Approach for Communication

People who experience psychotic symptoms find creative methods of self-expression. Clinicians who have worked for any length of time with this population can attest to the many such letters that they have received from individuals who experience psychosis. These letters are similar in quality. They have run-on sentences that often span several pages. The letters may include ruminative, nihilistic, persecutory, or existential themes with strong and distressing affect. Sentence structure is impaired. The writing instrument was obviously pressed excessively hard onto the paper, so that one can actually feel the writing on the backside of the paper. This *schizophasic* style of writing is discussed at length in Chapter 7, "The Relationship Between Neurobiology and Psychosis." Here is an example of one of these letters as it was exactly written, protecting confidentiality:

> Dear Sir's or Madam's: My Name is Rufus I 'am a Veteran out of the U.S. Marine Corp's I recently Lost my Mother The V.A. Police & The Western Security have treated me with so much disrespect among other things that are going on in my life I can see thing's before they happen please help me before these wholy entities open the gate this is a world wide universal spiritual emergency for my sanity sake please help me signed Rufus A child of god. (Personal Communication, Anonymous)

Gail Hornstein (2009), author of *Agnes's Jacket: A Psychologist's Search for the Meanings of Madness*, asserts that there are a number of people who experience psychotic disorders, hallucinations, and delusions who have had traumatic experiences. The meaning of the psychotic symptoms can be directly correlated with the trauma. Hornstein has paired her philosophy with the psychiatric survivor and other peer-recovery groups called Hearing Voices Network (see Appendix B for the website).

She advocates that this discovery-oriented and potentially liberating work should be offered in mainstream mental health treatment settings and not only whispered about in *church basements*.

Fromm-Reichmann (1954) suggests that the therapeutic approach to accurately understand psychotic communications is viewing it as an "expression of and as a defense against anxiety" (p. 419). She explains that the subjective experience of a person who has psychotic vulnerabilities creates tension when he or she feels dependent in a relationship, a fear of relinquishing that relationship, and the need to recoil from the relationship to avoid being rejected again. Interpersonal hostility becomes so highly magnified and overwhelming that it leads to unbearable degrees of anxiety for the vulnerable person; therefore, they begin to discharge it, or express the anxiety through symptom formation, such as experiencing auditory hallucinations of the other person's voice making distressing remarks. This thought is incongruent from the previously held belief that people who experience psychosis are incapable of participating in mutual relationships. Again, what Fromm-Reichmann was really saying is that people who experience psychosis are exquisitely sensitive to the fluctuating dynamics in relationships (Fromm-Reichmann, 1960). Because many people with psychotic experiences feel deeply rejected by people in society, she declares that they must be given a ripe social environment to which they *want* to come back.

Whereas many people who take their psychotropic medications as prescribed experience mental status stabilization, there is evidence that some of these people have had recurrences of psychotic symptoms. These symptoms may be caused by intrapsychic constructs, not biology; therefore, medications will have little to no impact. What I am suggesting here is that within a committed therapeutic relationship, in which the meanings of the psychotic symptoms are accurately understood and the client is appropriately responded to, psychotic symptoms can significantly, immediately, and permanently diminish without the use of psychotropic medications.

The practice of relying on psychotropic medication to relieve distressing symptoms is discussed by Siegel (2010a; b). He asserts that people with symptoms of psychosis can be helped with a concept he terms *mindsight*, which is the ability to see the internal world, to accurately notice what is going on inside of one's mind and inside the mind of others, and to effectively deal with this inner mind activity.

Read (2006), in his chapter "Breaking the Silence: Learning Why, When and How to Ask About Trauma, and How to Respond to Disclosures," offers the framework and direction of addressing trauma histories in psychiatric patients. First, compared with the general population, he acknowledges the overrepresentation of early and severe traumatic experiences, especially sexual and physical abuse, among inpatient psychiatric patients. Accurate trauma history collection is intermittent, as only sometimes clients volunteer this information, and there is a low rate of clinicians who directly ask about this history. Even after a new form and training was implemented by Read and Fraser (1998) in their study, clinicians still had a significantly low rate of inquiring about trauma histories at intake, selectively avoiding these questions. Clients deemed too psychotic to respond were especially less likely to be asked about their trauma histories. Second, even when trauma experiences were disclosed, there was a low rate of incorporating this information into treatment goals for the client. Without discovering such clinically important information that impacts every aspect of an individual's life, there is no opportunity to accurately conceptualize, contextualize, and address these experiences into the individual's resulting beliefs and behaviors. In Chapter 10, "Listening with Psychotic Ears Philosophy and Clinical Skills," you will find a review of Read's recommendations regarding how to ask about trauma history and effective clinical skills to manage trauma disclosures.

FINAL THOUGHTS

Upon asking about traumatic experiences among people with SMI, we find that a significant number of individuals respond with early and severe traumatic experiences and significant losses. Sexual abuse is one of the most commonly reported and the most damaging, impacting brain development and functioning, attachment styles, coping styles, and overall quality of life resources and decisions, including relationships, education, employment, finances, and medical health. In this chapter, we discussed possible new diagnoses that include the impact of early and severe trauma on the manifestation of psychosis, including obsessional psychosis and traumagenic neurodevelopment. With these new diagnoses, a more accurate understanding of trauma-induced psychosis can occur, also resulting in more accurate interventions that will increase quality of life for individuals who experience trauma-induced psychosis.

7

The Relationship Between Neurobiology and Psychosis

AS FAR BACK as the pioneer theorists Freud (1925), Kraepelin (1908), and Bleuler (1908), psychotic symptoms have been thought to originate from purely biological factors. Today, there is a near consensus among mainstream mental health practitioners and researchers that the origin of psychotic disorders, especially schizophrenia and schizoaffective disorder, lies in a biopsychosocial model, with robust emphasis on brain structure and the quality of neurotransmitter functioning. Furthermore, these brain alterations are best categorized in the professional literature by genetic transmissions and environmental influences during pregnancy, including obstetric adversities. The investigation of stress altering brain structure leaves off there. This chapter acknowledges and discusses the current evidence from the fields of medicine, and more specifically neuropsychiatry, that illustrates how the experience of psychosis may originate from brain structure, particularly the hippocampus, amygdala, and prefrontal cortex, and the metabolization of neurotransmitters, especially dopamine and cortisol.

The philosophy of *Listening with Psychotic Ears* is intended for an audience whose interests are in learning and practicing effective clinical skills that may or may not include prescribing neuropsychiatric medicine. The neurobiological explanations in this chapter are detailed but brief. I am not attempting to be a neurophysiologist. Instead, I am a social worker who has an appreciation for the medical advances and knowledge now publicly available. The bibliographic references include relevant

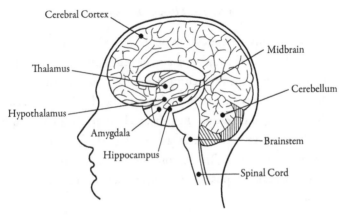

FIGURE 7.1 Brain anatomy.
Source: National Institute on Drug Abuse (1997). Mind Over Matter: The Brain's Response to Drugs, Teacher's Guide.

neuroscience literature for the reader who desires to pursue additional neurobiological information. We first explore how the brain generally works, and from this foundation, we can better understand how psychotic experiences are manifested in the brain.

(Image available at the website listed in Appendix B, https://science.education. nih.gov/supplements/webversions/BrainAddiction/guide/lesson1-1.html.)

The brain, an organ that can be held in the extended palm of one's hand, is made up of more than 100 billion tiny nerve cells called neurons. As small as it is, the brain dictates everything we do: talking, breathing, walking, feeling, contemplating the universe, creating theories and musical masterpieces, and so many more truly awesome exploits. The capacity of these behaviors depends on the number and quality of neurons and their potential for communication between one another. The electrical communication that occurs between the neurons in the synapse is termed *synaptic firing*.

When the brain is young and developing, the neurons have fewer connections. As the young child practices at something, like walking, these neurons develop connections. The connections develop pathways. As behaviors are repeated, these pathways become stronger, and the task becomes effortless. Whatever a person does frequently and repetitiously will develop those strong and numerous neuronal connections and pathways. Remember, what fires together, wires together. Once those behaviors have developed numerous and strong neuron pathways, the brain can communicate to the body to perform these behaviors automatically, gracefully, and on an unconscious level, while learning new behaviors and performing multiple tasks. This explains how our brains can handle a variety of tasks at once, such as driving in busy traffic and considering all the items that need to be discussed during the meeting to which we are driving.

Lower Survival Brain Development

The fetus and infant brains begin developing from the bottom, or brainstem, to the midbrain, or cerebellum, to the higher brain, or cerebrum. A baby is born with the whole brain tissue present, but the neuronal connections and pathways are not yet developed. The brainstem is almost fully developed at birth for survival activities such as breathing, hunger, digestion, heartbeat, sleep and arousal, and body temperature. In the first 6 years, with hardly any editing, the brain takes on all the information from its environment. The reason this occurs is so the brain can make as many neuronal connections as possible to learn to become independent and generally self-sufficient.

The creation of these connections at this stage of life is why it is important to expose infants and young children to many different sensations to develop as many neural connections and deep pathways as possible. As the child reaches adolescence, the brain naturally prunes away some of the neurons that are not needed. The adolescent brain is actually downsizing, as one might clean out a closet. Children who are not exposed to many different things and stimuli will have several neurons pruned away. Children who are traumatized again and again will have fear and threat magnified, as tenderness and exploration are pruned away.

Emotional Midbrain Development

Between the ages of 6 and 12, the midbrain, or emotional brain, is developing. The emotional part of the brain includes the hippocampus and amygdala, which process emotional activities such as rage, fear, tenderness, separation distress, nurturing, social bonding, exploration, contextual memory, and hormone control. The hippocampus, responsible for factual learning and intentional recollection of memory, is not developed at birth. It begins development and functioning at approximately 2 to 3 years old and is not fully developed until the age of approximately 15–16 years. The amygdala is responsible for long-term memory and the emotional tone of memories, which can be unconscious and without detail. Children of this age tend to experience limited capacity for emotional control and big feelings and are often termed *labile*, which means they quickly and frequently bounce between emotional states. The midbrain does do some editing of stimuli and information, but this editing is small in scope. Again, whatever experiences, stimuli, and information happen with frequency will cause even stronger connections and deeper pathways. Therefore, if a child is told that he or she is accurate at math, confidence develops to do more math, math will be practiced, and, as a result, the pathways that develop learning and logic will become stronger. The child will come to believe that he or she is good at math and, in fact, will be.

MAKING EMPATHY BOOKS—CREATING COMPREHENSIVE AND ACCURATE NARRATIVE AND NEUROPATHWAYS

The use of empathy books is a great example of how children can develop stronger neuronal connections and deeper pathways. More detailed information about how to make an empathy book is offered in the following paragraphs and in instructional videos, for which the links can be found in Appendix B.

Maison Creates an Empathy Book

At 3 years old, Maison was overwhelmed with her feelings. She was throwing a tantrum, kicking, screaming, and crying. Maison's mother got paper and a marker and constructed a book that they would draw together in. Maison's mother wrote the words of what had just happened to upset Maison, including the details and Maison's emotional reaction. Maison drew the pictures. Within minutes, Maison stopped crying and was engaged in the empathy book activity. Maison wanted to read the book over and over.

By engaging in the empathy book construction, Maison was able to create a comprehensive narrative. Her emotions were identified and validated. Reading the book created opportunities for endless future conversations, to which Maison could add her thoughts about this and other related emotional situations.

Maison and her mother made a habit of creating these empathy books. As Maison aged, she had a large vocabulary to describe her emotional life, felt validated, and was confident with her self-expression. As this activity was repeated, Maison's brain repeatedly made neuronal connections and deep pathways.

Higher Brain Development

With a growth spurt that begins around age 6, the higher brain gradually develops, mostly occurring between the ages of 11 and 26. Notice that the brain is not fully developed until around age 26. The higher brain is responsible for rational thinking and decision-making, impulse control, purposeful creativity, problem-solving, reasoning and reflection, self-awareness, kindness, empathy, and concern for others.

Always, the brain has the capacity to develop new neuronal connections and pathways. In a healthy brain, and in the absence of brain damage, with motivation and repetition, anyone can learn and excel at almost anything he or she chooses. Thoughts determine how we perform. If a person thinks he or she can lift the heavy chair or figure out a math problem, chances are that he or she will be able to do it. As Henry Ford said, "Whether you think you can or you think you can't, you're right" (Ford, 2016).

Sometimes, thoughts come in an unconscious and instantaneous manner. The brain in crisis will relinquish its abilities to make reasonable decisions (originating in the prefrontal cortex), and the focus of activity will reside in the survival brain, or brainstem. We are reminded of the parent who is able to lift a car to release her trapped child. She saw that her child was in crisis and did not use higher brain to say, "I can't possibly move that car." She just lifted the car and rescued her child. The brain communicated that a crisis was occurring, which alerted adrenal glands to produce cortisol, or stress hormones, to give her the necessary energy to lift the car that undoubtedly outweighed her strength capacity.

Left Brain, Right Brain, and Everything in Between

Whereas brain connections and pathways develop from the brainstem to the midbrain to higher brain areas, the left and right hemispheres and their communication modalities have distinct roles in behavior, cognition, and affect. The right-brain hemisphere is responsible for creativity, emotions, sensation awareness, intuition, and appraisal of safety and emotional self, which mostly occurs at an unconscious level (Devinsky, 2000; Nasrallah, 1985).

The left hemisphere of the brain is involved with language, linear organization, logic, and deliberate coping, mostly all of which occurs on a conscious level. The left hemisphere functions at its best when emotions are in the mid-to-positive range of stable and happy (Silberman & Weingartner, 1986).

A variety of activities and behaviors signify and facilitate left- and right-brain hemispheric communication. For example, people use hand gestures when talking for the purposes of organizing thinking and communicating, even when talking on the phone (Corina, Vaid, & Bellugi, 1992). If you identify as a *hand talker*, try sitting on your hands and talking. Pay close attention to your level of linear organization as you communicate your ideas. You might be surprised to see that linear thinking is decreased, as you are not able to access your left-brain hemisphere. Alternatively, as one is making a conscious effort to linearly organize thoughts into coherent communication, the use of intuition, creativity, and spontaneous affect may decrease, which are all right-brain actions.

Singing, another act that helps both hemispheres communicate, quiets the impaired conscious and linear left brain so that the affective, intuitive, and unconscious right brain can effectively take over and talk. Singing, or even learning to speak in different ways, such as a variety of pitches, whispering, or using a different accent, helps people who stutter or experience performance anxiety to communicate linearly (Healey, Mallard, & Adams, 1976).

Likewise, music, both a creative experience and logical exercise, involves both left- and right-brain hemispheric activity. Strong negative affect is soothed by pleasant music. The linear predictability and pleasant tone of the music is preferred by the left brain, which the Wernicke's area comprehends (discussed in detail later in this chapter) and communicates to the right brain, communicating an overall pleasant and safe feeling. This feeling translates into similar overall qualitative appraisals of the self and world, thus soothing the affect (right brain) of the listener (Levitin, 2006). We recall the German legend of the Pied Piper (Jacobs & Batton, 1894), who lures children and rats out of town with his soothing repetitious melodies. Whereas the heretic piper represents death or disease, in illustrations of this character, he is almost always playing a *magical* flute. The thought is that the music hypnotizes the logical left brain and attracts people and beasts, who then follow the origin of the music without tapping in to their logic and better judgment.

Similarly, the act of telling stories integrates both left- and right-brain functioning and builds strong connections and deep pathways from the brainstem to the higher brain cortex, especially the prefrontal cortex. The left brain comprehends the semantics of the words that are said, and the right brain comprehends the emotions that are associated with the words, such as tone of voice and facial and bodily expressions. Thus, both parts of the brain are essential for daily social interactions and functioning at all levels.

Neuroplasticity

Learning new information, tasks, activities, hobbies, languages, and unique experiences causes the brain to develop new connections, a capacity termed *neuroplasticity*. These new experiences cause the brain to interpret what is going on and learn for the purpose of repetition, surviving, and thriving. As previously stated, what fires together, wires together. As new information and activities are learned, the brain will make new connections, and these connections build new deep pathways. In the absence of damage to or malfunctioning of brain matter and functions, the brain has the potential to develop new connections and pathways until the moment of death.

How does evolution impact brain development? Do we have the same learning and functioning potentials today that humans did 500 years ago? Initially, for humans, survival was the name of the game. There was not much variety in human experiences. Each day was filled with the actions of finding food, staying warm, procreating, and defending the self or others from predators. Given this meek variety of experiences, compared with the contemporary brain, there were fewer neuronal connections, which resulted in fewer neural pathways. For the experiences that were repetitious, deep pathways were developed, and these behaviors were performed skillfully, rapidly, and unconsciously. In other words, the prehistoric person could skillfully and gracefully target, slay, and prepare a mean boar stew with the same ease as a person today might tie his or her shoe or combine ingredients to make a favorite and frequently eaten meal. As human experiences became more varied, more connections and more pathways were created over generations. The brain organ is actually bigger now than ever. Today, thriving, not just surviving, is the name of the game. We are not necessarily concerned with eating and dodging the fastest predator; humans have the luxury of maximizing our level of reward in a variety of experiences. We can choose from an overabundance of delicacies to enjoy, leisure activities in which to participate, music to listen to, types of books to read, fashion styles, places to visit, and more efficient ways to solve contemporary problems.

When areas of the brain have been damaged, such as a result from a stroke or accident, physical or occupational therapists have to reteach the person activities of daily living by having the person repeat the behavior over and over again. This repetition of behavior allows for the rebuilding of neuronal connections around the damaged area, developing new neuronal connections and pathways that can, again, have the capacity to become skillful, graceful, and unconscious.

Neurotransmitters

Another essential aspect to brain functioning lies in the quality and processes of neurotransmitters, which are chemicals that send messages between neurons.

The *monoamines* (dopamine, serotonin, and norepinephrine) are produced in the brainstem and serve a significant role in the regulation of cognition and emotional processing (Ansorge, Zhou, Lira, Hen, & Gingrich, 2004). Dopamine serves as a key component in motor activity, such as stamina, and reward experiences, such as learning, curiosity, pleasure, motivation, and vitality. Serotonin plays a role in the sleep–wake cycle and the regulation of mood and emotional experiences (Fischer, 2006). Norepinephrine plays a significant role in excitement and emergency alert and response, especially in traumatic and other stressful situations that require urgent decision-making and behavioral responses.

Neuropeptides include endorphins and oxytocin, among others. Endorphins regulate physical and mental pain and excitable pleasure. Oxytocin is released when social, especially caregiving, bonding occurs, resulting in deep rewards and soothing experiences. The release of oxytocin explains why a parent can soothe a crying baby again and again and not be bored or too irritated.

Cortisol, or the stress hormone, is produced in the adrenal glands in response to stressors.

Each brain, including tissue, cells, neurotransmitters, and their functioning, is as unique as a fingerprint because of its genetic coding and life experiences, including caregiving relationships and trauma. Life experiences are the result of neuronal branching and neuroplasticity.

BRAIN DAMAGE AND PSYCHOSIS

With all of this knowledge about basic brain functioning, we turn the attention to brain functioning in the face of anomalies and the origins of brain tissue and neurotransmitter impairment. This section specifically focuses on the areas of the brain thought to be most impacted as a person experiences positive psychotic symptoms.

The reader is reminded that the terms "psychosis" and "schizophrenia" are often used to refer to unique syndromes. Psychosis is intended to refer to a more general set of symptoms, not a specific DSM diagnosis. Schizophrenia is intended to refer to a specific brain syndrome and the progressive functional decompensation. We think of positive psychotic symptoms as symptoms that are there but should not be, such as hallucinations and delusions. Negative symptoms are those symptoms that should be there that are not, reflected in disorganization and decreased production in cognition, speech, and energy levels. The author will make every attempt, especially in this chapter, to use the specific word intended for the topic.

Genetic Influences Evidenced by Twin Studies

For approximately the last 40 years, most mainstream mental health treatment providers and researchers seem to agree, with degrees of variation and despite concrete evidence, that the origins of psychotic disorders, specifically schizophrenia, are genetically transmuted. This belief prompts the following question: What does it mean when we say a person has a *genetic predisposition*? Generally, when we say that one has a genetic predisposition, we are addressing the genetic code relatedness of family members who also have symptoms of a specific disorder. In this scenario, the risk is greater the closer the family member who manifests the illness is genetically to the predisposed person. For example, the risk of developing schizophrenia is greater if a grandparent has the illness than a third cousin. Similarly, the risk is even greater if a first-degree family member has the illness, such as a parent or sibling (Cardno & Gottesman, 2000; Kendler et al, 1985; McGuffin & Owen, 1995; Mortensen et al., 1999). However, even if there is no schizophrenia in first-degree relatives, the risk of manifesting schizophrenia is even greater as the number of affected blood relatives increases across generations, suggesting an emphasis on affected genes (Bleuler, 1978).

The medical world has come to understand genetic predisposition (bloodline) for schizophrenia and transmutation (manifestation) of schizophrenia from parent to offspring by exploring the research findings from twin studies, which began in the 1920s in Europe by Munich School members Luxenburger and Ruden (Strongmen, 1994). European studies found that manifestation of schizophrenia among both monozygotic twins (MZ) occurred in 46%, compared with 14% in nonidentical/dizygotic twins (DZ) (Gottesman & Sheilds, 1982). North American twin studies reflected slightly lower numbers of comparisons, with 31% of MZs both developing schizophrenia and 6% of DZ twins (Kendler & Robinette, 1983). Whereas much of the mental health profession relies on these studies to conclude that schizophrenia runs in families, when we think about the larger number, exemplified in these results, that do not manifest schizophrenia, the other factors that contribute to the manifestation of schizophrenia must be considered.

Around 1945, as the United States adopted more of a psychoanalytic explanation of mental disorders (the belief that families cause them), the etiological certainty of these twin studies came into question. These twin studies have received a great number of criticisms, including the subjective nature of diagnostic categorization, in which one clinician's diagnosis varies greatly from another's, and there may be a variety of contributing environmental factors that may have made the brain more susceptible to symptoms of psychosis (Gottesman, 1991).

Adoption studies were conducted on samples of individuals who had been removed from their mothers with a diagnosis of schizophrenia. One of the first of these adoption studies was conducted by Heston (1966). In a sample of 47 adopted adults, 5 developed schizophrenia spectrum disorders, whereas none of the 50 adults in the control group did. These results, again, are not in favor of a sweeping certainty that schizophrenia is solely a genetic phenomenon. Many other similar adoption studies result in unstable and noncompelling findings (Kendler, Gruenberg, & Kinney, 1994; Kety 1983; Rosenthal et al., 1968; Wender et al., 1974).

Many interested people and groups were hoping to find one single gene or several that were responsible for the genetic transmission of schizophrenia and other psychotic disorders. After several decades of this specific research, it was found that many combinations, not just a few, contribute to the possible explanation of genetic vulnerability that may contribute not only to schizophrenia but also to a variety of psychotic disorders that are identified in the DSM (American Psychiatric

Association, 2013). In fact, one significant meta-analysis found that as many as 3,000 genes (18% of all known genes) may impact the vulnerability of the manifestation of schizophrenia (Lewis et al., 2003). In *Schizophrenia: Fast Facts*, Lewis (2007) asserts there are likely to be 15–20 genes involved, and specifically, 4–6 susceptibility genes have been identified.

Researchers based at the Broad Institute in Cambridge and Harvard Medical School have pinpointed the gene (C4) that they found to be the biggest risk factor for schizophrenia (Sekar et al., 2016). They asserted that the gene C4 normally works in the immune system. However, with exposure to certain infections (toxoplasmosis, rubella, or influenza), the gene targets the brain and expedites the process of pruning away the connections between neurons made during early brain development. This pruning especially happens in the parts of the brain most affected by schizophrenia. Because of the 20-year translational science gap, mainstream mental health professionals do not have access to this finding yet. Still, this gene identification is from just one study, so an open mind must be kept about other factors that cause schizophrenia manifestation.

While there is strong evidence that genetics play a convincing role in the manifestation of schizophrenia spectrum illnesses, there is room for doubt in this reductionist certainty. In a detailed genome study of schizophrenia using a sample of 294 multiplex pedigrees (a family grouping of genetically related individuals) that met the criteria for schizophrenia, the findings were as follows. "Hard replication—implication of the same markers, alleles, and haplotypes in the majority of samples—is elusive. It is evident that these studies are inconsistent, and no genomic region was implicated in more than four of the 27 samples" (Sullivan, 2005, p. 7). The researcher continues by saying, "If correct, the implication is that (the data) contains a mix of true and false positive findings" (Sullivan, 2005, p. 10).

Now, if that sounded vague and unsubstantial to the reader, it was. Upon deep reflection and repetition of these twin, adoption, and genetic studies, these studies can be considered persuasive, but given that the gene or sets of genes have never been identified twice, these studies should not be taken as absolute proof (Gerhart & Marley, 2010). Of the hints of information that have been gathered from these effortful studies, the findings have serious limitations because the studies lack impressive consistency (Sullivan, 2005). In other words, the studies cannot be consistently repeated with similar findings. Additionally, the samples sizes are too small to assert completely generalizable statistical significance. Whereas these studies may be confusing or elusive and do not offer anything for us to hang our hat on, they do provide a starting point for the next generation of research (Sullivan, 2005).

"Schizophrenia is similar to other complex traits: it is possible that there are kernels of wheat, but it is highly likely that there is a lot of chaff" (Sullivan, 2005, para. 16). Sullivan summarizes that while the findings of this kind of research are not yet ready for "wholesale translation into clinical practice," they do provide a foundation for clinicians and affected persons in the areas of etiology, pathophysiology, and treatment" for the future (Sullivan, 2005, para. 18).

Environmental Influences

As discussed, family history plays some role in creating a higher risk for developing a schizophrenia or schizoaffective disorder; however, another factor that is just as important as family history in relation to brain functioning is environment. As asserted by Gottesman (1991), in a study of monozygotic co-twins, half of these twin sets presented with only one twin experiencing schizophrenia, and the other half presented with both twins experiencing schizophrenia. What, then, are some credible explanations of how the 50% of twins with only one twin experiencing schizophrenia came to be? Scientific exploration draws our attention to environmental impacts on the developing brain, both in utero and during the birth process. Provided next is a brief overview of the environmental risk factors that carry the most supportive evidence for the etiology of schizophrenia.

Obstetrical Complications

People who manifest symptoms of schizophrenia are highly likely to have experienced any number of obstetrical complications (OCs) at or during their birth process, especially fetal hypoxia (oxygen deprivation) and including preeclampsia (extremely high blood pressure in the mother), diabetes, or excessive bleeding in the mother (Buka, Tsuang, & Lipsett, 1993; Cannon, 1997; Dalman, Allebeck, Cullberg, Grunewald, & Koster, 1999; McNeil, 1988; O'Donnell et al., 2009; Sullivan, 2005; Takagai et al., 2006; Cannon, 1997). These medical phenomena impair fetal and infant brain development in areas similar to those impaired in schizophrenia.

Viral Infection

When the mother becomes infected with the influenza virus or rubella during the fourth, fifth, or sixth months, which are critical to fetal brain development, it is thought that the virus settles in the brain and central nervous system, specifically delaying the development of gray matter of the developing fetus (Barr, Mednick, & Munk-Jorgensen, 1990; Brown et al., 2004; Castrogiovanni et al., 1998; Limosin, Rouillon, Payan, Cohen, & Strub, 2003; Mednick, 1988; Murray, Jones, O'Callaghan,

Takei, & Sham, 1992; Selten, 1998; Short, 2010). Additional studies show that the birth dates of people with schizophrenia are highest in February and March, with March 6 being the peak day. These months fall after the months with the highest rates of influenza infection; thus, this correlation further supports the theory that something toxic occurring in the fetus's brain during the development months four to six may promote cognitive disorders later in life (Mortensen et al., 1999).

Analgesics/Aspirin

When analgesics or aspirin are taken most days or everyday by the pregnant mother, an increase in the risk in developing schizophrenia occurs in the fetus. Analgesics, aspirin, and similar medications cause a hormone-like reaction and impact smooth muscles, reduce inflammation, and affect the prostaglandin pathway, which impacts blood flow to the developing fetal brain (Gunawardana et al., 2011).

Nutritional Deficiency

During the first trimester of pregnancy, nutritional deficiency can influence the development of schizophrenia (Susser, Brown, & Matte, 1999). This deficiency may or may not result in low birth weight because the mother may have been able to gain better nutrition as the pregnancy progressed. However, the fetal brain may have previously experienced nutritional deficiency.

Extreme Stressful Events During Pregnancy and Early Childhood

Stressful events during pregnancy, especially spousal death (Huttunen, 1989) and military invasion (van Os & Selten, 1998), trigger maternal stress hormones (including cortisol), which cause alterations in fetal brain development, specifically in the hypothalamic-pituitary-adrenal (HPA) axis. Cortisol and the hypothalamus are two components of the brain that are specifically identified as showing significant differences among the brains of people with symptoms of schizophrenia and other psychotic disorders.

If extreme stress (increased cortisol causing increased dopamine, causing an inability to self-soothe) alters brain development in the fetus, contributing to a manifestation of schizophrenia, then why not equally consider similar extreme trauma (such as childhood sex abuse [CSA] or childhood physical abuse [CPA] and neglect) in very young children? These experiences also alter young brain development (HPA axis), contributing to the later manifestation of schizophrenia. Alterations and impairments in the brains of people diagnosed with schizophrenia are now additionally explained by those toxic events.

Born and Raised in Urban Environments

People born and raised in urban environments have more exposure to toxins, infections, pollutions, head injuries, certain illicit drugs, and social adversity (Mortensen, 1999). The more collective time a young person spends in urban environments before the age of 15, the more increased the risk is of experiencing a mental illness, especially schizophrenia (Mortensen, 1999). In one study, the incidence of schizophrenia was approximately 65 times higher among men raised in urban environments than among those raised in rural environments (Lewis et al, 1992). The constant mildly stressful overstimulation (i.e., moving and lighted signs, dangerous sound decibals, restaurants, and stores), increased incidents of severe stressful situations (i.e., violence and witnessing drug misuse), and excessive exposure to toxins have significant impacts on brain development.

Prenatal Exposure to *Toxoplasmosis gondi*

Toxoplasmosis gondi is a parasite found in the feces of some warm-blooded animals, especially cats (Brown et al., 2005); Webster, Kaushik, Bristow, & McConkey, 2013). Exposure to this parasite increases dopamine levels (Howes & Kapur, 2009; Torrey & Yolken, 2003) and decreases the ability to ward off predator vigilance behavioral traits, causing them to easily become victim to predators (Berdoy et al., 1995; Webster, Kaushik, Bristow, McConkey, 2013).

In summary, significant support has been provided to exemplify the variety of factors that impact the brain during fetal development that later manifest as schizophrenia or other psychotic disorders. These factors are listed in Table 7.1.

Does just one of these events lead to the manifestation of altered brain development causing schizophrenia and other psychotic disorders? From the advanced knowledge available today, scientists can confidently say that brain vulnerability for schizophrenia and other psychotic disorders does not rest on just one of these risk factors. Thus, a more complex situation is painted. Is it the ripe combination of these toxic influences during the most developmentally crucial time on the genetically vulnerable brain that later manifests in psychotic disorders, especially schizophrenia? Historically, mental health practitioners have seen that schizophrenia manifests in generations of families, so, without supporting strong empirical evidence, there has been an assumption that there is strong genetic predisposition transmission for schizophrenia vulnerability. Why not put more research emphasis on extreme adverse factors that occur from birth through early childhood? The answers to these questions are key to future prevention and more

TABLE 7.1

Environmental Risk Factors for the Development of Psychotic Disorders

Type	Risk Factor	Reference
Familial	Biological parent or sibling with schizophrenia	Cardno & Gottesman, 2000; Kendler et al., 1985; McGuffin & Owen, 1995; Mortensen, 1999.
Prenatal adversities	Prenatal influenza during 4th to 6th month	Barr, Mednick, & Munk-Jorgensen, 1990; Brown et al., 2004; Castrogiovanni, 1998; Limosin, Rouillon, Payan, Cohen, & Strub, 2004; Mednick, 1988; Murray, Jones, O'Callaghan, Takei, & Sham, 1992; Selten, 1998; Short et al., 2010.
	Prenatal rubella during 4th to 6th month	Gunawardana et al., 2011.
	Analgesics/aspirin most or all days of pregnancy	Read, Perry, Moskowitz, & Connolly, 2001
	Extreme stress during pregnancy, such as death of spouse or military invasion	Ross, Anderson, & Clark, 1994
	Childhood abuse and the positive symptoms of schizophrenia.	
Prenatal	Exposure to cats with *Taxoplasmosis gondi*	Webster, Kaushik, Bristow, & McConkey, 2013; Brown et al., 2005
	Toxic exposure: lead or pollution	
Obstetric adversities	Hypoxia, preeclampsia, diabetes, bleeding	Buka, Tsuang, & Lipsett, 1993; Cannon, 1997; Dalman, Allebeck, Cullberg, Grunewald, & Koster, 1999; McNeil, 1988; O'Donnell et al., 2009; Sullivan, 2005; Takagai et al., 2006.
Childhood	Nutritional deficiencies/low birth weight/starvation in mother	
	Time spent in urban environments before the age of 15	
Place/time of birth	Season of birth: late February to early March	

accurate and effective diagnoses and treatment of schizophrenia and other psychotic disorders.

Stress-Vulnerability Model

In 1977, the American psychiatrist Joseph Zubin formulated the stress-vulnerability model: a mixture of environmental, psychological, and biological factors that explain vulnerability to illness, specifically psychosis. The idea is that a person with low vulnerability needs a large amount of stress to experience illness symptoms. For example, the president of the United States likely has a low vulnerability to experience psychosis. Even in the face of daily extreme stress, little to no symptoms will manifest. Alternatively, a person with high vulnerability will need only a low level of stress to experience symptoms. The following example is all too common.

Stress-Vulnerability Steve

A man is hospitalized on an acute inpatient psychiatric hospital unit for the treatment of disorganized thinking and command auditory hallucinations. After just 2 days, his thinking becomes more linear, and his auditory hallucinations subside to mere sounds, such as soft footsteps. Because he no longer meets insurance reimbursement criteria, he is moved to a lower level of psychiatric care. He reports to the staff that he is feeling unsteady and requests to stay another night or two. His request is denied. He is discharged to his home, a single-room occupancy (SRO) in the neighborhood. That night, his rowdy neighbors cause his sleep to be disrupted. Two days later, after not getting enough sleep and anxious about a potential confrontation with the rowdy neighbors, he returns to the emergency crisis center with complaints of auditory hallucinations that are commanding him to jump in front of a train. This person, with an already high vulnerability to acute psychotic decompensation, was discharged from the hospital before he had a chance to adequately stabilize. Unfortunately, we see this repeated all too often in our current mental health treatment delivery system.

This stress-vulnerability model can be applied to both psychiatric and medical illness. People with high vulnerability (chronic medical conditions, such as bronchitis or nerve pain) experience dysphoric symptoms, especially when stressed. People who have no chronic medical situations (low vulnerability) can tolerate a lot of stress without manifesting symptoms. From the public health model, at some given stress exposure point, each of us, even the president of the United States, is vulnerable to medical illness or a psychotic break.

In 1997, Walker and Diforio updated this model of vulnerability to schizophrenia. The etiological impacts of schizophrenia are considered and point to *constitutional vulnerability.* Aberrant adolescent development is added to the formula. When stress is added, psychosis is the result.

While an earnest beginning, this model does not include all of the potential impacts that impact the manifestation of positive psychotic experiences, specifically schizophrenia, including early and severe adverse situations, such as childhood sexual and physical abuse. With new brain-scan and activity-tracking technology, our historical theories of wonderment can now be more confidently supported or denied. The medical branch of neurobiology has created some solid footing, but there is a long way to go.

In approximately 2007, and likely many times before and after this date, mental health consumers lobbied a branch of the APA demanding to identify the gene or combinations of genes responsible for schizophrenia that runs in families (Meldrom, 2003). These demands were not met due to a lack of supportive evidence. With the question of genetic predisposition still unanswered, researchers aimed to tackle the issue. The findings provided some sense of an explanation. For instance, Studies show that where an infant who is genetically predisposed to schizophrenia is born into a secure and mature family, the genetic effects may be neutralized and schizophrenia is not manifested (Tienari, 1992). Lewontin (1993), a renowned American geneticist, states that the current tendency is to overemphasize the role of genetics in human development. He points out that "genes affect how sensitive one is to environment, and environment affects how relevant one's genetic differences may be" (Lewontin, 1993, p. 30).

Other explanations for psychosis abound, including "Whereas normal states of awareness are comprised of an integration and balance of right and left hemisphere processing, psychosis may be a result of the intrusion of right hemisphere functioning into conscious awareness" (Cozolino, 2010, p. 108). When the right brain is overactive, the left brain, especially the left hippocampus and amygdala, and its inhibitory functions are diminished, causing the repression barrier to be less effective and allowing the unconscious and preconscious material to erupt (Shenton et al., 1992). The experience of hallucinations and delusions may be result of right-brain emotional and primary process activity and implicit memory that is popping through to the left conscious brain. People who have symptoms of schizophrenia "appear to openly struggle with shameful aspects of their inner world (likely stored in the right hemisphere) that the rest of us are better able to inhibit, repress, and deny" (Cozolino, 2010, p. 108). As stated previously, the etiology, or causes, for this decreased lower left-brain functioning may be rooted in genetic transmission, obstetric complications, and toxic environmental influences. The experience of psychotic symptoms, primary process thinking, is one in which thoughts and experiences erupt into the conscious logical process of the left brain, and the person makes attempts to logically interpret (left-brain activity) what is happening. As the left-brain functioning is impaired, so is the quality of logical interpretation, and this impairment is sometimes the conscious expression of implicit memory; thus, an elaborate or bizarre story is told (Maher, 1974). Diagnostic tests have shown that people who experience psychotic symptoms experience decreased lateral communication, often displaying stronger activity in the right brain. Furthermore, there is a strong correlation between decreased laterality and more severe psychotic symptoms (Wexler & Heninger, 1979).

EFFECTED PARTS OF PSYCHOTIC BRAIN

As previously stated, theories that attempt to explain the origin of schizophrenia have been based on visible characteristics, severity of symptoms, and deteriorating functioning over the life span. Now, with the availability of neuroimaging procedures, such as computerized axial tomography (CAT) scans, magnetic resonance imaging (MRI), positron emission tomography (PET), x-rays, and other specialized tests that involve imaging or chemical reaction, these inferences can be discredited, supported, or further explored, resulting in identifying additional findings. With this detailed information, the diagnosis could be more accurate than ever. This information is exceptionally hopeful news for people with psychotic symptoms, their families, mental health treatment providers, researchers, insurance companies, and policy makers. In fact, neuroimaging procedures have the capacity to have rippling positive impacts on everyone in our human race.

This section identifies and elaborates on what we know to be true about brain structure and neurotransmitters among people who have been diagnosed with psychotic disorders, specifically schizophrenia. Each area is identified, including the function it serves, ways in which the area may become impaired, and the manifestation of that impairment, including alterations of behaviors, cognitions, and emotions. The reader may refer to the images shown at the beginning of this chapter to serve as visual reference points.

Left Brain

As previously stated, the primary functions of the left-brain hemisphere are the *L* jobs: logic, language, linear organization, and de*L*iberate coping. The left-brain hemisphere typically operates in a conscious manner. Strong negative affect, such as fear and anxiety, impedes left-brain functioning. We have all heard hair-raising stories where, in the midst of a traumatic event, a person was rendered speechless and unable to scream for help. To a lesser degree, the phenomenon of stage fright occurs when the person is so scared that he or she is unable to perform the information that is known and could be comprehensively recited clearly when not scared (Cozolino, 2010). A major aspect of the left brain is Wernicke's area.

Wernicke's Area

Function

The primary function of Wernicke's area is to comprehend what is being said or read. This area relies on words stored in memory and their contexts. An innocent and sheltered five-year-old child said, "I want to be a 'double' for Halloween." What she meant to say was the word "devil," which she had only heard a few times, far less than the times she heard the word "double." Not having any previous experience with this word, thus no context in which to place it, for the purpose of recall, she relied on a word that she had stored many times in Wernicke's area.

Location

Wernicke's area is located in the temporal lobe and within the brain's communication loop that includes Broca's area, described later in this chapter. Wernicke's and Broca's areas are connected by long fibers called *arcuate fasciculus*.

Impairment

Wernicke's area may become impaired as a result of stroke, traumatic brain injury (TBI), heavy and long-term alcohol and other drug use, or extreme adverse experiences in childhood. Impairment of Wernicke's area results in aphasia or behaviors that include rambling speech or sentences that do not make semantic sense; furthermore, the person does not realize that he or she is not making sense. When questioned about the speech errors, the person may become frustrated and irritable because she does not realize she has made any errors and cannot understand why others do not understand what she is saying.

One video shows an interviewer talking to a man who has had a stroke and is now experiencing Wernicke's aphasia (see website listed in Appendix B). This man is using a lot of words, but he does not make much sense when answering the interviewer's questions. His comprehension of the interview is impaired, and his speech is also impaired, involving an abundance of tangential or unrelated ideas. It is nearly impossible to engage in a mutual and meaningful conversation with him.

Manifestation Among People With Psychotic Disorders

Damage to Wernicke's area can appear in people who are actively experiencing a psychotic episode. Speech, whether oral or in writing, can be abundant; however, the word choices and grammar often do not make obvious sense to the average listener. The person may make many attempts to communicate with others, but because the listeners are unable to comprehend what the person is attempting to communicate, the speaker begins to turn to writing to express his thoughts. We frequently see people with psychotic disorders writing pages and pages, filling one notebook after another with their thoughts.

Schizophasia is the term used to describe the impaired manner of speech or written communication common among people who experience acute psychotic episodes (Berrios, 1999, 2009). Schizophasia includes impaired access to correct and common words, which results in word approximation, neologisms, and alterations in speech rhythm.

Word approximation is when a person cannot think of the intended word and says a similar word or describes the essence of the word. The chosen word may relate to the intended word in sound or theme.

An example comes to mind. I am originally from southern and rural Indiana. Whereas my memory of the context of this conversation is fuzzy, I know I was trying to think of a word to describe a funky and distinguishable hairstyle. As soon as I said "Mohawk," I knew this was not the word I intended to say. After some stammering, I thought of it and hollered out, "Mullet!" Both, indeed, were unique hairstyles, but because of the closeness in lexicon (starting with the letter *m*), my brain offered the first word with that letter that fit the theme.

Likewise, children whose Wernicke's and Broca's areas are not yet developed say words that are similar in sound and meaning to the desired words. A child receives a new pair of cowboy boots. In her excitement, she yells out, "Now, I can do my *lime* dancing!" Of course, what she means to say is "*line* dancing."

Neologisms are words made up to represent something that already has a name or title, but the speaker has assigned the new word in its place. These words can be brand new, a combination of current words, or current words used in unorthodox ways. For instance, common and contemporary speech may involve the following statement when asking for the meaning or details of something: "Why don't you Google it?" or "Her photo is so perfect. It was definitely Photoshopped." In these examples, the existing words are being used in ways they are not meant to be used; therefore, new words have been created. Yet, in the acute psychotic experience, if a person does not understand or know of the real term for something, a random word or phrase will become identified as having the same meaning. The example of Chuck is representative of this occurrence.

Chuck, who was experiencing an acute psychotic episode, repeatedly said, "The hound dog makes me tired." At first, this phrase could be ignored as mere psychotic gibberish. However, upon closer listening, Chuck was explaining why he had not been consistently taking his antipsychotic medication, *Haldol*, which he knew as *hound dog*, because the side effects made him tired. Coming from a neurological perspective, Chuck may have been experiencing impairment in Wernicke's area and relied on words he knew well, for which he had deep neural pathways from hearing it so many times, to take the place of a term he either did not know or was not familiar with. Additionally, on further exploration, Chuck stated that the effects of Haldol made him feel like a "lazy hound dog on a hot summer day, only having enough energy to lie passively on a porch." So, the meaning of the phrase *hound dog* had strong association in sound and meaning to his feeling state, which is also likely why he did not question being given a medication called hound dog.

Rhythm of speech impairment is very common among people who experience episodes of psychosis. Between words, there are long pauses followed by attempts to resolve the lapse with rapid speech. This process is comparable to the cardiac condition of arterial fibrillation, where the heart skips a momentary beat and then rapidly beats in an attempt to make up for the missed beats. This skewed sense of rhythm is also seen in writing, where a letter in the middle of a word is repeated many times, emulating the break in thought.

Schizophasia is notable in speech and writing. Schizophasic writing may include 10–20 sentences or an entire document full of words connected only by associations. Whole sentences and pages of text are structured using these associations without a momentary deviation.

Communications tend to be preoccupied with themes of unusual thoughts, such as *evil forces at work*. The content repetition and affective pressure are visible, as a person will draw the same letter in a word over and over, or, as previously mentioned, press so hard that the words are indented over multiple pages. These characteristics represent an alarming sense of affective urgency being communicated. This sense of urgency is understandable if evil forces are indeed at play. A person could be trying to warn others about it.

Finally, concrete use of language, or language taken in the extreme literal sense, is another example of the manifestation of damage to Wernicke's area and is prevalent among people who are experiencing an acute psychotic episode. The following is an example of concrete language use.

"Where did you work when you were a dentist?" The man points to his opened mouth. He is correct in his response, but the spirit of the interviewer's question was to prompt him to talk about the geographical area of his dental practice. The impairment of Wernicke's area leaves his word comprehension impaired and extremely concrete, which results in an inability to meaningfully communicate with others. We use our psychotic ears to imagine what else could he possibly have heard and interpreted when pointing to his open mouth. How can the question be asked in a manner that is concrete, such that he has the capacity to understand? Examples of other ways this question could be asked more concretely would be, "What town did you have your dental practice? Was your office in a professional building or was it a stand alone building?" He might ask me the difference between a professional building and a lay person's building. We must be careful how we use metaphors in our everyday language.

Another example is a letter written by a woman experiencing an acute psychotic episode. She wrote, "Barbara and I split up and I fell apart at the seams (mentally)." The writer made a special point to note that her "falling apart at the seams" was a metaphor; her seams had not really fallen apart, but rather, she had lost control of her mind. In her three-page letter, which was ultimately one sentence, she pointed out on several occasions the concrete meaning of her metaphors. While the writer may have needed these metaphors to be interpreted, a reader without psychosis would have easily been able to understand what she meant to communicate.

The mental status exam (MSE) is a tool used by most mental health professionals to assess and organize ways in which mental status may be altered. There is a question in the MSE that prompts the clinician to say a cultural metaphor and ask the client to make an interpretation. The metaphors are usually philosophical and generalizable.

Whereas these sayings can be interpreted in a variety of ways, the client who is experiencing a psychotic episode will likely give a concrete or other unexpected response outside the range of usual responses. The following story is an example.

The psychiatrist said to the client, "You cannot have your cake and eat it, too." The client responded, "Why would I want to eat my cake in this hospital? I will save it for when I am discharged and can really enjoy it!" The MSE tests for and can identify these types of alterations in cognitive responses.

Ways to Improve Wernicke's Area

When the brain is damaged and impairments are manifesting, neuroplastic efforts can be made to perform *neural work-arounds*, which can, with time and repetition, develop new neuronal connections and pathways. Because speech and written language are disrupted in their natural processes due to damage, the use of sign language may allow for communication of thoughts and feelings that *work around* the parts of the brain responsible for language, themes, and feelings. Encouraging a person to talk with their hands while talking with you can activate communication pathways between the left- and right-brain hemispheres.

The act of singing, mentioned previously, can activate communication pathways between the left- and right-brain hemispheres, as well. Granted, a person may feel especially self-conscious when asked to sing out their concerns, as if they were in a Mary Poppins musical: "I need to speak with a mental health professiooooooooooo oooonaaaaaaaaalllllllll." Thus, a more adaptable method is to encourage the person to whisper or speak in a variety of pitches, as opposed to a monotone expression, which is commonly observed among people who experience episodes of psychosis. The right-brain act of accessing the tonal essence of what is being communicated could work around the impaired left-brain language loop and could coherently and logically express what is on a person's mind.

Wernicke's Area in Action

Wernicke's area processes that which is heard and what it expects to hear. We can understand that what it expects to hear is based on what it has heard (with strong emotion or repetitiously) in the past. Furthermore, because of Wernicke's area impairment, the person also has alterations in the logic and conclusions of the origin and processing of these unsafe feelings.

Are You Happy to See Me or Is That Your Seatbelt?

Brenda, a woman who experienced episodes of psychosis, was called to another state to say her goodbyes to her dying grandmother, who had raised her from birth. Her own mother did not raise Brenda because she was in the process of addiction and could not protect Brenda from sexual abuse at her boyfriends' hands. This particular trip, in and of itself, was extremely stressful and emotionally overwhelming for Brenda. On the airplane ride, because she was seated next to a man, she became increasingly fearful. As the man attempted to obtain and fasten his seatbelt in the compact seat space, he unintentionally touched her leg. Already in emotional overload and with this physical touch in a tight space, she perceived his touch as a sexual advance, which she and her brainstem knew all too well. She stood up and shouted for him to "STOP!" She called for the attendant. They spoke in the aisle, which was also quite compact. Another man's newspaper unintentionally grazed her bottom. Already in sexual threat mode, she yelled at him, too. When the attendant attempted to calm her, Brenda smacked the attendant's face. Ultimately, the local police were notified, and, awaiting landing, they swiftly took her to an inpatient psychiatric facility, where she stayed for 7 days. She was controlled with both physical and chemical restraints. Her grandmother died while she was in the hospital.

In Benda's case, because of her early, severe, and repeated sexual abuse, her brain had developed deep and pervasive perception pathways that perceived the world through the lens of sexual violation and threats of abuse. Because Brenda was so emotional and feeling threatened, her capacity for considering the logical turn of events was severely impaired. Also, because of a lifetime of early and severe trauma and cortisol and dopamine overload, she experienced HPA dysregulation and was unable to be soothed. She perceived the accidental touching by the men as sexual violations. She perceived the female flight attendant as condoning these sexual violations.

Broca's Area

Function and Location

The main function of Broca's area is to control language output. Broca's area is located in the frontal area of the left-brain hemisphere and is an essential part of the language loop. Whereas Wernicke's area helps to understand contextual speech and writing and construct a coherent response, Broca's area is involved with the coherent planning of writing and speech expression, including muscle movement of the lips, tongue, and mouth. The arcuate fasciculus, a threadlike portion of the nerve cells that transmits impulses, facilitates the combining of these processes. Because of this additional area that electrical brain currents must pass through, we think faster than we talk. Thus, talking is often associated with brainstorming, and many people benefit from talking so they know what is on their minds. Another example of Broca's area involvement is the repetitiousness of hearing and repeating speech with geographical accents, which allows the neuronal connections and deep pathways to develop, resulting in an unconscious speech accent that can come out of hibernation after many years of being away from accents and speech styles that are familiar.

Impairment

Damage in Broca's area can be the result of stroke, brain tumor, trauma, lack of social opportunities, or drug use. People with impairment only in Broca's area can understand speech and written forms of communication but have a reduced capacity to speak or write complete sentences to accurately express what is on their minds. The thoughts are there, but the impairment in Broca's area prevents the words from coming out. With severe Broca's area injury, speech will often become truncated, with a person saying only one or two words of a whole sentence, for example. Some people sustain so much damage that they can only produce a few words and use them repetitively for every type of communication.

One elderly woman, Dora, who experienced a stroke that left her with severe physical damage, including Broca's area impairment, could only say the word "Chevy," which she uttered for everything she wanted to communicate.

DAUGHTER: Hi Mom! How are you doing today?
DORA: Chevy.

DAUGHTER: Did you eat breakfast already?

DORA: (affirmatively shaking her head) Chevy.

DAUGHTER: Oh good. Then you are ready for me to take you to the doctor now for your check up?

DORA: (negatively shaking her head and pointing to her shoes that she needed to be put on her feet) Chevy.

DAUGHTER: Ok, Mom. I will help you with your shoes.

DORA: (smiling) Chevy.

Dora seemed to understand the context of her situation, evidenced by appropriate affect and other body language, but because of her impaired Broca's area, she could not come up with any words other than "Chevy" to express herself.

A video example of a man who manifests Broca's aphasia can be found at the link listed in Appendix B (https://youtu.be/f2IiMEbMnPM). The man is attempting to describe to a clinician a medical condition in his legs but is having difficulty. There are exceptionally long pauses between words, and he only speaks a few important words, leaving out verbs and embellishments. He clearly understands what is being said, and his affect is appropriate, but he cannot construct complete and conversational sentences, making meaningful communication difficult.

We all make speech mistakes. These mistakes are commonly made when we first wake up and our synapses are not yet efficiently firing. Mistakes are made when we are experiencing strong emotions and the right-brain activity is overshadowing the left-brain activity. On the occasion of *Freudian slips*, speech mistakes are made when we are defended against a situation that is in conflict with our values, resulting in strong feelings, such as embarrassment or fear of abandonment. Here, the affect—strong, present, unconscious, and having no outlet—finds its way out, sneaking past the language loop and out the mouth.

In the discussion about brain development, mentioned was the circumstance of extreme moments of terror that may render a person speechless. What exactly happens in the brain when we experience speechless terror? Why does Broca's area become inhibited during trauma? Why would evolution select silence in times of crisis? Perhaps the explanation is the fight or flight response: When one is severely threatened, the reaction is to run, fight, or simply keep quiet (freeze). The freezing reaction of animals, being still and quiet when they sense a predator, allows them to be less visible because a still and silent target is more difficult to detect (Cozolino, 2010, p. 278). In a threatening situation, the brain regards only what is moving. When there is threat, brain activity is significant in the brain-stem to allow for enough energy to fight or flee. In other words, evolution has taught the brain to "shut up or do something" when in danger (Cozolino, 2010, p. 278).

Manifestation Among People With Psychotic Disorders

People who are experiencing an acute psychotic episode often display Broca's area impairment. This person will likely have a reduced capacity to express himself or herself through speech and writing. As previously stated, the laws of evolution and survival dictate how extreme fear impacts brain functioning. "Strong affect, especially anxiety and terror, result in high levels of right hemisphere activation and appears to inhibit the left hemisphere and language—hence, the experience of stage fright and speechless terror" (Cozolino, 2010, p. 96). Since a significant portion of people who have been diagnosed with psychotic disorders, especially schizophrenia, have experienced early, ongoing, and severe trauma (Davidson & Smith, 1990; Ellason & Ross, 1997; Goff et al., 1991; Jacobson & Richardson, 1987; Masters, 1995; Mueser et al., 1998; Read, 1997; Read, Perry, Moskowitz, & Connolloy, 2001; Ross & Joshi, 1992), these early and severe traumatic experiences stunted the growth of the language parts of brain (Wernicke's and Broca's area). Has fright caused a strong and deep pathway to develop that hinders language and focuses activity in the brainstem on survival, constantly regulating the fight or flight response? The answer to this question is *yes*. Because the early traumatic experiences began during a time when Broca's area was not yet developed, these horrific experiences occurred *before* the child had the brain capacity to understand and put words to what was happening to them. Thus, the brainstem could sense threat because of physical pain, abandonment, and deprivation. These threatening experiences resulted in the person becoming terrorized and speechless, as activity in the language loop was paralyzed. Speechless terror ensued. Therefore, even if there were some comprehension and language capacity developed, this person's emotions were hardwired to be in survival mode, albeit conscious of the effects of right-brain activity and reduced activity in the left brain.

Right Brain

The left brain stores logic and language. The right brain stores creativity, emotion, and holistic appraisal. The young brain connections and pathways first develop in the right brain. This is why a young person can draw a picture, with all the details, for a long time and not truly understand the importance of being somewhere on time. In this example, the right brain eclipses the processes of the left brain. The right brain develops around the age of 2; then, the development of the left brain picks up. When a part of the brain is impaired, the synapses create new pathways for connection. Thus, as the left brain shuts down, the right brain (creative and emotional) strengthens.

Damage to the right brain results in impairment in grasping interpersonal cues, nonverbal communications such as facial and hand expressions and body language, and the emotions of others. Consider the following example.

Caroline Knows All

Caroline, 39 years old, has symptoms of Asperger's disorder. At social gatherings, Caroline will thrust herself into preexisting conversations, being the connoisseur on every topic, and always efficiently work the conversation around to her knowledge of her many favorite college sports teams. She talks incessantly about specific players and their associated player and team statistics. Her conversation is impressive at first because of her detailed knowledge of so many players. Soon, this conversation feels as though she is talking *at* others, resulting in others feeling left out or oppressively trapped in conversation. Caroline lacks the capacity to pick up on her audiences' social cues and physical cues, such as the wandering of bored eyes. The listener makes kind efforts to reinstate mutual conversational footing, but these efforts are not recognized. As a result, people tend to respond to Caroline by walking away and avoiding her in the future. Caroline's social relationships and network are extremely limited.

Adults who have experienced childhood trauma show unbalanced left- and right-brain thinking. Some show a higher rate of right-brain activity and less left-brain activity when asked to consider the unpleasant memories (Schiffer, Teicher, & Papanicolaou, 1995). These individuals need help learning coping skills that access left-brain logical and linear activity, such as those taught in dialectical behavioral therapy (Linehan, 2014). Alternatively, in alexithymia, the ability to logically tell the details of a story, which is a left-brain activity, is impaired by right-brain activity such that the person expresses poverty of emotions while telling the story. This phenomenon is commonly observed in 911 operators, police officers, some athletes, and gang members who are frequently involved with high emotions. People who experience alexithymia have difficulty in traditional talk therapy because they have difficulty accessing emotions to bring to the session and impaired imagination about alternative possible outcomes, leaving the person's actions concretely repetitious.

Not Too Bad . . .

Nathan, a 44-year-old man, has been in psychotherapy for 7 months. Each week, when the therapist asks how his week was, he replies, "Not too bad." The therapist has to ask pointed and concrete questions to prompt Nathan to share details. Because of Nathan's emotionally reserved style, he reports feeling socially distant and lonely but has no imaginative ideas about what to do differently to change his situation.

Corpus Callosum

Function and Location

The corpus callosum is a thick bundle of white matter neuron fibers that connect the left- and right-brain hemispheres. This bundle is located on top of the brain stem and under the cerebral hemisphere.

Impairment

The corpus callosum can become impaired by way of a birth defect, known as *agenesis of corpus callosum* (ACC), intentional psychosurgery, or traumatic brain injury. With ACC, the infant is born with little to no corpus callosum and is easily diagnosed within the first year or two of life. Agenesis of corpus callosum causes impairment in muscle coordination (e.g., the inability to hold the head up, feed oneself, or walk), vision depth perception, pain perceptions, and sleeping. Research has shown that children with symptoms of dyslexia have a smaller corpus callosum (Hynd, et al, 1995).

In situations of reduced corpus callosum fibers, the brain thinks in concrete (literal) ways. The following is an example of a man who had a severed corpus callosum. Two words were flashed on a screen, one on each side of the screen. The word was the compound word "toadstool." He was asked to figure out the meaning of the words on the screen. He could not determine that the word meant *mushroom*. He, first, had to draw a toad and then a stool; after that action, he could visually see what was documented on the paper looked like a mushroom, hence providing the meaning.

Manifestation Among People With Psychotic Disorders

Studies have shown low corpus callosum connectivity in brains of people with schizophrenia and increased brain activity in one side of the brain hemisphere or the other. Some are more creative, emotional, and social, showing more right-brain hemisphere activity. Others are more logical, know trivia detail, and understand the intricate workings of systems, showing more left-brain hemisphere activity (Innocenti, Ansermet, & Parnas, 2003). In times of threat or emotional activity, the brain will abandon higher brain thinking, leaving more energy for the brainstem for fight or flight behaviors. Additionally, as this person with schizophrenia is already living on the right (emotional) side of the brain, the perceptions and reactions to threat will be magnified, and left-brain (linear and logical) activity will be reduced.

Ways to Improve Corpus Callosum Functioning

A great amount of empirical evidence exists that supports ways to improve corpus callosum functioning. One example is taking up any kind of musical performance, which uses both left- and right-brain hemispheres. Music appreciation (melody and tone) is mostly a right-brain activity, whereas musical performance (linearly playing the correct notes) involves more left-brain activity. The corpus callosum has been shown to be significantly larger among musicians, specifically among children who had at least 15 months of musical training before age of 6 (Steele, Bailey, Zatorre, & Penhume, 2013). In addition, compared with right-handed people, left-handed or ambidextrous people have an overall 11% larger corpus callosum (Witelson, 1985; Driesen, Naomi, & Raz, 1995). There has been a myth that women have a larger corpus collusm than men, but Bishop and Wahlsten (1997) debunked this myth in their metaanalysis.

Limbic System

Function and Location

The limbic system is a collection of midbrain structures located on both the left and right brain and under the cerebrum—responsible for conscious and higher brain activity. Whereas there are many tiny structures that make up the limbic system, the main structures include the amygdala, cingulate cortex, hippocampus, and hypothalamus. This complex system is responsible for survival impulses such as emotion (especially fear, anger, and pleasure), behaviors (especially motivation for sex and hunger), memory, and learning. The limbic system has direct communication with the frontal lobe, impacting decision making and reward, and the brain stem, which links emotions to smells.

Impairment

The limbic system can become impaired as a result of degenerative diseases, viruses, or infections. Variations in the limbic system are also observed in some brains of people with mental disorders, including depression, anxiety, dementia, schizophrenia, and bipolar disorder. Psychological trauma can also impair the limbic system.

Limbic system dysfunction can result in the following behaviors (Amenson, 1998):

- Limited comprehension of social conversations and situations, especially if the conversation includes strong affects.
- Limited ability to learn from and generalize situations. As a result, each situation seems unique; small changes in the environment can cause emotional reactions of confusion, frustration, and anxiety.

- Disruption between current thoughts and feelings and current situations and long-term goals.
- Impairment in learning new complex tasks or learning new tasks from the beginning.
- Difficulty organizing thoughts and feelings into a coherent sense of self. Identity is fragmented, confused, and inconsistent.

Many of these items are learned by reflective relationships and socialization. People with psychotic disorders are usually deprived of these rich social and reflective relationships, which leave them deprived of such opportunities and continually impaired.

Hippocampus

Function and Location
The function of the hippocampus is the formation and recall of memories and spatial awareness, acting like the brain's librarian, taking in short-term memories and judging what to store into long-term memory. The hippocampus is located in the midbrain and is bilateral.

Impairment
The hippocampus may become impaired as a result of any of the following occurrences: starvation of oxygen (hypoxia), encephalitis, epilepsy, stroke, traumatic brain injury, depression, or Alzheimer's disease. In addition, general anesthesia medications temporarily impair the retention of memories.

Manifestation Among People With Psychotic Disorders
Damage to the hippocampus can cause impairment in creating new, lasting memories. Thoughts are only retained for a short period of time, which obstructs learning new ways of doing things, such as how to get to a new restaurant or operate a new computer program. The hippocampus is one of the areas that looks different on the brain scan of a person with schizophrenia versus that of someone without (Adriano, Caltagirone, & Spalletta, 2012; Schmajuk, 2001). Studies comparing these brain scans suggest that deterioration is caused by a disease process and not by genetic transmutation (Baare et al., 2001; Borgwardt et al., 2010). Brain scans are important for determining impairment to this part of the brain, because positive psychotic symptoms are often so severe that a lapse in memory or other signs of hippocampus impairment are not noticed or given attention. The problem is that impaired memory can have significant consequences for people living with symptoms of

psychosis. If a person forgets to maintain certain benefits, such as Medicaid or Social Supplemental Income (SSI), he or she could lose much-needed funds or support services as a result. Similarly, forgetting to take medications could have dire affects for someone on psychotropic medications, causing symptom relapse or worse. These types of consequences lend to the stereotype that people experiencing psychosis are comprehensively lower functioning, when, in fact, they may be experiencing legitimate issues with their memories.

Explicit and Implicit Memory

Scientists, physicians, philosophers, and artists have been concerned with explicit and implicit learning and memory since the beginning of time. Two psychologists, Peter Graf and Daniel Lawrence Schacter, introduced the concepts of *explicit and implicit memory* in their 1985 article, "Implicit and Explicit Memory for New Associations in Normal and Amnesic Subjects" (Graf & Schacter, 1985).

Explicit memory is learning that occurs during repeated task-driven activities. Memory is conscious, fact driven, and requires intentional recollection. The more one interacts with facts and stimuli, the more one will be able to remember and use the information. For example, migratory birds have a large hippocampus aiding their spatial memory. Macquire et al. (2000) found that the grey matter volume in the posterior hippocampi of London taxi drivers is greater than age-matched brains, reflecting the intricate detailed representation of the city. Furthermore, they found that there is a correlation in the more time spent taxi driving and the greater hippocampus volume size.

The brain structure called the hippocampus stores explicit memories. The hippocampus is not developed at birth, begins functioning development between the ages of 2 and 3, and is fully developed by age 15–16. Additionally, explicit memory depends on nearby neural structures in the temporal lobe, including the amygdala, rhinal cortex, and the prefrontal cortex. Connections between the prefrontal cortex and temporal cortex are made through the thalamus. Neurotransmitter systems that are active in explicit memory are acetylcholine, serotonin, and noradrenaline.

Explicit Memory Impairment

In 1953, surgeons performed neurosurgery, or transorbital lobotomy, on patient HM, removing his hippocampus. As a result, HM could not form new memories and was unable to create short-term memories that informed long-term memories.

At the point when the hippocampus is damaged, tasks that rely on memories prior to the damage are unchanged as they have repetitively been stored in the amygdala. However, no new memories are formed.

Implicit Memory and Learning

Implicit memory consists of unconscious associations based on previous experiences. One of the first written acknowledgments of implicit memory was in 1649, when Descartes wrote about adverse childhood experiences that remain imprinted on the child for the remainder of his or her life (cited by Perry & Lawrence, 1984). Additionally, implicit memories are formed with repeated tasks that are stored as short-term memories in the hippocampus and then into long-term memory and emotional tonality through the amygdala (Schacter, 1987). Repeated tasks, such as driving to work, can be accurately conducted without conscious effort. Familiar words and images are more easily perceived. Additionally, as something seems familiar, there is more of a chance that it is associated with correctness or affirmation, whether or not the person consciously agrees with the statement, song, or image. Additionally, this familiarity is congruent with positive affect. For example, a person who recognizes a song from years may experience positive affect, even if he does not know the meaning of the lyrics or did not like the song back when it was popular.

Implicit Memory and Impairment

The mechanism of hypnosis bypasses the hippocampus as detailed memories and neural pathways are created and stored in the amygdala. Information seems to come out of the blue, as the amygdala is unconsciously and unintentionally activated (Hull, 1933).

When emotional or physical (including sexual) trauma occurs to individuals whose hippocampus is not yet developed (under the age of 3), she may not have explicit memories of the incident, but because of physical pain and a resulting fear response, she may have implicit memories of the tone of this and other similar situations. These individuals may unknowingly develop avoidant behaviors, including phobias, and hallucinations and/or delusions from the traumatic material.

Janet, along with Freud, observed adult hysterical amnesia from traumatic events. Janet (1893) wrote of a woman who developed an unconscious avoidant reaction following a traumatic event. A man appeared at her doorway and mistakenly reported that her husband had died. While she could not remember the events of the report, she became frozen with terror each time she passed this door.

In another situation that resulted in the observation of implicit memory, a woman was told about the death of her mother. While she could not consciously remember the details of the report, the details manifested through the mechanism of hallucinations.

In traumatic situations, individuals may develop an enlarged amygdala and experience physiological and psychological symptoms of threat, including hypervigilant (fight), avoidant (flight), and dissociative (freeze) reactions to similar and even generalized stimuli. These symptoms today may explain neurobiological symptoms of PTSD. With the enlarged amygdala, the person views the world from a fear/threat perspective.

Another common phenomenon of bypassing hippocampus and creating long-term memories is that of childbirth memories. How many times have we heard women telling of the horrific pain of childbirth, yet remember this event so very positively, rationalizing by saying, "You just develop amnesia for the pain and remember that sweet angel baby."

The hippocampus and amygdala work together to store factual and emotional explicit and implicit memories that consciously and unconsciously motivate behaviors.

Ways to Improve the Hippocampus

There are several ways to improve hippocampus/memory functioning. In recent years, there has been an upsurge of programs that market the strengthening of brain structure and neurotransmitter functioning, termed *neurobiotics*. Dr. Bob Bilder, a neuropsychologist at UCLA who created Brain Gym, stated that brain cells do reproduce and reposition. Brain Gym is a space for visitors, students, and faculty to learn about the scientific potentials and limitations of brain muscle training (see Appendix B for Brain Gym website). In addition, designed by neuroscientists, Lumosity.com is a computer gaming program with the purpose of scientifically training brains through gaming to be more flexible and increase attention, speed, memory, and problem-solving abilities.

Top Seven Ways to Improve Memory

1. Exercise
2. Drink less alcohol and less frequently.
3. Take more naps.
4. Break your routine. Be adventurous.
5. Eat more vegetables.
6. Meditate and participate in mindfulness activities (listening to relaxing sounds, breathing, and counting exercises).
7. Drink one to two cups of caffeinated beverages.

(For more ways to improve memory, see the website listed in Appendix B, http://www.discovery.com/tv-shows/curiosity/topics/10-ways-to-improve-memory.htm.)

Amygdala

Function and Location

The amygdala, another bilateral component of the limbic system, monitors and reads all emotional signals, especially registering fear and threat, and trigger-relevant safety behavioral responses. For example, one can glance at a lost stranger, and the intuitive gut reaction says that the person is scared. Almost immediately, the amygdala reads the facial expression and has an impulse to comfort the person. The amygdala has strong neural pathways to many parts of the brain, including the prefrontal cortex; this part is where the brain makes a decision about the safety and social appropriateness of talking to the scared person.

Impairment

Because what fires together, wires together, as the person experiences fear and threat, more activity to the amygdala will occur. As more activity occurs, this area of the brain will strengthen and grow, just like any other muscle in the body. For a person who has experienced ongoing significant stress or trauma, increased blood flow to the amygdala has occurred. People who have symptoms of PTSD will have an enlarged amygdala. This means that the neuronal connections are strong and the pathways are deep. Through the lens of this person's perspective, many situations, benign or malignant, will be perceived as threatening; thus, the person might respond to a harmless situation with either fight, flight, or freeze, which impacts their capacity to regulate stress reactions, including fear, vigilance, and cardiovascular responses (Davis, Suris, Lambert, Heimberg, Petty, 1997). Research shows that Vietnam, Iraq, and Afghanistan war combat veterans are vulnerable to a high frequency of threat perception (autonomic arousal) and subsequent impulsive reactions; therefore, these veterans probably have enlarged amygdalas (Lasko, Gurvits, Kuhne, Orr, & Pitman, 1994; Elbogen et al., 2010). With the high incidence of early and severe trauma among people with symptoms of psychosis, it stands to reason that this sample population will show enlarged amygdalas, resulting in high frequency of perceiving many situations through a fear/threat lens and reacting accordingly.

Another way that the amygdala may be altered is through psychosocial surgery or lobotomy, which, as has been discussed in previous chapters, was used toward the end of the 19th century until the mid-20th century, at which time it greatly fell out of favor. Today, psychosurgery is still, but rarely, performed on select patients who suffer from the most severe and otherwise untreatable seizures and symptoms of Parkinson's disease, obsessive-compulsive disorder, and major depressive disorder (Lapidus, Kopell, Ben-Haim, Rezai, & Goodman, 2013). The procedures are much more scientific and targeted and are conducted with more precise instruments than an ice pick. Furthermore, many of these patients receive deep brain stimulation treatments and show significantly positive effects with very little side effects.

Manifestation Among People With Psychotic Disorders
Amygdala impairment is found among people who experience depression, autism, PTSD, phobias, antisocial personality disorder, obsessive-compulsive disorder, mood disorders, and schizophrenia. Mirror neuron reaction activity, found in the amygdala, is what enables humans to, almost instantly and without words, be able to repeat survival behaviors and feel the pain of another, otherwise known as empathy, thus triggering socially mutual behaviors.

The Face of Amygdala Impairment
Tony, a 36-year-old man, endured early and ongoing physical and emotional abuse from his single mother. Before his father abandoned the family when Tony was 7 years old, Tony was the recipient of severe physical abuse. As Tony grew up, he began bullying vulnerable children at school. By the age of 20, he had developed a prostitution ring that included several young males and females and single mothers who were in desperate need of extra cash. When he did not receive his cut from the profits, Tony would severely beat his workers. When asked about this, he casually reported he was simply getting his needs met. The innate empathy with which he was born was socialized out of him. He learned to ignore the social and emotional cues, and this impaired the potential for future mutually beneficial social behaviors and relationships. As he was afforded little to no connection with his caregivers, he repeated the behaviors that were modeled to him; thus, his expression and communication of need and attachment pain were bypassed. Logically, he knew that preying on vulnerable people was immoral, but he attempted to justify his behaviors as getting his own needs met.

People with symptoms of PTSD have had ongoing and intense experiences of fear and threat, which floods the brain with the stress hormone cortisol and activates the amygdala, causing it to overread and overreact to experiences perceived as threatening, again resulting in an enlarged amygdala.

Ways to Stabilize Amygdala Functioning
Hormones affect amygdala reactions. For example, oxytocin, the hormone released when one is caring for another, minimizes fear, experiences of threat, and anxiety. The more a person can be in connection with another (pets, strangers, children, patients, students, loved ones, etc.), especially with caregiving and bonding intentions, the more oxytocin will be secreted by the pituitary gland in the brain, resulting in a mildly euphoric effect and minimizing fear perceptions and reactions.

In the last 20 years, Western culture has been inundated with the word "mindfulness," which refers to being aware of or present in the mind, body, and spirit.

Mindfulness interventions have made their way into a variety of evidence-based interventions that attempt to manage anger, self-mutilation, addiction, psychosis, and anxiety, such as dialectical behavioral therapy (Linehan, 1993; 2014) and trauma-focused cognitive-behavioral therapy (Cohen & Mannarino, 2012). The purpose is to be aware of that which is present.

Mindfulness interventions make attempts to intervene at the primary, secondary, and tertiary levels (Siegel, 2010b). Primary mindful interventions attempt to maintain the brain's natural opiate neurotransmitters, thus being able to absorb stress with minimal dysphoric reactions. Secondary mindfulness interventions attempt to minimize amygdala and HPA activity when risky threatening situations are identified. After a person is in a fight or flight reaction, the tertiary mindfulness interventions, such as nasal breathing and sensory-focused activity (chewing on ice, tasting a sweet apple, or singing), attempt to bring regulating brain chemistry and cognitions back to emotionally stable and linearly logical processing by reducing amygdala activity and regulating HPA functioning. Mindfulness interventions help at the tertiary level to teach calming and present-orienting behaviors, calming the overstimulated amygdala and HPA, after a person has had dissociative episodes that interfere with quality of life. Mindfulness interventions are being widely embraced and taught to a variety of special populations, including elementary-aged children in a program called Mind Up (The Hawn Foundation, 2011) and veterans, trauma victims, and people with a variety of symptoms of mental illness (Vujanovic, Youngwirth, Johnson, & Zvolensky, 2009).

Neurotransmitters

Each person has had a different set of experiences, which result in variations in the number and strength of neuronal connections and pathways. Regardless of the nature of these experiences or the behaviors developing connections and pathways, these processes will continue until the day we die. Of all the many etiological theories, the neurotransmitter dopamine has played the most significant role in explaining schizophrenia and other psychotic disorders. Cortisol is also noted as a major player in these explanations. Both neurotransmitters are discussed in this section.

Function of Dopamine

The purpose of dopamine is to give a person a sense of pleasure, such as when listening to a soothing piece of music, eating one's favorite soup, or participating in an enjoyable activity, such as riding a bicycle or wanted sexual activity. The brain offers various amounts of dopamine, depending on the stimuli. One cannot take a synthetic or man-made dopamine substitute. However, one can do activities or take prescription or illicit drugs to induce a varying push of this desired neurotransmitter. In the instance of drug use to induce a surge of dopamine, the first use or first use after a long period of abstinence will release a large amount of dopamine because the reserve has not been heavily accessed recently. This relationship is why people report that the first drug use is the greatest and why subsequent uses do not create the same effect. Perhaps, the phrase *chasing the dragon* is a familiar one. This phrase represents the circumstance of continual use, in that the dopamine reserve depletes with every use and the amount released can never be as great as the first time. The person continues to use frequently, in hopes that there will be a rush of dopamine to match the first, thereby creating a psychological addiction. When the person significantly slows down or stops using, the dopamine reserve has an opportunity to replenish again.

Considerations

The field of psychiatry initially became interested in the role that dopamine plays in the manifestation of psychosis because of the following findings: (1) Neuroleptic medications that reduce the amount of available dopamine in the synapses also reduce the manifestation of positive psychotic symptoms and (2) neuroleptic medications that increase the amount of dopamine also increase the manifestation of positive psychotic symptoms (Casslon, 1988). These medications include those used to treat Parkinson's disease and illicit drug use, such as cocaine and crystal methamphetamine. Later, it was discovered that these medications block the dopamine receptor, specifically the D2 receptor, which is most common among people who have been diagnosed with schizophrenia. Other antipsychotic (or antidopamine) medications block other dopamine receptors. This variation in receptor blocking is why multiple neuroleptic medications are tried when one does not work. There is no systematic way to know which dopamine receptor is problematic or which medication to prescribe to address the issues.

Manifestation Among People With Psychotic Disorders

Early dopamine research studies, particularly the study in 1967 by the Dutch scientist Jacques van Rossum, asserted that among people with schizophrenia and other psychotic disorders there was an abundance of the neurotransmitter dopamine found in the brain synapses (Baumeister & Francis, 2002). Yet, upon examining bodily fluids and through postmortem autopsy procedures, excess dopamine was not found among people who had been diagnosed with schizophrenia (Bowers, 1974; Post, 1975; Haracz, 1982). This surprising finding propelled researchers to continue to explore this dopamine–psychosis connection. First, it was found, in the autopsies of 20 schizophrenic brains, that there were 70% more D2 receptors compared to a nonschizophrenic brain (Howes & Kapur, 2009; Lee et al., 1978). Initially, this finding fell on skeptical ears, as other studies showed that neuroleptic medications could alter the density of dopamine receptors (Seeman, 2011). This theory was first tested in the brains of rats, which were fed neuroleptic medications, finding an increase of dopamine receptors (Burt et al., 1977). Then, there were multiple studies on the autopsies of people with schizophrenia who had been given neuroleptic medications. These studies consistently showed a significantly higher density of dopamine receptors, thus increasing the sensitivity to dopamine (MacKay et al., 1982). All these studies showed that people with schizophrenia were not born with too much dopamine or an overabundance of dopamine receptors. Instead, the neuroleptic medications they were given were causing both an overabundance of dopamine receptors in an attempt to override the drugs' effect and oversensitivity to dopamine.

However, the elevated dopamine receptor density theory was once again strongly supported by the findings of studies involving the following two populations: people who carried a diagnosis of schizophrenia and were never medicated and the prodromal, or first-episode schizophrenia, populations (Post, 1975; Haracz, 1982). The findings showed that the dopamine levels and amount of receptors were similar to the brains of people who had never been diagnosed with schizophrenia (Martinot, 1990). Higher rates of dopamine production can be explained by childhood sexual and physical abuse (Read, Perry, Moskowitz, & Connolly, 2001) or cocaine or crystal methamphetamine use, which have all been associated with symptoms of psychosis. What all this suggests is that, rather than a biological explanation for excess dopamine, other factors, especially the influence of neuroleptic medications, could cause the number of dopamine synapses to increase. Therefore, as the person continues to take these medications for years, the effect will diminish. In an attempt to manage the presenting psychotic symptoms, the individual will be prescribed heavy doses or different antipsychotic medications. As a result, the person will have more intense psychotic symptoms and episodes, which will land him or her in the hospital for longer periods of time because of impairment in independent living functioning, causing them to be unable to live in the community.

Function of Cortisol

As stated, cortisol is produced in the adrenal glands in response to stressors. This stress hormone breaks down lipids and proteins to make immediate energy available to muscles, thereby managing stress by fight or flight (Cozolino, 2010). The adrenal gland cannot distinguish between threatening stress, such as a tornado, or enjoyable stress, such as receiving an award. In both kinds of stressful situations, adrenaline and cortisol are released. Even with extreme excitation, the release of these substances interferes with immune functioning, higher brain processing, and decision-making. As cortisol is released, so is dopamine released. These chemical reactions have been observed as quickly as within minutes or delayed by hours in studies that generate perceived stressful situations including loud noises, restraint, real or imagined separation from loved ones, public speaking, or watching horror movies. Levels of glucocorticoid secretions are obtainable through cerebrospinal fluid (CSF), urine, plasma, and saliva. Overstimulation of cortisol results in an atrophy of the hippocampus, impairing explicit memory (van Eck, Berkhof, Nicolson, & Sulon, 1996). Overstimulation of cortisol and dopamine can cause a chronic over or under response of the HPA axis, (termed HPA dysregulation) causing hyperautonomic arousal or needing excessive stimulus to feel a basic amount of pleasure, as in addictions to behaviors (sex, shopping, video games, X games, etc.) (Read, Perry, Moskowitz, and Connolly, 2001).

Glutamate Versus Dopamine

Glutamate is another neurotransmitter shown to play a role in the brains of people diagnosed with schizophrenia. Glutamate neurons are essential in connecting the pathways that include the hippocampus, prefrontal cortex, and thalamus, which are all areas of the brain identified as dissimilar in the brains of people with schizophrenia, showing reduced glutamate activity. Negative psychotic symptoms (i.e., social withdrawal and reduced emotional expression) and cognitive impairment (i.e., paranoia) are the manifestations of reduced glutamate activity. Atypical antipsychotic medications that indirectly improve N-methyl-D-aspartate (NMDA) receptor functioning result in recuperation of negative psychotic symptoms (Leo & Regno, 2000). Here are the most commonly prescribed atypical antipsychotic medications on the US market today: haloperidol, clozapine, risperidone, olanzapine, quetiapine, and clozapine, which carries a black box warning because of the potential fatal risk of agranulocytosis, or lowered white blood cell count (Alvir, Lieberman, Safferman, Schwimmer, & Schaaf, 1993). This hypoglutamate theory is noteworthy and consistent with the hyperdopamine theory of explaining schizophrenia. The thought is that the decrease of one neurotransmitter triggers an increase in the other and vice versa (Kantrowitz & Javitt, 2010). This causal relationship explains the delicate balance of why stimulant medications that improve the symptoms of the negative psychotic symptoms would potentially induce positive psychotic symptoms in a brain with schizophrenia. The use of antipsychotic medications causes a decrease in dopamine and positive psychotic symptoms and an increase in negative psychotic symptoms.

Basal Ganglia

Location and Function

The basal ganglia sits deep in the midbrain, near the thalamus, and its parts are located both on left- and right-brain hemispheres. The parts that make up this circuit are the striatum, globus pallidum, thalamus, substantia nigra, and subthalamic nucleus. The main functions of the basal ganglia have to do with *behavior switching*, or determining which behaviors to initiate or repress at the right time. Current research findings suggest much more complicated and pervasive impacts on automatic behaviors of sequencing, attention capacity, filtering, and implicit learning and memory (Raunch & Savage, 1997).

Within the direct and indirect pathway circuitry, excitatory and inhibitory neurotransmitters are released (specifically dopamine, gamma-amino-butyric acid [GABA], acetylcholine, and glutamate), resulting in hyperkinetic (physically overactive) and hypokinetic (physically lethargic) reactions. In other words, given the neurotransmitter release and subsequent chemical reaction, voluntary movements are inhibited, causing decreased ability to move (lethargy), or involuntary movements are uninhibited, causing an exacerbation of movement (akathisia, tremors, or as severe as Huntington's disease). To further elaborate, people who have been diagnosed with Parkinson's disease have deteriorating voluntary movement and may have difficulty swallowing and talking. Alternatively, people who have symptoms of Huntington's disease cannot stop moving.

Impairment

How does neurobiology help explain why so many people with psychotic disorders use and misuse street drugs? We can look to the basal ganglia circuitry, specifically dopaminergic pathways, for some of the biological explanation to this question, as it has an important role in reward and movement behavior.

Rewards serve as positive reinforcements, causing a person to want to perform a certain behavior repeatedly. The release of dopamine causes an increased capacity for behaviors to be repeated. The frontal cortex plays an important role in discriminatory decisions, such as whether a behavior is in a person's best interest. As previously stated, there is decreased activity in the frontal cortex of schizophrenic brains (Andreasen et al., 1997). This decrease helps us understand why a person with a psychotic disorder might crave and use drugs continuously despite the almost certain negative consequences, such as increased positive symptoms of psychosis or impulsive self- or other-destructive behaviors that result in police involvement or, possibly, eviction from housing.

Manifestation Among Those With Psychotic Disorders

Among people with schizophrenia, the volume of the basal ganglia has been shown to be larger and have varied shapes (Mamah, Wang, de Erausquin, Gado, & Csernansky, 2007). When the basal ganglia are impaired, a number of brain activities become dysfunctional. The following is a list of the ways that basal ganglia impairment manifests:

- Distortions of perceptions of sound, brightness of color, and size of objects, so sensations seem overwhelming.
- Inability to filter out background noises that others can ignore (distracted and overwhelmed).
  Example: Henry and his case manager met in an interview room at the community mental health center. Henry was distracted by the sound of the air conditioning unit and felt that it was squeaking so loud, like "sneakers on a basketball court," although it was barely noticeable to others. They had to change rooms for the conversation to continue.
- Reduced focus on important items (paying rent or traffic); increased focus on irrelevant items (the buzz coming from a fluorescent light bulb).
  Example: Eva was taking classes at a community college. She was convinced that the lighting in the classroom was purposefully set to a hue that made her sleepy and unable to pay attention in math class. Ultimately, Eva failed the class.
- Limited ability to relax and rest; being physiologically and emotionally aroused much of the time; mind is racing but accomplishing nothing.
  Example: Lucas, 19, presented to the mental health center during his first psychotic break. He had periods of stability and then decompensation. He was not able to sit still in individual or group-therapy sessions. He would often lose track of his thoughts and would respond to the sounds and voices he heard. He would frequently get up and leave the room and come back in. His psychotic episodes became more regular and bizarre.
- Desperate attempts to reduce anxiety, arousal, and stimulation; attempts are ineffective, bizarre, and create additional problems (a makeshift hat from a pizza box).
  Example: Gavin experiences extreme social anxiety, and when he does go out into public, he wears his hoodie up (in warm weather), sunglasses, and headphones. Gavin is fearful of the judgments of others, but, inadvertently, he calls attention to himself because of the way he dresses, which just feeds into his anxiety.

Gray Matter

Function

Gray matter contains most of the brain's neuronal cell bodies. The gray matter includes regions of the brain involved in muscle control, sensory perception such as seeing and hearing, memory, emotions, speech, decision-making, and self-control.

Impairment

Gray matter can become impaired as a result of smoking (Almeida et al., 2011), viral infection/influenza during pregnancy (Allen, 1998; Barr, Mednick, & Munk-Jorgensen, 1990; Brown et al., 2004; Castrogiovanni, 1998; Limosin, Rouillon, Payan, Cohen, & Strub, 2004; Mednick, 1988; Murray, Jones, O'Callaghan, Takei, & Sham, 1992; Selten, 1998; Short et al., 2010), and the overwhelming stress of childhood maltreatment (De Beli et al., 1999).

Manifestation Among People With Psychotic Disorders

The gray matter brain functions seem to relate precisely to how the person with schizophrenia manifests impairment: sensory perception such as seeing and hearing things that are not there, memory loss, overwhelming emotions, speech disturbances, decision-making impairment, and lack of self-control/impulsiveness. Additionally, people who have been diagnosed with schizophrenia have enormously high rates of both smoking cigarettes and childhood maltreatment. Researchers have significantly documented reduced gray matter among people who have been diagnosed with schizophrenia (Agartz, Andersson, & Skare, 2001; Job, Whalley, Johnstone, & Lawrie 2005).

White Matter

Function

White matter is made up of the bundles of nerve cells that connect the gray matter areas. Each nerve cell is covered with myelin sheath, an electric insulator that increases the speed of nerve signal communication.

Impairment

There are a number of ways that white matter can become impaired, including multiple sclerosis, inflammation, Alzheimer's disease, alcohol abuse, and age (Marner, Nyengaard, Tang, & Pakkenberg, 2003; Monning, Tonigan, Yeo, & McCrady, 2013). Demyelination, or a breakdown of the white matter around the nerve cells, can occur because of genetics, infectious diseases, autoimmune reactions, smoking, stress, and chemical agents, such as insecticides, weed killers, and neuroleptic medications. The reduction of communication can cause reduced sensation, cognition, movement, and more, depending on the area of the brain that is affected. White matter can re-generate, whereas gray matter cannot.

Manifestation Among Those With Psychotic Disorders

Among schizophrenic brains, there are some white matter differences (Lim et al., 1999). Only certain parts of the brain, specifically the prefrontal cortex, show decreased volume. This decrease may be a result of acute head injuries (Wolf et al., 2001; Arundine et al., 2004). However, the most significant white matter difference in schizophrenic brains lies within the decreased *anisotropy*, or the value of electrical transmission. In other words, the white matter volume is similar to general brains, but schizophrenic brains significantly lack integrity and show lower rates of electrical transmission.

Ways to Improve White Matter

White matter naturally regenerates until midlife and then slowly degenerates with age. The myelination, or the growth of white matter around nerve cells, process is improved with ongoing breast milk and whole milk between the ages of 1 and 2. Healthy lifestyle choices including eating nutritious foods, exercising to maintain healthy weight and increase blood flow to the brain, learning a new skill, and interacting socially.

Frontal and Prefrontal Lobe

Function

The frontal lobe of the brain is considered the *home* of the personality, as it dictates many aspects of an individual's unique functioning. These functions include motor function (including facial expression, hands, fingers), problem-solving, spontaneity, short-term memory, language comprehension, and motor expression, initiation (drive for personal goals), judgment, impulse control, and moderating social and sexual behaviors (Yang & Raine, 2009).

Impairment

The frontal lobe is considered to be the most vulnerable because of its frontal un-protected location. Traumatic brain injuries are the result of open or closed injuries. Open injuries are when the skull is punctured, such as gunshot wound, falls, and construction accidents. Closed wounds occur when the brain collides with the skull and brain tissue is damaged or breaks down integrity and can occur from child abuse, war combat, domestic violence, contact sports, and automobile accidents. Heavy alcohol use and age results in frontal lobe shrinkage (Kubota et al., 2001).

Dysfunction Manifestation

Among the brains of people who have been diagnosed with schizophrenia, the frontal cortex reveals reduced blood flow, which manifests the following behavioral manifestations (Brown & Thompson, 2010):

- Depressive affect;
- Negative psychotic symptoms, such as avolition (lack of drive to pursue personal goals);
- Memory and comprehension of complex and abstract information processing;
- Reduced capacity to plan, especially with a sequence of steps to achieve a goal;
- Limited problem-solving ability;
- Difficulty understanding the consequences of behavior, repeating the same mistakes;
- Difficulty seeing situations from other points of view;
- Limited ability to recognize social cues and expectations.

Temporal Lobe

Function

The temporal lobe is located in the bottom middle cortex, just behind the temples. Its primary function is to process auditory, visual, language recognition, and memory formation. The temporal lobe includes the hippocampus and accesses the amygdala.

Impairment

There are a variety of ways the temporal lobe can become impaired, causing temporal lobe epilepsy, including stroke, infection (meningitis or encephalitis), brain injury, or brain tumor (Cirino & Willcutt, 2017; Brown & Thompson, 2010). Individuals who display these kinds of symptoms can easily be misdiagnosed with schizophrenia because hallucinations (especially auditory) and delusions are a common result.

Dysfunction

- Hallucinations or false perceptions (auditory, visual, olfactory, tactile)
- Delusions (persecutory, thoughts taken from mind, situations having special meaning (radio speaking to the person)
- Actions are based on hallucinations and/or delusions

Manifestation Among People Who Experience Psychosis

Among the brains of people diagnosed with schizophrenia, the gray matter is reduced in the temporal lobe (Shenton, et al, 1992). Additionally, the amount of reduction of gray matter is congruent with the degree of thought disorder.

Some MRI studies have shown that the primary auditory cortex, which is within the temporal lobe, is active in those who hear voices (Dierks, Linden, Jandl, Formisano, Goebel, Lanfermann, & Singer, 1999). The primary auditory cortex is likely being activated by some other mechanism in a way that gives the sensation of hearing voices, although they are internally generated inside the brain. *Real sounds* must come in through the auditory nerve, but eventually the information reaches the primary auditory cortex and is likely processed in a similar way. It is no wonder people experience voices as being real because they, in fact, are real and generated by their brains.

HOW DOES NEUROSCIENCE IMPACT NONMEDICAL MENTAL HEALTH TREATMENT DELIVERY?
New Mental Phenomena: Traumagenic Development

Indeed, the advances of medical technology have afforded us the benefits of documentable trends in brain alterations among people who have psychotic experiences, and specifically a diagnosis of schizophrenia. These alterations include the integrity and volume of both brain structure and functioning. There is near consensus of genetic explanations for these brain differences, despite conclusive and repeatable empirical studies whose findings show otherwise. It is indeed observed that psychotic disorders *run in families*, so the erroneous and overgeneralized conclusion is that the cause of schizophrenia must be genetic. The studies that are most commonly cited to support the genetic etiological argument include topics such as family genetics (twin studies), prenatal (during pregnancy), and postnatal (during birth) impacts. Then, etiological studies focus on recent (within the last month) environmental stressors that contribute to psychotic decompensation. In this lineage, here is a glaring gap. Only until recently (since the late 1990s) have there been scientific conversations and studies that look at the significance of early and severe child maltreatment (CSA and CPA) and their impact on brain development and altered functioning. Researchers have paired these brain structure changes to people who are diagnosed with PTSD, but only recently to people who experience positive and negative psychotic symptoms (Grillon, Southwick, & Charney, 1996).

If all the findings presented in this chapter are empirically supported and repeatable, at what point do we recategorize schizophrenia as a brain disorder and treat it as such without all the associated stigma? What about those people who experience the positive psychotic symptoms of hallucinations and delusions and have little to no evidence of any of the above findings? Are they accurately diagnosed with schizophrenia or shall we keep exploring to pursue a diagnosis that more accurately identifies the symptoms and pinpoints the origin of the symptoms? Read, Perry, Moskowitz, and Connolly (2001) suggest a new diagnostic category termed *posttraumatic dissociative psychosis*.

Once a person has inherited the genetic vulnerability of developing a psychotic disorder, as described in the twin studies, he or she is not guaranteed a manifestation of the disorder. Why is this variability the case? Think of fruit seeds and plant life. Not every seed grows into a thriving, fruit-producing tree. So, what makes the seed grow? The answer includes the optimal amount of water, sunlight, nutrients, and oxygen, otherwise referred to as environment. Yet, everyone knows that a mistreated puppy will grow up to be a wounded and often an aggressive and defensive animal to ensure its own protection. Most people have a basic understanding of *object relations*; the wounded animal has internalized and repeats hurtful and harsh *object introjects*. As previously mentioned, a significantly high number of people, but not all, who develop psychotic disorders have experiences of early childhood severe trauma. Is it the traumatic experiences that impact the brain and subjective meaning system (mind), manifesting the same abuse content in hallucinations and delusions?

Because most people logically accept these common explanations of environmental impacts (as given in the examples of fruit trees and puppies), what is strange is that people will not afford these same environmental explanations to mental illness in people? We go back to Fromm-Reichmann's term *defensive countertransference*. The stories that our clients tell about their early experiences of abuse by the people who should have been their protectors may just be too much for our minds to bear. Mental health clinicians often do not even ask these essential questions about early traumatic experiences during the initial assessment.

According to a purely biological model of explaining SMI and psychosis, the following myth is still prevalent: *Talking to seriously disturbed people about their feelings and experiences is counterproductive* and should be avoided (Hornstein, 2009). People have subjective perceptions that are based on the quality of their environment, and these perceptions come with strong emotional reactions. Even including the neurobiological advances that are currently available, this does not mean that feelings are gibberish and cannot be made sense of. Every person makes conclusions about what is happening to him or her within an environment. People with psychotic disorders are hardly exceptions.

Appropriate and conscious administration of psychotropic medications often works quickly in quieting the most distressing psychotic experiences. Appropriate and conscious dosage refers to using no more than an effective dose, including zero to very low dosages. In addition to psychotropic medications, individuals should also be offered a full range of recovery services. Additionally, psychotropic medications should not be used to punish or quiet people whom others fear, including men, people of color, individuals from lower socioeconomic levels, and people who are physically large.

A great deal of scientific enthusiastic interest and exploration of the early psychotic or prodromal episodes has occurred in recent years. One significant belief is that with every psychotic episode, a neurodegenerative process occurs. Given this belief, there is a thrust to explore early and effective intervention to improve long-term functioning and prognosis. Additionally, as one can guess, almost all early episode studies involve the use and efficacy of psychotropic medications, and an earnest research consumer would investigate funding sources (i.e., pharmaceutical companies) of these studies. The practice of instantaneous psychotropic medication prescription as an intervention for early episodes of psychosis is continuous, at the least, from the philosophical argument involving the unethical practice of withholding effective treatment or administering a placebo (Rothman & Michels, 1994; Wyatt, 1997). However, with so few high-quality scientific nonmedication early episode interventions being conducted, supported, and published, we are again in a similar situation as before (flash back to the mutually benefiting relationship between the APA and Big Pharma) of overvaluing psychotropic medications over other recovery methods and being saturated and socialized with an abundance of pharmaceutical propaganda, making the use of other recovery methods scarce, unfamiliar, insecure, and *alternative*. While appropriate and conscious administration of psychotropic medications may show efficacy in early psychotic episodes, we must remain open to long-term findings and valuing additional recovery methods.

FINAL THOUGHTS

Understanding the workings of the brain and how impairment to a certain part facilitates or exacerbates symptoms of psychosis offers insight into why people living with these symptoms express certain behaviors. This knowledge allows for a different perspective on the origin of psychosis beyond the static belief that an inherent, marginalizing dysfunction exists in people living with psychosis. Taken with the knowledge of how trauma and environmental factors attribute to the development of psychosis, we can start to see that there is no clear boundary between those who experience symptoms and those who do not. With this insight, we can recognize the genuine nature of psychosis as an impairment that can and should be approached with treatment in the same fashion as other physical impairments are approached.

Summary of Unit II

THIS UNIT PROVIDED a look into the lived experiences and possible biological and psychological origins of symptoms of psychosis. Rather than merely seeing a person as a representation of their mental illness, we can acknowledge that looking deeper into a person's past and indentifying the specific origin of his or her mental impairment allows for deeper understanding of this person in their environment and the types of treatment options available beyond the standard fare of institutionalization and psychotropic medications. The narratives provided throughout this unit help us embrace an inclusive perspective about what people with symptoms of psychosis have been and are going through. There are many options for how this inclusive perspective can be developed, and *Listening with Psychotic Ears* is at the foreground of beginning this process.

Ethical and Professional Obligations Impact Macro, Mezzo, and Micro Levels of Treatment Delivery

8

Consumer/Psychiatric Survivor/Ex-Patient (C/S/X) Movement

AS FAR BACK as history is documented, individuals who have suffered the iatrogenic trauma of mental health treatment have come forward and spoken about their treatment experiences in an attempt to advocate for themselves and others who feel trapped in the mental health treatment system. This chapter explores the needs and accomplishments of this movement, the status and goals of the movement in contemporary times, and the needs of the future.

HISTORICAL NEEDS AND PROMINENT INDIVIDUALS AND GROUPS

Over the years, many individuals in mental health treatment facilities suffered abuses (including electroconvulsive treatment [ECT], lobotomy, physical restraints, isolation, forced medication, denial of human and civil rights, powerlessness, and oppression) and severe neglect. These individuals began to organize outside the hospitals and talked about their shared experiences. As we explored in Chapter 5, "Historically Ethical and Effective Mental Health Approaches for Healing the Distress of Psychotic Experiences," Clifford Beers was just one prominent example of the psychiatric patient turned activist.

There are countless individuals who interfaced with the mental health treatment system and wrote an autobiography detailing the iatrogenic abuses they experienced while in treatment. One list of these many bibliographies of first-person narratives can be found at the ISPS (The International Society for Psychological and Social Approaches to Psychosis) website (see Appendix B). Many peer-run organizations include these narratives on their website, such as the National Empowerment Center (Appendix B). These autobiographies are invaluable as they document the very real and unimaginable experiences faced by individuals who found themselves in the mental health treatment system.

1960S–1970S

During the 1960s and 1970s, the civil rights movement was organizing and benefiting several underrepresented groups, such as African Americans, women, and LGBT individuals. Psychiatric survivor groups were also inspired. They partnered with pioneering groups and took on their philosophies and strategies, and they also began to enjoy widespread population increase, organization, and political momentum.

In the early days, there was so much work to be done to turn the *mental health treatment system ship* to a different, more humane, ethical, and effective course. Activist efforts, mostly consisting of antipsychiatry principles, were aggressive and militant, starting with their confrontational names, such as Network Against Psychiatric Assault (established in 1970 in Portland, Oregon), Insane Liberation Front, and Mental Patient Liberation Front (founded by Howie the Harp in 1971 in New York). Their choice in names was intended to cast off the passive stereotype of mental patients and communicate a fight against the oppression and abuse of the mental health treatment system (Reaume, 2002; 2008). Individually, they referred to themselves as *psychiatric inmates* to reflect the feeling of pervasive powerlessness in a system by no fault of their own. Given the history of severe abuses by individuals, groups, and institutions who proposed to help, these groups insisted on maintaining their independence and refused external funding, fearing the invisible and delayed obligations that may be associated with funding sources.

Hundreds who represented thousands met at campgrounds and university campuses, completely unfunded by corporate sources. They identified and defined their goals, values, and positions (philosophical and political) on the most mainstream and egregious mental health treatment practices. Beginning with small and local groups on the east and west coasts, these groups began to communicate and organize with each other, forming the Annual Conference on Human Rights and Against Psychiatric Oppression. Their communication validated and fought against the systematic iatrogenic trauma of mental health treatment. They provided mutual support and consciousness-raising groups. The members came together and shared their respective experiences of treatment or witnessed atrocities in treatment facilities. Through a realization of the pervasiveness of these behaviors, they helped each other understand how to advocate and be part of the movement that would be taken to lawmakers to create a change in policies related to mental health treatment.

Principles

Specifically, these psychiatric survivor groups advocated the following principles:

- They stood against any *forced* treatment.
- They stood against any *inhumane* treatment, including psychotropic medications that (1) leave a person incapacitated and (2) have long-term and permanent impact on the body, ECT, social seclusion, and physical restraints.
- They stood against *sanism*, which is the pervasive prejudice and discrimination against individuals who live with symptoms of mental illness or are labeled as such. Stigma and discrimination had become strong barriers to resources that significantly impact quality of life, such as safe and affordable housing, employment, social friendship and helping networks, and much more.
- They stood against the medical model, which maintains that the professional is the expert and will assess, diagnose, and prescribe treatments for the problems they have identified and prioritized. Methods of treatments were decided on by mental health professionals and were focused on solely stopping symptoms with psychotropic medication. In the medical model, the patient is in a submissive power position and must comply with all prescribed treatments. Since psychiatry is the branch of medicine that most interacts with recipients of mental health treatment, much of the movement's efforts were toward the field of psychiatry, and was appropriately termed *antipsychiatry*.
- They advocated for collaboration in their own assessments, including identification and prioritization of the issues that would be the focus of treatments.
- They advocated for choices in mental health treatment, including talking, holistic methods (exercise, creative expression, employment), peer support, and conscious use of psychotropic medication (including identifying medications with the most efficiency and fewest side effects, the fewest medications, and using the lowest dosage of medications.)
- They advocated for peer involvement in *every* aspect of the mental health system, including policies, treatment implementation, boards of directors (51% of any governing and decision-making body), and more. (Mead, 2003).

Beginning in 1972, a newsletter called *Madness Network News (MNN)* was written and published as a means for communication among psychiatric survivors. Beginning in the San Francisco area, *MNN* quickly evolved into a quarterly newspaper with a national and international readership. *Madness Network News* became the unapologetic voice for factual reporting and personal expression (art and stories), advocating for "full dignity, self-expression, and civil rights of people diagnosed and labeled as mentally ill" (to learn more about the *MNN* newsletter, go to the website listed in Appendix B). This historical source of communication was and still is invaluable among those who find themselves oppressed by the label *mentally ill*. As the movement began to realize its goals and policy changes were addressing the major principles of the movement, the group did not pursue other contemporary issues related to mental health treatment and, thus, the *MNN* publication ceased in 1986. The *Madness Network News Reader* was compiled by Sherry Hirsch (1974), one of the original *MNN* editors, and is currently available from booksellers. Individual volumes are available online.

Another ex-patient/antipsychiatry newsletter was *Phoenix Rising*, published in Canada between the 1970s and 1990s. The newsletter was founded by Carla McCague and Don Weitz, former mental patients, and written by individuals who referred to themselves as ex-*inmates* and no longer as ex-*patients*.

Judi Chamberlain was one of the most renowned activists for the psychiatric survivor movement. An ex-mental patient, Chamberlain was a cofounder of the Mental Patients Liberation Front. Chamberlain was an accomplished author, publicizing many articles and books. In 1978, Chamberlain published her most influential book, *On Our Own: Patient Controlled Alternatives to the Mental Health System* (Chamberlain, 1978). In this book, she candidly criticizes the mental health treatment system, asserting that the prejudice, discrimination, and oppression that systematically pervades the profession not only is not helpful but also robs individuals of their independence and demoralizes people in a system whose intentions are to help with recovery. Additionally, she asserts that the patients themselves believe these crushing messages. She asserts that individuals with mental illnesses need help, but the help that is offered is very different from the kind of help individuals with mental illnesses want and need. Chamberlain is a self-reported noncompliant patient. She stated, "Well, I've been a good patient, and I've been a bad patient, and believe me, being a good patient helps to get you out of the hospital, but being a bad patient helps to get you back to real life" (Chamberlain, 2013, para. 1). (To read more from this book, see the link in Appendix B.)

The psychiatric survivor movement targeted three groups that were most responsible for forcing and coercing individuals into treatments that were the most harmful. These groups were the American Psychological Association (APA), the National Alliance on Mental Illness (NAMI), and the Office of the Surgeon General of the

United States. Supporter and psychiatrist Loren Mosher said, "In contrast to every other medical specialty, psychiatry is very much about force, coercion, and control. There is no other specialty of medicine that can force you to take a treatment that you refuse" (Meldrum, 2003).

Wanting to draw attention to the power of the psychiatrist over vulnerable patients, psychiatric survivor members organized and demonstrated outside APA conventions. And NAMI was targeted because of their overarching evangelizing for families to legally remove all legal rights of their mentally ill family members, including financial and healthcare decisions. Additionally, NAMI had been known to collaborate with pharmaceutical companies in their biologically based etiological explanations of mental illness and forcing psychotropic medications. The US surgeon general was targeted, as this department is responsible for all medical specialties, under which the field of psychiatry is situated.

1980s

The 1980s brought transition in the psychiatric survivor community. The passionate organizing efforts and militant demonstrations and protests resulted in great changes. The paradigm was shifting from a mental health treatment world that would systematically abuse its imprisoned customers to a world that was beginning to listen, make and revise laws, and be open to additional necessary mental health treatment reform that would protect and benefit its consumers. The goals and actions of the movement were evolving. Many of the aging militant activists were left behind, as their trauma made them unwilling and unable to turn the page. The remaining activists would now reenter and be invited into the mental health treatment system that had once injured them, as both consumers and providers. The federal government, community support program, and NIMH provided significant funding and support to construct drop-in centers (realizing a total of 13) and numerous self-help groups that were facilitated by and for individuals with mental health concerns. Even the terminology has evolved from psychiatric survivor and ex-patient to other terms. There are a variety of terms that refer to the unique and specific population of individuals who live with symptoms of severe mental illness (SMI). Here, the more common terms are identified, and their unique differences are described.

Accurate and Respectful Nomenclature

Psychiatric survivor. Psychiatric survivor is a self-identified term for individuals who identify as having experienced any range of iatrogenic trauma as a result of human rights violations at the hands of the mental health profession, specifically the field of psychiatry. These traumatic experiences range from not being valued enough to be listened to, being spoken down to, and having food and toileting rationed, to the coerced or forced use of psychotropic medication, physical restraints, solitary confinement, ECT, lobotomies, and even death. Individuals who self-identify as psychiatric survivors are making a statement that they have survived the personal and social oppression and marginalization that results from being labeled a mental patient. This can be seen as a self-empowerment term.

Some reject the term "psychiatric survivor," asserting that it suggests that a person has faced a life-threatening situation and escaped. Some suggest that because of the lingering damaging impact of iatrogenic trauma from the mental health treatment experience, many have not escaped or survived. Others say that the term "survivor" is still a reaction to oppression and some prefer a more neutral term.

Patient/ex-patient. "Patient" was used to designate a person who was sick and impaired and sought out professionals for purposes of treatment and healing. This term has generally lost favor, as its use has come to designate the disproportionate power between patient and professional. This term may still be used among practicing old school mental health professionals.

Client. Mental health clinicians commonly use "client" in an attempt to defer power that had been inherent in the patient/professional relationship. Yet, despite the illusion of a more equal position in the therapeutic relationship, the reality of us/them is still pervasive. Extremist recovery-oriented people continue to bring this insight and are still working to cause not only a language shift but also a shift in philosophy within the treatment setting.

Individuals. California state psychiatric hospital staff use "individuals" to offset the oppressive relational hierarchy between mental health recipients and professionals. However, the use of this word is a forced requirement based on a lawsuit brought by patients toward the state of California, rather than an actual shift in beliefs or attitudes by the treatment staff; therefore, the philosophy has not changed toward a more respectful practice.

Members. "Member" commonly refers to individuals who belong to a clubhouse model of treatment. Here, individuals with mental illnesses participate in a supportive work framework, and their commitment, participation, and reward from the job is the treatment. There is often an egalitarian power spread among members and staff, and these roles are blurred.

Persons with lived mental health experiences. "Persons with lived experiences" is a more neutral phrase that simply communicates that the person possesses insider knowledge about the unique experiences of living with symptoms of mental illness. This phrase is outside the marginalized and disabled identity of what someone with mental illness is assumed to be and that of someone who has been victimized by the mental health treatment system.

Consumers. The word "consumer" (of mental health treatment) was offered by mental health professionals in their attempt to shift labeling from the oppressed mental patient to individuals who receive mental health services. Some people preferred this term for a short time in an attempt to regain power from mental health professionals, just as one would be a valued customer of a retail store, recognizing that customers have choices and keep the store alive. This term was so embraced by some, that the National Mental Health Consumers' Association, a conservative group that represented individuals who had interfaced with the mental health treatment system, was formed in 1985.

The term "consumer" has lost favor and has been rejected by people with lived experiences, as the term implies only the taking action and no individual prefers to be seen solely as a self-absorbed taker. Additionally, the term is in the same vein as "capitalism," and this term is associated with the mutual financial benefits enjoyed by pharmaceutical companies and psychiatry, which maintains the power differential over individuals who find themselves in the mental health treatment system.

Still, some individuals completely reject the idea of mental illness and all categorizing labels.

Because of the wide diversity of individual experiences of this group, there has not been a democratization of the mass self-identify. There are times when a general term is needed, such as in this book, for instance, when referring to the group of people with lived experiences. Furthermore, depending on the setting in which people with lived experiences congregate for a shared purpose, more distinctive identities, such as artists, workers, students, or residents of a treatment facility, are used that reflect this wide diversity within this population. Overall, when choosing a term, the subtle implications should be considered. "This is a very diverse group of people with vastly different views of terminology" (Reaume, 2008, p.?? or 2002).

Ask the person to whom you are talking which terms he or she prefers. This may invite a conversation of the pros and cons of each term. If you have to make a guess, consider which is most respectful to the individual and the general population.

In 1986, the National Mental Health Consumer's Self-Help Clearinghouse (NMHCSC) was constructed through the Mental Health Association of Southeastern Pennsylvania. The Clearinghouse is peer managed and staffed. Their goals are directed at peer information and empowerment through their website (see Appendix B for link), directory of peer-driven services, electronic and printed publications, training packages, and consultation. The Clearinghouse works with peers to organize and establish high-quality peer-run services, as well as organizations that are interested in planning for and evaluating ethical and effective recovery services. Additionally, the NMHCSC maintains an extensive library on topics that are essential to the C/S/X community.

The National Empowerment Center (NEC) is a peer-run organization that advocates for recovery-based treatment for symptoms of mental illness. The organization's website is full of treatment and advocacy information for those who live with symptoms of mental illness. The NEC's founder, Daniel Fisher, now a board-certified psychiatrist, once experienced hallucinations and delusions, for which he was psychiatrically hospitalized three times, and diagnosed with schizophrenia. The activist Judi Chamberlain was also an NEC employee.

Fisher (2006) and the NEC has put forth a list, compiled from a qualitative study, of characteristics that contribute to one's own recovery.

- Trusting oneself and others;
- Valuing self-determination;
- Believing that one will recover and having hope;
- Believing in the person's full potential;
- Connecting at a human, deeply emotional level;
- Appreciating that people are always making meaning;
- Having a voice of one's own;
- Validating all feelings and thoughts;
- Following meaningful dreams;
- Relating with dignity and respect;
- Healing from emotional distress;
- Transformation from severe emotional distress;
- Recovery from mental illness.

Additionally, Fisher's (2006) research study identified a list of dichotomous characteristics that distinguish those in illness and those who are in recovery.

- Dependent versus self-determining;
- Mental health system support versus network of friends support;
- Identify solely as consumer or mental patient versus identify as worker, parent, student or other role;
- Medication essential versus one tool that may be chosen;

- Strong emotions treated by professionals as symptoms versus worked through and communicated with peers;
- Weak sense of self, defined by authority and little future direction, versus strong self, defined from within and peers and a strong sense of purpose and future.

In 1985, the first Alternatives conference was held. This conference is organized by the NEC and aims to turn around the mental health system through peer advocacy at the macro, mezzo, and micro levels. This conference and its efforts are alive and well today. Videos of the conference can be viewed at the NEC's website.

As peer-run groups were beginning to be funded by the government and other self-oriented groups, Support Coalition International was formed and renamed Mind Freedom International in 1988. This was an independent and grassroots organization that was run by and for people who found themselves in the mental health treatment system. Mind Freedom International is still alive today. More information about Mind Freedom can be found at their website.

THE 1990S

On July 26, 1990, the American Disabilities Act (ADA) was signed by George H. W. Bush, with amended changes signed by George W. Bush on January 1, 2009. The ADA prohibits and protects from discrimination based on disabilities. Additionally, the ADA requires employers and public areas to provide reasonable accommodations to those with disabilities. Persons who live with mental illness were able to enjoy these legal protections and accommodations based on their disabilities.

In 1991, a group of network users and psychiatric survivors gathered in Mexico and formed the World Federation of Psychiatric Users (WFPU). In 1997, their name changed to the World Network of Users and Survivors of Psychiatry (WNUSP). The WNUSP, an international psychiatric user and survivor group, whose membership is managed by and represents psychiatric survivors worldwide, has goals that include promoting international human rights; developing psychiatric survivor networks, especially among those countries that have little to no representative networks; developing long-term funding; developing treatment knowledge beyond the medical model; and creating a user/survivor oral history library (accessible through the WNUSP website; see Appendix B).

In 2004, at the Second General Assembly held in Denmark, there were 150 participants and 50 countries represented. In 2007, the WNUSP was granted special consultive privileges with the United Nations (Mezzich, 2007).

THE 2000S
Metropolitan State Hospital Lawsuit

In 2002 (*U.S. vs. California*), patients of Metropolitan State Hospital (MSH) filed a lawsuit asserting that the hospital was in violation of meeting basic civil rights. Specifically, in this lawsuit, many care areas were noted as inadequate, neglectful, punitive, and abusive. Patients at MSH were not offered adequate, complete, and consistent social and psychiatric assessments and individual treatment based on their behavioral, psychological, and neurological symptoms. The assessment process and treatment goals failed to incorporate the individual's strengths, skills, and interests. Individuals were detained at a higher level of care than was warranted, without supporting evidence. Individuals did not receive preparation to transition to, or succeed in, a new sustainable living situation. Individuals were given inappropriate medication prescriptions and lacked side-effect monitoring. Individuals were not provided with adequate general medical interventions and care. Basic infection control protocols were not followed, putting individuals at risk. Individuals were not given adequate dental care. Individuals were not provided adequate nursing care and special care services including physical, occupational, and speech therapy or dietary services (especially aspiration-risk monitoring). Noted was excessive use and lack of monitoring of restraints, seclusion, and PRN ("as needed") medication. Noted was a lack of protection from harm, including patient on patient physical and sexual assault, staff assault, elopement, and self-harm. There were inadequate incident reporting, investigation, and tracking and trending practices. Noted were poor environmental conditions including inappropriate temperatures, eroding and unmonitored physical materials, and poor air quality including constant urine and fecal odors (for more about the lawsuit, see the link in Appendix B). This is just one of many civil lawsuits that have been filed to legally demand and enforce increased quality of conditions and care for people who are at the authoritarian mercy of mental health treatment. The combination of these formal lawsuits and psychiatric survivors intentionally and systematically telling their stories to the public set in motion mandatory transition to better mental health treatment conditions and the foundation of what we now know as the recovery model, presented later in this chapter.

Hunger Strike

In 2003, a well-experienced panel, representing psychiatric survivors, went on a hunger strike to draw the general public's attention to and protest the abusive, authoritarian, and harmful practices of psychiatrists whose clients perceive these practices as humiliating and ineffective. They then demonstrated in front of the

APA's Pasadena, California, office. The group demanded to be shown the scientific proof that schizophrenia was a biologically based disorder, implying that effective treatment would be, in kind, biologically based (i.e., psychotropic medicine). The APA did not (suggesting "could not"?) respond with scientific evidence but demanded that they disperse and cease contact with their staff. "These efforts got more attention than expected and less than what was deserved," said UCLA professor of social welfare in the School of Public Affairs, David Cohen, author of *Mad in America* and over 120 articles (Meldrum, 2003, video). The entire conversation was captured in a 38-minute documentary, *Where's the Evidence? A Challenge to Psychiatric Authority*, which can be viewed on Vimeo (see Appendix B for the link).

The tireless efforts of these groups and individuals speaking out about their experiences in the mental health treatment system have resulted in many significant changes in law/policy and practice in the mental health system.

PRESENT

Today, leaders in the peer recovery movement are active at every level of mental health treatment delivery, making changes that ensure treatment choices, efficacy, respect, and civil liberties. Employing individuals with lived experiences is now common practice among mental health treatment agencies to make revision suggestions and to keep these agencies and professionals honest in language, attitude, practice, and policies. However, mainstream mental health treatment system reform still has a long way to go.

In a 1986 report, noted in the newsletter *Phoenix Rising* (McKinnon, 1986), three contemporary C/S/X movement positions were identified: conservative, moderate, and radical.

- Conservative, represented by National Mental Health Consumers' Association
- Moderate, represented by the National Alliance of Mental Patients (National Association of Psychiatric Survivors)
- Radical, represented by the Network to Abolish Psychiatry

Many websites, books, and publications recount the personal narratives of individuals who continue to be traumatized by mental health treatment. Spending any length of time in a mainstream mental health treatment facility will uncover any number of mental health treatment practices that are still in need of reform.

Hearing Voices Network

The Hearing Voices Network was founded in 2010 by Patsy Hage, a *voice hearer*, and her psychiatrist, Dr. Marius Romme (http://www.hearingvoicesusa.org/about-us). Patsy's voices escalated, commanding her to hurt herself, and the psychiatrist continued to pressure her to believe they were only symptoms that should be stopped. Patsy begged Romme to consider his Christian beliefs, asking if he thought Jesus Christ, who also heard voices, was mentally ill. Romme reconsidered, and together, the quality of their conversations about Patsy's voices took a turn. They took their inquiry to a public talk show and had voice hearers call in to share about their personal experiences. Their discovery was that many people hear sounds and voices that are not distressing. Dr. Romme stated on the Hearing Voices Network, "Many voices can be unthreatening and even positive. It's wrong to turn this into a shameful problem that people either feel they have to deny or to take medication to suppress" (http://www.hearingvoicesusa.org/about-us, para. 2).

Between 1987 and 2010, there had been many efforts to organize groups of voice hearers all over the world. It was not until 2010 that the first Hearing Voices Network would convene in the United States, joining 26 other countries. Today, there are 54 official Hearing Voices Network groups in the United States. More information can be found at the Hearing Voices Network website (see Appendix B). Additionally, first-person narratives of voice-hearing experiences and recovery can be found on the website and on the website of a collaborative international organization, the International Hearing Voices Network (see Appendix B).

Full Recovery From Mental Illness

So, we ask, why is recovery from mental illness still so unthinkable today? The majority of individuals who experience SMI, especially psychotic disorders, are still told by their treating professionals that the illnesses with which they are diagnosed leave them impaired for life and a full recovery is not possible. In addition, they are advised to take psychotropic medications for the remainder of their lives. We are reminded of the long-term impairment that psychotropic medications have on the brain's capacity to optimally function. We are reminded of Fromm-Reichmann's spirit. It is not that individuals and illnesses are untreatable, it is that the professional is not offering an effective treatment (Fromm-Reichmann, 1960).

No one is rushing down to the community mental health center for assistance with early symptoms of mental illness. No one wants the prejudice, discrimination, oppression, and marginalization that always comes with the label of being a mental patient. Besides, even today, the mainstream mental health treatment practices are so far from what the National Empowerment Center asserts as effective in the recovery process. Without effective and humane treatments, people find themselves in bizarre and hopeless situations with very limited resources, resulting in layers of trauma and serious losses. Additionally, individuals who are in emotional distress for long periods of time often turn to substances or behaviors that change the way they feel. Continued misuse leads to physiological and psychological dependence and causes a lifestyle of demoralization, poor choices, and mental illness. It is these individuals who are being told, in mantra/drill format, that they are untreatable and incurable. This population is growing, so society believes this mantra, too. However, we are seeing a growing number of individuals and groups who access these recovery practices and are creating a self-determined life worth living, including stability, self-confidence, and productivity and pursuing and realizing life dreams. Plentiful stories of recovery from mental illness, and even psychotic disorders, can be accessed by any of the C/S/X Movement organization websites and their conferences.

FUTURE

Advocacy groups are seeing their goals become realities. These groups continue to assert their revised and rephrased goals. More individuals who live with symptoms of mental illness are invited to serve on panels of decision-making bodies, ensuring human rights and protections. Peers are evaluating mental health treatment programs and making reform suggestions. These individuals are being employed by private corporations and federal- and state-operated agencies.

Social and professional attitudes about mental illness and the possibility of recovery continue to be revised. More peer/survivor-run programs, employment, and educational opportunities are developed and maintained. In kind, the quality of life for people who live with symptoms of mental illnesses continually increases.

So, what does the future bring for people with lived mental illness experiences in the mental health treatment system? People with lived experience need to discuss and agree on relevant, contemporary issues within mainstream mental health treatment. Advocacy groups, including representation by people with lived experience, need to have a voice at all levels of care and legislation so more effective policies and humane and effective mental health treatment will be prioritized to provide increased quality of life for people living with SMI.

Advocacy and Recovery Model Principles

Advocacy principles are similar to the militant ones that were shouted in the earlier days of the peer recovery movement. However, the language is asserted in what is expected, rather than that which is being fought against. The following contemporary principles are common assertions:

- Self-determination and choice
- Rights protections
- Stigma and discrimination reduction
- Services responding to multiple life needs of individuals, including friends, housing, jobs, and community
- Self-help/peer-support programs
- Involvement in every aspect of mental health system
- "Nothing About Us Without Us."

Finally, one overarching principle that is to be included in all recovery work is that recovery is a real possibility.

Peer-advocacy and support groups continue to use the most effective organization theories, philosophies, and strategies (Davidson et al., 2006). Goals continue to be relevant and productive. Goals continue to be evaluated and revised so that the most relevant and clear goals can be established. These organizations continue to access sustainable funding that honors their goals. Peer advocacy and support groups continue to systematically and pervasively reach out to more mental health practitioners, especially those in the mainstream mental health treatment system (Davidson, Chinman, Sells, & Rowe, 2006; Mead, 2003).

Systems that interface with mental health treatment, reimbursement, and policies continue to incorporate individuals and groups who advocate for people who experience symptoms of mental illness. These systems include Recovery and Wellness Centers in the mental health treatment system, and medical insurance companies including commercial, state (Medicaid), and federal (Medicare) insurance. Peer certification is a professional training standard that is now implemented in 34 states. Caps on job responsibilities and salaries for peers continue to be challenged.

FINAL THOUGHTS

There are growing numbers of opportunities for people with lived experiences thanks to the work of the advocacy groups and individuals discussed in this chapter. Training programs developed by peers for mental health practitioners are greatly needed. Publication of research and evaluation of programs and evidence-based interventions are needed. Peer-run respite care programs are being developed across the United States. Such facilities are promising in effectiveness and aim to prevent the financial burden and social disruption of psychiatric hospitalization. More investment in peer-run facilities is needed in the United States and across the world. "The scope of our achievements of the past is an indicator of the possibilities [for] our future," says accomplished activist, Sally Zinman, executive director of the California Association of Mental Health Peer Run Organizations (CAMHPRO). (Zinman, 2015, slide 35).

9

Existential and Spiritual Philosophy for Healing
the Distress of Psychosis

IN THIS CHAPTER, we explore the personal subjective workings of psychotic behaviors and symptoms and explore more accurate conclusions of common behaviors seen among people who experience psychosis. We also explore subjective perceptions of mental healthcare, social interactions, and the surrounding world.

EXISTENTIAL/SPIRITUAL MEANING SYSTEMS

The concept of existentialism, or spirituality, is concerned with one's personal subjective meaning system that transcends the daily grind of survival. This concept has to do with making meaning and the purpose of one's own existence and working toward one's own human potential and personal growth. Concepts that are common among existential/spiritual conversations include human interconnection; authenticity, genuineness, and congruency; awe and wonder; and self-actualization. Existentialism/spiritualism has to do with making personal sense of the vicissitudes of life, such as developmental milestones (development and maintenance of relationships, social competition, school, and employment), hardships, and tragedies (ending of relationships, illnesses, accidents, and death). Finally, existentialism centers on the subjective angst, as a person falls short of achieving his personal potential in these mentioned areas.

The age-old concept of free will is an existential/spiritual one. The concept of free will considers one's true freedom or personal power to make choices, in light of multifaceted influences, including social (macro, community, family), spiritual, conscious/unconscious, and neurobiological influences, to name a few. While there are many conscious and unconscious forces that contribute to one's ability to make choices in one's own best interest, existentialism views these choices as a personal responsibility, and one should be held accountable to the choice that is made.

Existentialism emerged following World War II. Some of the most significant existential philosophers of the nineteenth and twentieth centuries have included Albert Camus, Simone de Beauvoir, Martin Heidegger, Soren Kierkegaard, Rollo May, Friedrich Nietzsche, Jean Paul Sartre, and Paul Tillich. These philosophers wrote an abundance of papers and novels that were absorbed with existential themes. They enjoyed public and private philosophical debates. While most religions contain philosophical assertions about these existential/spiritual occurrences, it is noteworthy that one can be fully immersed in his or her existential/spiritual life and not be involved in any religion in the very least.

Victor Frankl was both a neurologist and psychiatrist. His survival experiences as an Auschwitz concentration camp inmate moved him to develop logotherapy, an existential theory and practice of identifying and nurturing personal meaning, which he argues is the most primitive human drive (Frankl, 1946). Frankl asserted that logotherapy could be effectively applied to people with severe mental illness (SMI), including schizophrenia. Frankl believed that the cause of schizophrenia was physiological in nature, with no available effective treatment. Given this, Frankl believed that people with schizophrenia should look beyond their symptoms and harsh self-observations. Additionally, Frankl's prescription for existential health was to engage in meaningful activity, which brings with it all the unconscious social influences (i.e., stigma) and personal accountability. Does this sound familiar? The recovery model's mantra is creating a self-determined life worth living, and Frankl might add, "to the very end." Victor Frankl touted the principles of the recovery model, well before its time.

Consider the existential and psychological explanation of the following example.

Jekyll and Hyde Sara

Sarah's first acute and intense psychotic episode occurred later than most, at the age of 42. She had three grown children. Sarah considers herself a family-oriented woman who prides herself on generously helping others. Sara was employed as an office manager at her church parish. In an attempt to keep up with her increasing work demands, Sarah began drinking more coffee, which initially provided energy and focus.

Within 2 months, Sarah began feeling increasingly irritable and having thoughts that her pastor was making sexual advances toward her. Soon, she began believing that her sister-in-law was talking negatively about her and turning her close-knit family against her. Thinking that her food was being poisoned, she ate as little as she could and would do so in secret and ritualistic ways (i.e., only eating food she had prepared, in private, and with plastic utensils).

Sarah began experiencing disturbing sounds and hearing the harsh voice of her deceased father. At one family gathering, Sarah, who was naturally a quiet and nurturing woman, physically assaulted her sister-in-law. She ran away from the family and survived on the street for 3 weeks. Seeing that this behavior was extremely out of Sarah's character, her family continued to look for her. Eventually, they were able to locate Sarah, who had been taken in by an elderly farming couple. Sarah's family brought her to the community hospital, where, after a full medical workup, she was first diagnosed with schizophrenia at the age of 42.

Any sharp clinician would question this late-onset schizophrenia diagnosis. Unlike most, Sarah reacted to the diagnosis with relief and fully accepted all the treatment, support, and resources she was offered.

Beyond an accurate diagnosis, let us consider the existential/spiritual perspective of Sarah's situation. Sarah had a rough life. Being the eldest girl of a sibship of 11, her childhood was overshadowed by daily caring for her younger brothers and sisters. She stopped going to school after the fifth grade. She reports that she does not remember much about her childhood. While she does not report sexual abuse, she has some prominent risk factors including not remembering much about her childhood, delusional themes of inappropriate sexual advances, excessive shyness, submissiveness, avoidance, and rage.

Sarah's embracing reaction to her late-onset diagnosis is curious. Unlike many people who receive a diagnosis of schizophrenia, and given her questionable circumstances, Sarah did not protest. The schizophrenia diagnosis was acceptable to her identity. The experiences of physically assaulting her sister-in-law and accusing her pastor of sexually inappropriate gestures were extremely incongruent with her identity. She would rather accept the diagnosis of schizophrenia than consider these thoughts and behaviors her own. Sarah was delighted to have the support that her mental health treatment team provided. She liked taking the antipsychotic medications because they made her feel somewhat emotionally numbed and calmed her rage.

Being a generous person who prioritizes the needs of others, Sarah struggled to incorporate this piece of her identity in making (existential/spiritual) sense of her schizophrenia diagnosis and mental health treatment. She was invited to a speaker training, where she would learn to do community speaking. Sarah learned to tell her story for the purposes of reducing mental health stigma and advertise the benefits of mental health treatment to newly diagnosed individuals. Sarah accepted her new schizophrenia diagnosis to explain her unthinkable behavior and congruently used it to help improve the lives of others with SMI.

For Sarah, accepting treatment and using her experiences to help others accept their diagnoses provided her with a sense of relief during her existential crisis. However, because the origins of the existential crises are not being accurately identified in her treatment, Sarah will likely not discover the underlying elements of her identity now that she is pacified by the comfort of the mental health treatment system and psychotropic medications.

WHEN ONE IS NOT UNDERSTOOD, WE SHOULD LISTEN DIFFERENTLY

In the acute phase of psychosis, people often speak in a manner that makes them seemingly indecipherable. We have a great deal of new empirical support about the workings of the psychotic brain through brain-imaging technology that can identify alternative brain functioning and behavior among people who experience symptoms of psychosis. We know that the communications of this person who has something to say often gets jumbled through the malfunctioning Broca's area, which makes him or her unable to get the thought out of the mouth. Just because we cannot understand, do we ignore the intentions of the person who is attempting to communicate? We should not be ignoring these communications, but all too often, this is what happens.

The following conversation occurred during group supervision where clinicians present individuals on their caseload and receive feedback and guidance about their work. The clinician gave the following details about Dave.

Goodbye Dave

Dave was a 37-year-old male who was new to this clinician, this visit being only the third visit together. The clinician stated that Dave was disheveled and rambling but present and asking for mental health help. When the group members asked about the content of Dave's rambling, the clinician had no idea. The clinician was asked further about what Dave was saying, as if to say, "Come on. Really. What was Dave trying to say?" The clinician really did not have any thoughts about what Dave was expressing. Upon further inquiry, the clinician said he was so frustrated with not being able to understand Dave that he ended the session 30 minutes early and dismissed Dave. He had not one single plan for Dave, not even another appointment. This quality of mental health treatment was egregiously neglectful. Unfortunately, this is not an uncommon interpersonal experience for people who

experience symptoms of psychosis. Because the person's communications are difficult to understand, they are often ignored or just medicated with no attempts to understand their expressions. With or without a formal diagnosis, the individual who
experiences hallucinations or delusions constructs his or her own meaning system
or personal explanations of the new experiences and has related concerns, opinions,
and reflections. Mental health professionals often overlook this meaning system; instead, the symptoms and strong emotionally laden communications are *managed*,
primarily with medication, which sometimes works for some people some of the
time and not for some all the time.

Everyone has a meaning system, including individuals who experience psychotic
symptoms. The skills of *Listening with Psychotic Ears* go beyond attempting to quiet
or stop the psychotic symptoms. Instead, when one is not accurately understood, we
listen differently, attempting to accurately understand and effectively deal with this
meaning system. This fresh perspective will reduce the manifestation and distress of
psychosis and other symptoms of mental illness, thus increasing quality of life.

Let us consider a different example where the person with psychotic expressions
is actually listened to, heard, and communicated with, resulting in a much better
outcome than what Dave experienced.

Breakfast With Aki

A student asked to talk with me in my office about her paper being late. When asked
what stressors or obstacles were occurring in her life, she explained that she was suddenly fraught with caring for her mother, a 50-year-old Asian woman who had been
in excellent health. For the last 2 weeks, her mother could not walk, was vomiting
on herself, and had to be fed, showered, and helped to the bathroom. All medical
tests were inconclusive, and no origin of the acute paralysis was detected. Prior to
this, the mother was hard working and was the middle manager of an international
corporate bank. In the course of our conversation, the student mentioned that her
mother's last day of work was the day before this conversation occurred. The company had laid off 10 middle managers. Given that all medical tests were conducted
and there was no scientific medical explanation for the acute paralysis, that last sentence captured the existential meaning of these paralyzing symptoms. The corporate
bank had laid off this woman, and her last day was yesterday. Her symptoms had
acutely worsened as the last day approached.

This hard-working woman, whom we will call Aki, upon losing her employment,
also lost her identity and life's purpose. Aki perceived this life event as an identity
injury, as though the company were firing her because she had not performed up
to expectations, which was not true. Aki's identity was grounded in her work. She

wondered what else she would do with herself. Where did she belong? What would become of her without working? Aki was experiencing an existential crisis.

Aki was not accustomed to reflecting about her emotions and sensations and had difficulty identifying and expressing what was on her mind. Given her Asian culture, she was more in the habit of holding back her expressions, exercising stoicism, and presenting a pleasant manner through even the most difficult times. This situation was more severe than she had ever experienced, and Aki had few adaptive coping skills with which to manage this situation.

Aki was experiencing classic symptoms of conversion disorder. She expressed herself with her body, and what her body was saying was, "I feel disabled. I need support in the most basic sense."

During the course of the conversation with the student, Aki's adult daughter, this meaning of Aki's behavior was interpreted. I asked the student if she could have a conversation with her mother to bring awareness to the meaning of these somatic expressions. At first, the daughter said, "No way! I do not have those kinds of conversations with my mother!" I pointed out that her mother likely does not know how to have those kinds of conversations and could really use her help to overcome this disabling crisis. The student thought about it and agreed that she would find a way to talk about it with her mother.

The next week, the student was waiting for me outside the classroom. She looked tired, and I worried what news she might have for me. "How is your mother?" I asked.

She told me that she thought about our conversation and had slept on it. The next morning, as she fed, toileted, and bathed her mother, she reflected on how much (or little as it were) energy she had in her to care for her paralyzed mother. As she put her mother in her clean clothes, she mustered up the courage to say the following to her mother.

Mom. Getting laid off by your employer was a real blow to you. You have always been a hard worker and enjoyed your work. Part of you must be thinking that you did something wrong to be laid off. The fact is that nine other highly paid middle management also got laid off, not just you. Not working has left you wondering a lot of things; how will you explain this to your friends; what you will do with yourself; what will become of you without work, how will you define your daily structure, what meaning will you have in your life? Mom. The fact is that you have a great employment history and, in time, will be able to find another job that you really enjoy. You have a lot of skills to offer, and you have a lot of people who tell you that you are a pleasure to work with. Mom! I am wondering if losing your job makes you feel disabled, and BEING paralyzed is the only way you know to express yourself. I love you, Mom, and will support you in whatever way you need.

Stunned at her eloquence and poignancy, I asked, "What did she say or do next?"

The student said, "She said nothing. I thought maybe the physical problem had more impact than any of us had ever expected and that she did not have the capacity to even understand what I was saying. I put her in her bed and went on to my afternoon class."

I felt so sad for this family. My mind began to race about getting Aki the most advanced comprehensive testing that was available. Then, suddenly, the student's face lit up like a Christmas tree!

She said,

"The next morning, I had to go to my internship very early. When I woke up, I smelled bacon frying and hot coffee. With eyes wide open and curious, I went into the kitchen and saw my mother busy at the stove. She said, "Good morning, Sweetheart!" I was so amazed that I could not say anything! My mother put my breakfast on a plate and poured coffee into my favorite cup. She said, "Hon, I heard what you said yesterday and thought about it. I am sorry that I put you through all this. You were right. I have a lot of work to do to get back to work and moreover, to find out who I really am." Dr. Dunn, I was so stunned that I could not even eat my breakfast! Tomorrow, she even has a job interview!

This is the power of truly hearing what a person is communicating and helping with whatever those needs are. Aki had heard and verified the interpretation of feeling existentially paralyzed by her job loss. She no longer had the need to communicate with her body what she was feeling because she was now deeply understood. She felt unconditional support from her daughter. Aki's symptoms resolved almost immediately, never to return.

WHAT IS A MEANING SYSTEM?

What is a meaning system, and how does it develop? A meaning system is the collective pattern of psychological and emotional attachments that develop as a result of lived experiences over a lifetime, the most robust and pervasive originating from early childhood experiences. The choice of food is a tangible and simple example of one's personal meaning system. Each of us can identify foods that we eat that provide emotional reactions, especially comfort, from our childhoods. For me, being from rural Indiana, on the border of Kentucky, I get excited and comforted by a pot of green beans boiling with bacon fat, or as my grandmother used to call it, *hog jowl*. Whenever I get a whiff of this aroma, immediately, I am affectively and cognitively transported to an innocent time when all the cousins were running around playing imaginary games, while the adults were in the next room, howling with laughter and playing cards. These associations are forever part of my personal meaning system.

Meaning systems include all kinds of associations within the range of lived experiences and the emotions that come with them, including joy, fear, loneliness, excitement, desperation, disappointment, and pride. The list is endless. Every human being has a personal meaning system that contains conscious, preconscious, and unconscious associations layered with affect. You can identify some of your personal meaning associations by telling a story from your past and identifying points in the story that contain strong feelings. Whenever you come across these situations, people, names, places, or things, your associated affect will impact your thoughts; thus, your decisions and behaviors will be impacted.

Visiting the Magic Portal to Receive My Special Powers

Juan is a 39-year-old man who presented to a mental health center after the recent passing of his mother from cancer. He is unemployed and lives alone in an apartment in a busy part of town. He previously lived with his mother and worked as her caretaker until her death. Juan never knew his father and does not have any siblings. Juan had been supporting himself from money that his mother left him after her death, but he ran out of money 2 months ago. Juan has been in a financial crisis for the past 10 months, but he recently received a letter stating that his appeal to receive Social Security benefits was approved and he will be receiving $15,000. He strongly had the urge "to go to Venezuela to visit a magic portal to receive his special powers."

Juan states, "I want to develop amnesia so that I can forget everything that I know. I want to think like other people." Juan believes that he was sent to Earth as a punishment and that "I am basically here to suffer." He also wants to understand why he enjoys walking around in bad neighborhoods after dark, likes to ride the bus, and is soothed by the voice that announces the stops.

Juan presents with auditory hallucinations that tell him that his life is not worth living and bad things are going to happen to him. He states that he hears multiple voices, which he believes to be lost souls. He states that he has heard voices on and off since the age of 5, although the auditory hallucinations have increased in frequency and intensity since the death of his mother. He denies visual, tactile, olfactory, and gustatory hallucinations. Juan also presents with paranoid thoughts that people are going to kill or torture him for his Social Security money, as well as his belief that his presence on Earth is a reparation for a malicious thought his mother had in their previous lives on "the green planet." Juan learned these beliefs from his mother, who he believes had spiritual gifts. The beliefs appear somewhat delusional, but Juan considers them to be his spiritual beliefs that he learned from his mother.

Additionally, Juan presents with symptoms of depression, including depressed mood, lack of energy, and feelings of hopelessness. He states that he has been depressed since the age of 13, when his grandmother died. Juan states that his depression worsened significantly after the death of his mother 2 years ago.

Juan also presents with symptoms of anxiety and is unaware of when his anxiety began. He reports constant worrying that bad things are going to happen to him. He states that the worrying impacts his sleep, and he takes Xanax that had belonged to his mother to help him sleep at night. He also experiences social anxiety and does not have any social support in his life. Juan reports being unable to trust other people because "this planet is cloaked in evil." Although Juan has not had enough money to buy groceries, he reports being unable to go to a food pantry for fear of catching diseases from other people. Juan also states that he has anxiety about taking showers and brushing his teeth, and, thus, presents with very poor hygiene. At the initial session, he stated that he had only taken one shower in the past month and had not changed his clothes in several weeks.

All people who have and have not been formally diagnosed with mental illnesses and psychotic disorders have complex personal meaning systems (affect-laden cognitions and associations) that live in the conscious, preconscious, and subconscious. Juan experiences themes of fear of being hurt by malicious people and a deep and pervasive sense of sadness. Juan's mother often told him of the world being a scary place and that all people are out to get him. Juan had no other relationships by which to confirm or deny this, so this scary belief became firmly embedded in his meaning system. From this, Juan developed a delusion that his Social Security money would be stolen. Additionally, given Juan's mother's low opinion of others, he was not able to access many supports, such as the food pantry and friendships, which caused extreme loneliness and depression.

Juan came to the community mental health center because he was in a financial, social, and mental health crisis. He was penniless, hungry, and alone. In crisis, people are sometimes more available to help and open to suggestion than any other time, and this was the case with Juan. He began telling his concerns to a crisis worker, who helped him get some food, assisted him with a Social Security application, and gave him social relationships to turn to for mutual support, which also gave him opportunities to debunk his mother's myth that "all people are bad and will hurt you."

PRIMARY PURPOSES OF MENTAL HEALTH TREATMENT

What are the primary purposes of mental health treatment? For what purposes do people seek out psychotherapy? These answers might differ, depending on whom you ask. How might a clinician answer this question? How might a person seeking mental health services answer this question? Initially, and with any client, any skillful and ethical clinician would assess for danger to self or others and then provide the highest level of care for safety. Beyond that, generally speaking, a mental health clinician provides outpatient mental health services for the purposes of self-understanding, stabilization, and improving quality of life. These goals might be achieved by any combination of the following modalities: individual therapy, short-term structured curriculum therapy (CBT, solution-focused therapy, problem-solving therapy), long-term open-agenda psychotherapy (psychodynamic or psychoanalytic psychotherapy), art therapy, drama therapy, medications, meditation, and many others.

MAINSTREAM MENTAL HEALTH SERVICES FOR PEOPLE
WITHOUT PSYCHOSIS

Mental health treatment services look one way for people without a diagnosis of SMI or psychosis. A comprehensive assessment includes safety risks, questions about suicidal and homicidal thoughts, and observations about ability to care for self and protect self and dependents from harm, especially in the first session. While always on the mental health clinician's radar, after the initial session, these issues are not the focus of the therapeutic work. Typically, a great amount of time is spent collecting information about early childhood relationships and experiences and understanding these attachments and associations, both from the client's and clinician's perspectives, and current manifestations of these experiences. The unconscious and preconscious, maladaptive behavior and thoughts are brought to the conscious level so that a rational choice can be made. Here lies the focus of most of the remainder of the therapeutic relationship.

ADDRESSING PSYCHOTIC SYMPTOMS IN MAINSTREAM
MENTAL HEALTH TREATMENT

Mental health treatment services take on different treatment goals for people who have been diagnosed with SMI or psychosis. During the assessment, lots of exploratory questions are asked to consider the need for inpatient hospitalization, including suicidal and homicidal impulses and the ability to protect self from harm. Self-understanding is not a mainstream treatment goal for people with psychotic experiences. The curious person would ask, "Why are these treatment goals so different for people who experience psychosis?" The answer includes a few different components.

Historically, as stated, among people who experience psychotic symptoms, clinicians do not explore feelings and deep-seated psychological connections for fear of disorganizing effects and inducing an acute psychotic decompensation. This kind of mainstream clinician may not want to uncover past experiences that open up big and unresolved feelings because the necessary resources to manage these feelings and reactions are rare or nonexistent. These resources may include time or additional clinicians, as hearing about and effectively helping someone cope with these kinds of experiences will take additional time, sensitivity, and skill. In addition, it is extraordinarily difficult to hear about the deep, deep hurt caused from early childhood trauma and then wrap up that conversation and move to the next client who needs help with a housing application. The goals of mental health treatment with people who experience symptoms of psychosis are simplistic: to decrease symptoms and link with resources such as housing and financial benefits. Along with these simple treatment goals, low expectations of client capability follow. Many, many people believe that people who experience psychosis are not capable of reflection and relationships, including therapeutic ones. So, for people who experience symptoms of psychosis, the therapeutic treatment goals are primarily focused on stabilization and connecting to resources that improve quality of life. Does this feel like enough clinical attention is being offered? What do you see missing?

We seem to conveniently *forget* that people who experience symptoms of psychosis are embedded in our day-to-day lives. This person is quite possibly your work colleague, your child's elementary school teacher, the person who helps you with your computer needs, your neighbor, or others. People who experience psychotic symptoms are among us. Taking this perspective, the person WITH the illness, becomes *the person*. Some individuals are disabled by the illness and some are not. Regardless of ability, why would we not extend hope for a meaningful life and offer all interventions and supports that we know to be effective in improving quality of life to any and all people?

Now, we pull the curtains back and explore the subjective experiences of people who experience symptoms of psychosis.

Gene

At the age of 20 and in his senior year of college, Gene had his first psychotic episode and was diagnosed with schizophrenia. He had been studying engineering and living in the university dorm. At that time, he was hospitalized and prescribed Thorazine. His psychiatrist told Gene and his parents that because of his psychotic illness, he would not be able to complete his college degree or work because both would be too stressful. The psychiatrist advised that Gene return to live with his parents, where he could be monitored and completely cared for. Additionally, Gene was to enroll in Social Security benefits (cash and medical reimbursement); since he would not be able to work, he needed these benefits to sustain himself. Finally, Gene and his parents were told that he would need to take the medication for the rest of his life. His parents followed the doctor's recommendations, removed Gene from college, moved him into a basement room of his own, and enrolled him in state and federal benefit programs.

After living in the basement of his parent's apartment for a few months and becoming anxious and depressed, Gene took his Social Security check and moved into a SRO hotel, where he had his own room and shared a bathroom down the hall with other residents. He did not like the antipsychotic medications that he was prescribed because they left him feeling numb, disorganized, lethargic, and sexually impotent. He lost hope and flushed the medications down the toilet. He spent his days listening to the radio, fixing other people's electronics, visiting the library, and hanging around the SRO. While he knew many of the residents in the SRO, he was cautious of their partying behaviors, referring to them as "pimps, prostitutes, and needlers" and did not socialize with them. He was also cautious to get close with anyone for fear that they would find out about his mental illness and reject him, as all of his other friends from college had done. He did not have even one friend. He lived in this SRO for 20 years. One day, Gene received an eviction notice because the building was in such disrepair that it was planned to be demolished.

Can you imagine what existential/spiritual themes may regularly come up for this person over the 20 years that he lived with a psychotic disorder? Can you imagine how these themes manifest in day-to-day life for this person? What do you suppose Gene felt after receiving this eviction notice? I am not suggesting that every person who experiences psychosis is haunted by all of these issues. I am suggesting, though, as Goffman asserted, people who experience symptoms of psychosis are, by society, generally and systematically treated in similar ways. We will now explore these social dynamics and resulting subjective experiences that Gene and other people with mental illnesses, specifically psychotic disorders, commonly experience.

COMMON EXISTENTIAL EXPERIENCES OF PEOPLE
WITH PSYCHOSIS
Desperate Denial

Having a mental illness impacts every aspect of a person's life. Psychotic disorders tend to manifest in the adolescent years. This is a time when peer relationships are the most important kind of relationship, and they are fragile. When friends notice a serious and pervasive change in their friend's personality, out of fear, not knowing how to help, and being invested in their own needs, they often back away. Since these peer relationships seem so essential, this isolation is devastating to the one being excluded. No one wants this rejection. The symptoms of mental illness are real and can get in the way of productive thinking and behaviors that are necessary to be productive in school and work. As a person is feeling marginalized and left behind in social relationships, school, career, and community, outside of admitting to having a mental illness and an open discussion, there is nothing that can be said or done to remedy these relationships. No one wants these experiences. In the face of such essential deterioration and losses, sometimes people will respond with desperate denial.

Vladimir, a 36-year-old man with a long history of disabling mental illness and frequent hospitalizations, resided in a locked residential facility. He would pace in the halls, muttering, "Just call me Coca-Cola!" What he was saying was that he wanted the pleasures of everyday life, including a simple Coca-Cola.

Young people with the newest onset of symptoms of mental illness can be some of the most difficult. No one wants these symptoms and their results. As clinicians make attempts to educate the client about his or her illness, the client may have difficulty paying attention. What he or she is paying attention to is his or her own internal thoughts of, "This is not happening! I am not mentally ill!" Any coping skills that could be used are not because he or she does not think there is anything to manage. He or she makes every attempt to carry on with life as usual, focusing on everyday things, friends, hanging out, and fashion and fantasizing about a desired life.

Abject Loneliness

Remember the movie Cast Away (Zemeckis, 2000) with Tom Hanks? The main character, Chuck Noland, is stranded on an uninhabited island. Included in the many efforts to survive, he draws a face on a volleyball and names it Wilson, who becomes his daily companion. With found items, he constructs a raft to try to save his own life. On the expedition, the volleyball falls overboard, and then Chuck is overcome with abject loneliness.

Fromm-Reichmann and many other subjective-oriented theorists have commented on how deeply isolating the experiencing of living with mental illness is because of the strong social dynamics of fear, shame, and rejection (Fromm-Reichmann, 1948; Goffman, 1961). Even family members subtly and overtly ignore the person with the mental illness. We are hardwired for relationships. Even people in solitary confinement in prison will naturally use their imagination to be in relationship with something living for survival. Why do we deprive this basic human need of being in relationship from people who live with mental illness, especially symptoms of psychosis?

Without relationships, symptoms of physical and mental illness increase. The attachment theorist and social worker James Robertson noticed John Bowlby's detachment process (protest, detachment, despair) that occurred in young children who were medically hospitalized for long periods of time (Robertson, 1952; Bowlby, 1979). He noticed that the hospital visiting hours were quite brief, lasting anywhere from zero to 2 hours, and some hospitals only allowing brief viewing through a glass partition. He noticed that the longer a child is separated from her parent, the more altered the attachment style, often forever resulting in mood and behavior changes and her future relationship potentials. Robertson made a movie, *A Two Year Old Goes to Hospital* (1952), based on his findings of these children and their process of detachment following separation from the parent, especially the mother. Because of the social expectations of the fathers during the 1950s, we can imagine that most of the caregiving responsibilities and relationships were assigned to the mother, leaving the father with a very different type of relationship and attachment style with the child.

We see a similar attachment/detachment process among many people who live with mental illness, especially psychotic disorders. Protest is similar to the denial phase of a person with mental illness: "I do not have a mental illness!" In this phase, people will not follow mental health treatment recommendations. These recommendations could be life-preserving if the person is able to continue with close relationships and life dreams, and some do. However, because of relationship disruptions and brain misworkings, these efforts are often impaired. Living with profound despair is overwhelming and often can only be tolerated for short periods. In an illusional effort to soothe oneself, individuals with mental illness often turn to substances and behaviors to self-medicate the resulting despair. This extended experience leaves the individual disconnected with others, the world, and his or her own psychological pain and existence. We term this *detachment* in the most extreme sense.

With unparalleled empathy for human suffering, Gabor Maté, a medical physician, wrote the book *In the Realm of the Hungry Ghost: Close Encounters with Addiction* (2010), about his work with drug-addicted and homeless men and woman who reside in the east side of Vancouver. In the Buddhist tradition, there are 10 realms of life: the enlightened realm of *Buddha* being at the top and the realm of *Hell* being at the bottom. The realm of the *Hungry Ghost* sits at the number nine position, just before *Hell*. Maté asserts that these women and men who have lived a lifetime of horrific abuse, neglect, emptiness, and inadequacy use heavy and constant doses of drugs to self-medicate themselves out of the *Hell* stage. It is ironic that a person could use detachment as a coping style to live with detachment. Detachment begets detachment.

Mary Ainsworth constructed the famous social experiment termed the *Strange Situation* (Ainsworth et al., 1978). Following a separation, a baby's reunification effort with the mother is observed. Ainsworth noted the following attachment styles: secure, anxious, avoidant, ambivalent, and disorganized. Disorganization, or aloofness toward relations with others, is an attachment style that naturally develops as a style/skill to cope with the absence of consistent and timely caregiving. The experience of psychosis can serve as the ultimate disorganized attachment style that some people consciously or unconsciously use to cope or position themselves one realm up from *Hell* to the realm of the *Hungry Ghost* in the absence of the caregiver and other major attachment losses.

Major Loss of Dreams

Adolescence and young adulthood are times when a person begins to make serious strides in his own career. Often a process of an emotional mixture of trial and error and related feedback, he fine-tunes his interests and skills, emerging in his late 20s and early 30s with an image of what life path he will forever follow. Mental illness, often beginning in late adolescence, impacts an individual similar to a "traumatic warp" (Fromm-Reichmann, 1948, para. 4) that impacts this process with disruptions in education, work, and intimate relationships. During this time, dreams of a career in graphic design are interrupted, desires for a life partner and a couple of children are seemingly untouchable, and more basically, being able to financially support oneself is unimaginable. Instead, the world of acute episodes of illness, hospitalizations, disrupted relationships, and neuroleptic medications makes the age of *30-somethings* a very different reality. No one in high school imagined his own reality of living in the realm of the *Hungry Ghost* or even terrorized in *Hell*.

Vulnerabilities Exposed

Upon initial assessment, patients are barraged with questions about their every thought and its intensity. Many of these thoughts are quite personal and sensitive. "So, how long have you been feeling like taking your life?" "Why have you not told anyone about these thoughts?" "What sounds do you hear?" "What does the voice say to you?" "What associations do you have with a cough?" This laundry list of private questions is often asked by a person who has never before and never will again interact with the person. Often, the clinician has this *transient* understanding of the relationship, as well, and makes very little attempt to be sensitively attuned to the delivery and handling of these exchanges. Privacy is rare, or almost impossible to find, in mental health assessment facilities. Questioning is often done in open day rooms, for safety purposes, where other people and staff can hear what is going on or in front of several clinicians (anywhere from three to 20) at a time for teaching purposes.

Inpatient or residential psychiatric facilities that house people with SMIs often create an environment where sleeping, eating, using the toilet, and showering are in open areas where individuals can be supervised. How would you feel if you had to do your business in a room with no door and where everyone could see everything? Many facilities do not have doors or, in fact, have cameras that peer into these private areas.

In public psychiatric facilities, where the majority of people receive mental health treatment, other clients/patients are exposed to the private material of others. I do lots of presentations and consultations with audiences in public community mental health centers. To manage my anxiety, I usually arrive early. I end up standing in the waiting room, witnessing the *goings-on* at each facility. It is not uncommon for a clinician to open the door and holler out a person's name for everyone to hear. Sometimes there is a thick piece of glass separating the staff from the patients. There is often a lot of background noise, including televisions with dinging sounds familiar in shows such as *Sponge Bob Squarepants*, people arguing, background Muzak, sirens, intercoms making announcements for groups to begin, among other random sounds. Patients must revert to screaming through the glass to have their requests heard. "I need to see a psychiatrist! I am having trouble with my medications!" When asked about the nature of the trouble, how does a person discretely say through bulletproof glass that he is experiencing sexual dysfunction? Recently, I heard a man yelling, albeit quietly, through the bulletproof glass that he was just discharged from a psychiatric unit the day before and needed to see someone about his medication. How do you imagine he felt about receiving this kind of *help*?

Stacy, a 26-year-old female, made her first attempt to get help for her long-standing anxiety and depression. Her treatment consisted of meeting both a psychiatry resident and a therapist, both asking about her history, each hand-ling the information differently. The therapist paced the sessions carefully and slowly as Stacy's story unfolded, containing detailed memories of sexual miscon-duct at the hands of her father. The psychiatry resident, needing to complete internship assignments, requested Stacy to be interviewed in front of six other psychiatry residents and their two supervisors. The psychiatric resident did not take Stacy's well-being into consideration before making this request. Stacy was asked to tell the details of her story with nothing more than a thank-you to follow. Immediately after the interview, Stacy became acutely suicidal and expe-rienced panic attacks. Is it no wonder that patients have vulnerability exposure on their minds?

Hans Prinzhorn, originally trained as an art historian, then psychiatrist, requested the artwork (drawings, paintings, sculpture) from untrained inmates of several European insane asylums. Of all of the works that were submitted, he chose some 5,000 pieces for his own collection. Some were photographed and published in his book, *Artistry of the Mentally Ill* (Prinzhorn, 1922), which is now out of print. You are able to see photographs of this fascinating work online (see Appendix B for the link).

Subsequent books, such as *Beyond Reason: Art and Psychosis Works from the Prinzhorn Collection* (Busine, Brand-Blaussen, & Douglas, 1998) borrowed and published these images. By doing an Internet search for "Prinzhorn Collection," you will find an abundance of websites that contain these images and some associated text. By flipping through these images, you will find monsters/trolls, juxtaposition worlds, distorted people, devastated faces, gagged mouths, obsessively repetitive orderly writings, ethereal images, lonely fragile trees, and, again and again, images of nude people and body parts. Most of these artist inmates lived and died in the European insane asylums (Tausk, 1933).

These common themes manifest in people with SMIs, especially psychotic disorders. Are some themes more pronounced among people with psychotic mental illness who have had traumatic experiences? As discussed at length in Chapter 3, "Brief History of Iatrogenic Trauma from the Mainstream Mental Health Treatment System," a high proportion of people who experience psy-chotic symptoms have experienced early and severe trauma, such as sexual abuse; parent abandonment; witnessing physical violence onto himself or someone he deeply loves, such as a mother or sister; or severe emotional and physical neglect. These traumatic themes will expectedly emerge in art, language, behaviors, and delusions.

Emotional reactions to traumatic experiences are unique and can be com-plex. The following is a brief list of common emotional reactions to traumatic experiences: feelings of emptiness; inadequacy; vulnerabilities exposed; shame; guilt; personalization—"I think everything is my fault"; projection—"I think everything is your fault"; hypervigilance; emotional numbness; interpersonal disconnection; difficulty trusting; loss of personal power; rage; restlessness/agitation; hopelessness; fear; social withdrawal and isolation; stubbornness; difficulty sleeping; and compulsively turning to behaviors or drugs to soothe or dissociate.

We explore further into the lives of people with SMI to discover their stressors. In 2002, I conducted my doctoral dissertation, a qualitative and quantitative retrospective medical record analysis, to discover what kinds and quantity of factors contribute to a person's acute psychotic episode from the patient's perspective (Dunn, 2002). The first subject availability sample (*n* = 100) found the following top six most frequently reported categories and the most frequently reported examples of each. Each are listed in frequency order (Table 9.1).

Do any of these stress-inducing categories resonate with you? When you stop to think about what kinds of stress-inducing themes might be on the minds of people who experience mental illnesses and symptoms of psychosis, are they any different than what is on your mind? Many of the stressors were similar to a general population, such as changes in primary support group, medical changes related to healthcare matters or services, and housing changes. Other stressor categories differed from the general population, such as changes in mental health treatment and self-sabotaging behaviors.

Compared to a life events stress list used in related literature for the general population (i.e., Holmes & Rahe, 1967), there were several noteworthy stressors that were *not* mentioned by any subjects (all with SMI) in this research study. These items included pregnancy, having a baby, retirement, sexual difficulties, large mortgage (although debt was mentioned), partner reconciliation, and son or daughter leaving home. It is noteworthy that 65% of this sample of people with SMI were under the age of 40. Upon pregnancy, women with SMI are almost always counseled to have an abortion or adopt out their babies. If the woman decides to carry the pregnancy to term, their newborn babies are often taken into *protective* custody immediately after birth or soon after out of fear that the mother would not have the capacity to adequately care for the infant. Therefore, this common practice and the age of this sample limits the probability of a person with mental illness experiencing the stressors of having raised a child in their custody or having a child leave home to pursue greater independence. Finally, these common life events stress lists imply lifestyle situations that are typically not characteristic of people with mental illness, which implies that the lifestyles of people with SMI are uncommon, missing out

TABLE 9.1

Top Six Most Frequently Reported Factors Contributing to Acute Psychotic Decompensation

Reported Category and Examples	Frequency (n = 100)
Changes Related to Primary Support Group	64
– Real or perceived motives of *evil* from family	
– Real or perceived rejection by family of origin	
– Poor social support—isolation	
– Real or perceived rejection (negative shift in support) by friend	
– Real or perceived rejection by significant other (argument, infidelity)	
– Family conflict	
Medical Changes Related to Healthcare Matters or Services	42
– Stress of symptoms of mental illness	
– Recent onset of painful physical condition (sore throat, dental problems, rash, exacerbation of illness)	
– Real or perceived obstacle in healthcare services	
– Recent diagnosis of terminal illness in significant other, child, family member	
– Chronic medical problems	
Changes Related to Mental Health Treatment	42
– Discontinued medication as prescribed	
– Disagreement with therapeutic staff	
– Disagrees with diagnosis	
– Discussing painful issues in treatment	
Self-Sabotaging Behavior	25
– Drug/alcohol relapse	
Problems Related to Incarceration with Legal System, Crime, Trauma	22
– Victim of violence	
– Victim of robbery	
– Victim of sexual assault by acquaintance, family, significant other, police/security	
– Victim of physical assault by stranger, family, significant other, police/security	
Housing Changes	21
– Homelessness	
– Conflict with neighbor	
– Moved in with significant other or family	
– Eviction	
– Loss of utilities	

on many common personally rewarding situations that afford others opportunities for deep interpersonal connection and socioeconomic comforts and securities. We listen for these themes of significant losses or desires in the vernacular of people who are actively experiencing symptoms of psychosis.

People with experiences of psychosis can and do enjoy a variety of positive experiences and rewards. These pleasures can result from joyful rewards of relationships, seeing and experiencing the wonders of the world, spontaneous surprises, volunteer and paid employment, toys of all sizes, the power of money, mysterious synchronicity, the concrete manifestation of increased quality of life (i.e., housing, friendships, and clothing), and a variety of explicit and subtle life winnings. To accurately understand and communicate with a person who experiences symptoms of psychosis, these rewards should also be listened for in the spoken stories, conversations, and other expressions.

Perhaps we all have experienced some form of stigma and marginalization in our lives, some significantly more than others. What characteristics do you have that have marginalized you? Your answers may include situations where your family did not have as much money as the other families at school, or your height, religious practices, medical conditions, hair texture, eye shape, and family make-up (i.e., having two fathers and no mother) made you different. Perhaps you have a learning disability, are the son or daughter of a preacher, have a disabling accident or medical condition, or are living with family violence, mental illness, abuse, or addiction. The list is endless. People who experience SMI often feel very different from other mainstreamed individuals. We listen for these themes in the roots of delusions and hallucinations.

Consider the following poem, written by Debbie Sesula (2013). She emphasizes how people with psychotic symptoms are more harshly judged and marginalized by common stressors (see Appendix B for link to poem).

You and Me

If you're overly excited
You're happy
If I'm overly excited
I'm manic.
If you imagine the phone ringing
You're stressed out
If I imagine the phone ringing
I'm psychotic.
If you're crying and sleeping all day

You're sad and need time out
If I'm crying and sleeping all day
I'm depressed and need to get up.
If you're afraid to leave your house at night
You're cautious
If I'm afraid to leave my house at night
I'm paranoid.
If you speak your mind and express your opinions
You're assertive
If I speak my mind and express my opinions
I'm aggressive.
If you don't like something and mention it
You're being honest
If I don't like something and mention it I'm being difficult.
If you get angry
You're considered upset
If I get angry
I'm considered dangerous.
If you over-react to something
You're sensitive
If I over-react to something
I'm out of control.
If you don't want to be around others
You're taking care of yourself and relaxing
If I don't want to be around others
I'm isolating myself and avoiding.
If you talk to strangers
You're being friendly
If I talk to strangers
I'm being inappropriate.
For all of the above you're not told to take a
pill or are hospitalized, *but I am!*

How is the stigma of mental illness different from other potentially dishonoring situations? Like some experiences mentioned, the very situation like mental illness often changes the course of life. The altered mode of brain functioning causes episodes of misperception and inability to linearly communicate one's thoughts. Furthermore, these episodes may cause behaviors that are humiliating and even cause the person to be kept in a controlled and supervised environment, such as a hospital or jail, which has the exponential effect of stigmatization and social marginalization.

Whether or not the individual experiences symptoms of mental illness, we all have some similar general concerns. We are all attempting to straddle the basic human need balance of fitting in and yet being an individual. Everyone has a moving wave of moods, and some moments are higher than others. We all enjoy making an impact in our own experiences and having a range of aversive emotional reactions to being told what to do. And, sometimes, we enjoy taking our seat on the bus and watching the world go by. We like familiarity, as much as variety. Each of us finds our own niche in the world; the comfort zone size of that niche varies from person to person and is larger for some and more microscopic for others. Along we all go.

PRACTICING EXISTENTIAL/SPIRITUAL ACCURATE UNDERSTANDING

Existential psychotherapy is the exploration of one's lived experience, especially early childhood experiences, and the pairing of these experiences to one's current perceptions. The essence of existentialism is that lived experiences create our perceptions. Psychoanalytic psychotherapy is the exploration of these lived experiences and the conscious, preconscious, and unconscious manifestations of these experiences, bringing associations of lived experiences and meaning patterns to the conscious level so that a person has the capacity to make conscious choices. Dynamics of transference and countertransference are exactly this—bringing associations of past significant individuals to conscious awareness so that the person has the capacity to regulate her reactions toward this person. There are no particular intervention methods in existential therapeutic work—more of a general searching for and congruently manifesting authentic meaning and purpose. Tenets of psychoanalytic psychotherapy and existentialism are a perfect marriage for accurate understanding and effective communication with individuals who experience symptoms of psychosis in present time and episodically.

Now, we have a general understanding of the kinds of things that are and are not on the minds of people who experience SMI and psychosis. This is a rich opportunity to more accurately understand what these individuals are attempting to communicate. However, there is more to this process of accurate understanding and effective communication.

Hypergraphia is the behavior of excessive writing. People with SMI sometimes experience episodes or partake in the ongoing habit of writing. The writing is dense, full of personal expression, and often involves themes such as spirituality, morality, and fears. Usually, people who participate in hypergraphia write in one notebook after another or save piles of notes. Others write on anything to which they have access.

An example of this writing involves a petticoat called Agnes's Jacket (Hornstein, 2012). Agnes Richter was trained as a seamstress before being committed to an Austrian psychiatric hospital in the 1890s. Richter was not allowed to have a pen for fear that she would harm herself. Instead, she was given a needle and scissors because of her previous professional training. She stitched her thoughts, feelings, and images into the lining of a petticoat. This petticoat was preserved in the Hans Prinzhorn collection (see Appendix B).

Born in 1927 in Rome, Fernando Oresete Nannette experienced hypergraphia. He spent most of his life in psychiatric and criminal institutions. Nannette wrote stories, drawings, and postcards to imaginary relatives. In the one institution, Volterra "Ferri" unit, he wrote elaborate futuristic stories on every possible inch of the wall and railing. Oresete died in Volterra on November 24, 1994. Images of his work can be found at the link in Appendix B.

These examples of hypergraphia are offered to identify and normalize a common experience among people who experience psychotic disorders. Individuals who need to write should be allowed and given the tools to do so.

FINAL THOUGHTS

In this chapter, we addressed existential and spiritual considerations for addressing individuals who experience symptoms of psychosis. Existential and spiritual experiences are important to consider among this population because these experiences are often pathologized or considered a symptom that should be suppressed, rather than a normative human experience. In this chapter, we identified common existential and spiritual meaning systems. We explored how these experiences really have no legitimate room in mainstream mental health treatment and are not customarily addressed, especially among individuals who experience symptoms of psychosis. Finally, in this chapter, we identified some common experiences among individuals who live with symptoms of psychosis and how these experiences negatively impact existential and spiritual beliefs. Practicing the philosophy and techniques of *Listening with Psychotic Ears* allows for individuals to identify their own existential and spiritual experiences and for the development and progression in these normative areas of human existence. These clinical skills enable clinicians, family members, and individuals themselves to "emerge with the capacity to render the unimaginable storms a little more imaginable" (Jackson & Williams, 1994, p. xi).

10

Listening with Psychotic Ears Philosophy and Clinical Skills

THROUGHOUT RECORDED HISTORY, and even today, people with mental illness have been deeply discredited and written off by society and by individuals in their inner social circles. People with mental illness are deserving humans with an illness that is no fault of their own. People who are experiencing psychosis are making attempts to communicate, but because the result of altered neurobiology is *formal thought disordered*, their words come out in ways that seem mysterious and bizarre. We have not had the tools and philosophy by which to understand these meaningful communications. Because of this dearth, we do not make attempts to understand and communicate with people with mental illness, which leaves them shut down and living a frail, marginalized life.

The work of the sociological anthropologist Goffman and others has given us the structure and language by which to explore both the broken mental health treatment delivery system and the impact of iatrogenic trauma on people who experience symptoms of mental illnesses. Goffman terms this dynamic *interactional sociology*, describing how one system interactively negatively impacts the other (Goffman, 1961).

We can and should make attempts to understand the communications of people who are actively experiencing symptoms of psychosis. The skills of *Listening with Psychotic Ears* facilitate the therapeutic relationship that is required to accurately understand and effectively communicate with people who are actively experiencing psychosis, thus empowering people and improving quality of life.

What is the meaning of *Listening with Psychotic Ears*? Many people speak in various languages: Mandarin, Spanish, Japanese, French, Farci, and others. As we hear another speaking in a recognizable language, we focus our attention, wanting to understand every word and cultural dynamic. Even in the English language, there are cultural dialects that influence accurate understanding of social situations. Sometimes on a television program, a person from a rural part of the United States will be speaking, and English subtitles will be necessary because the dialect is so difficult to comprehend. Being from rural Indiana, I am able to hear rural speech and understand unspoken social nuances from this distinct culture. The same dynamics are at play when a different language, such as Spanish, is spoken. People who experience symptoms of psychosis are also speaking in a unique language pattern with a context of unique cultural experiences that can and should be understood. When we hear someone speaking in a psychotic dialectical pattern, we should perk up our *psychotic ears* so that we might have every opportunity to understand every word and cultural dynamic. This action is the meaning of *Listening with Psychotic Ears*.

Friends, family members, and clinicians cannot know where and how to intervene unless the client is first heard, so others must actively listen until the other is accurately understood. Sullivan (1955) suggests that a lengthy interpersonal relationship is required to accurately understand the person's life, meaning system, and difficulties because the person at the center of concern may not be able to fully communicate these points. Active listening involves listening through the person's current and past life context, in that order, and sensitively asking for elaboration and clarification. We listen not solely on a linear path, but also from a holistic perspective, as the symptoms themselves alter (in brain functioning) the method of content expression. To accurately understand this individual, we must listen within the context of this alternative pathway. If a person speaking Spanish is listened to with Korean language ears, he or she will not be accurately understood because *both parties must be communicating within the same language* to bring about clear understanding. Otherwise, both have a high potential to be misunderstood. With accurate understanding, we have more of a chance at effective communication, which can result in successful problem solving and increased quality of life.

Examples of Psychotic Metaphors

I have softening of the brain, and I will soon be dead.

5,000 years ago, I walked with God.

There is a monster in my throat.

There is a tiger in my ass.

I want to be your hot dog.

The rabbit needs a job.

Just call me Coca-Cola. Who has the French fries?

I am a husband's wife!

I am a bird with broken wings.

BEGIN BY GROUNDING ONESELF IN COMPASSION
Philadelphia Cream Cheese Treatment

Deondra was approximately 32 years old. Because she was mentally and physically un-stable, she frequented the hospital where I worked for many years, so I saw her many times over those years. She had been diagnosed with schizophrenia and could not stay away from crack cocaine. She would do anything possible to get a hit of crack, in-cluding having sex with anyone, anywhere. Because of her addiction, she was HIV pos-itive and had given birth to several children, all of whom had been taken away by Child Protective Services (CPS). One particular day, Deondra presented to the hospital emergency department as a *hot mess*. She could not sit still, writhing and getting up and down from the gurney. She had not showered in weeks. As a result of shooting up crack cocaine, she had a sizable infected abscess that she was treating with Philadelphia cream cheese. She repeatedly hollered that she had to get back to her *friends*, the guys in the abandoned building on the corner of Ontario and Wells Street. She was about 8 months pregnant. This would be her sixth child taken at birth by CPS.

The extreme situations that a person finds herself in can unconsciously trigger negative and painful emotional countertransference reactions. What do you feel in reaction to Deondra? Do you feel sorry for her? Do you blame her for her situation? No matter the feelings, they are likely strong ones. Commonly, clinicians have strong emotional reactions to their own feelings because these feelings are in conflict with what is thought should be believed about the clients that are being helped. So as to avoid these unbearable feelings, people sometimes blame and judge, with thoughts like the following: "How could she get herself in this situation, again?" or "One more person using up our tax dollars." This condemnatory path further marginalizes and alienates Deondra and leaves the clinician feeling ineffective and resentful. As a more humanistic and effective alternative, we (friends/family members/clinicians) can begin by grounding ourselves in compassion.

What is compassion? Compassion is acknowledging that people's behaviors or circumstances may be dictated by influences we are not able to be aware of and accepting them completely regardless.

Deondra had over 2 months of intensive psychiatric work, and upon her hospital discharge, she immediately relapsed by using crack cocaine, became pregnant again, and continued to use while her baby was growing inside her. Deondra only had the dissociation of drug intoxication and the people who shared a drug-using life-style as coping methods for the hellish life she led. Mental health workers or family members with higher expectations for Deondra could perceive her behaviors in a negative light, one that would shame or blame her. Yet, there are other ways to accurately understand Deondra's behaviors and intentions.

Without anger, we take the firm stance that is needed and proceed with love and kindness, even if negative behavior occurs. Proceeding with a truly compassionate attitude with Deondra (and her unborn child), we see that she is unable to make decisions to keep herself and her unborn child from harm and must do what is necessary to legally hold her in the hospital, even if it is against her wishes. She was kept in the hospital until her baby was born, and she was medically stabilized. When she returned to the hospital after relapsing again and again, she was welcomed with compassion by some staff.

One easy way to orient one's self in this truly compassionate attitude is the following: "If this were me or someone I love, how would I want to be handled?" Many would answer with qualities of gentleness, sensitivity, soothing, protection, guidance, unwavering commitment, and forgiveness. What other ways would you or someone you love desire to be handled when at your most vulnerable?

BE AWARE AND MANAGE DEFENSIVE COUNTERTRANSFERENCE

Intimate and therapeutic work can stir up a variety of feelings for anyone. If unmonitored, our reactions to our loved ones and clients can be an obstacle to the client's progress. Consider, again, Fromm-Reichmann's idea of *defensive countertransference*. The client tells his story. The therapist cannot tolerate the client's despair. She flees from and dismisses the experiences of the client (Fromm-Reichmann, 1950).

Also, remember the many individuals from the Cabrini Green Housing Projects who came to the psychiatric emergency room for crisis help. Each woman told her story filled with multiple sexual assaults, chaotic attachments, addiction, and a variety of other ongoing traumatic situations. The common response from many mental health workers, especially psychiatrists, was "she is making it up." The mental health workers experienced a classic defensive countertransference reaction, as they could not bear to hear these horrid details experienced by these Cabrini Green residents and fled from the pain of the interpersonal connection and the story.

These unregulated defensive countertransference reactions cause iatrogenic trauma for the client. We often hear of even more severe stories, in which the client is severely injured or even killed because the clinician or police had such strong and unregulated defensive countertransference reactions. As with any type of counter-transference, the matter is *when*, not *if*, it is going to happen. We should all be aware

of and manage our defensive countertransference reactions so as to not be an obstacle in the person's opportunity for psychological and spiritual growth.

Weiden and Havens (1994) identified five dynamics that interfere with alliance
building with individuals who live with schizophrenia, including paranoia, denial
of the illness, stigma, demoralization, and terror from the experience of symptoms.
Strategies that cut through these defensive countertransference reactions include
empathizing with mistrustful and guarded clients, reframing for those who deny the
symptoms and illness, using empowering affirmations to those who feel demoral-
ized, and normalizing emotional reactions and behaviors (Weiden & Havens, 1994).

ASK ABOUT BOTH CURRENT COMPLAINTS AND EARLY LIFE

Of course we want to know the nature of the person's current complaints, for this
is the focus of much of the work. However, to accurately understand the origin
and meaning of these current complaints and situations, we must ask and understand the qualitative details of significant people, places, and situations that have
impacted the person's early life. With this understanding, we have the opportunity
to connect the psychological dots for the person.

Consider this example. Marcus wears a yellow dish glove on his right hand to
"keep away the bugs under his skin." The dish glove has to be yellow or else it does
not work for him. The goal now is to determine what the significance of the glove is
and, more importantly, why it needs to be yellow. Is there a relationship between the
glove or the color yellow with something in Marcus's early life? Once we can decode
the significance of the glove and its color, our therapeutic work becomes offering
these interpretations to Marcus so these behaviors become choices, rather than unconscious actions that could marginalize him or create more serious repercussions,
including mandatory detainment or treatment.

Read and Fraser (1998) remind us of the high rate of childhood sexual or physical
abuse among people who experience mental illness, specifically psychosis. In their
study of 100 subjects interviewed at psychiatric hospitalization admission, only 17%
were asked about childhood abuse (Read & Fraser, 1998). Of the subjects who were
asked, 82% affirmatively answered, once again confirming high rates of abuse among
people with mental illness. Read and Fraser (1998) also noted that males and the
more disturbed or disturbing were less likely to be asked about childhood abuse.

That said, just as in the general population, people do not always want to *go there*,
meaning going back to discuss the original sources of psychological pain. Some
people do not have psychological insight; others do not have the coping skills or
interpersonal support. For some, the pain is so uncomfortable, overwhelming, and

present that connecting the dots between past trauma and current manifestation of symptoms seems obvious, and not attempting to connect those dots for these people would be neglectful. Therein lies the opportunity for newfound strength (Terr, 1991).

Alternatively, Read (2006) suggests that all clients should be asked about possible histories of trauma, despite the insecure and avoidant countertransference reactions the clinicians might be experiencing. Regardless of whether the clinician is worried about upsetting the client or that they may not know what to say in response, clients who present to mental health treatment settings expect to be asked about traumatic experiences, and when they are not, they feel disappointed, dissatisfied, and thwarted (Read, Hammersley, Rudegeair, 2007; Read & Ross, 2011; Read, van Os, Morrison, & Ross, 2005).

Familiar, Soothing, and Hazardous

Janine was a 22-year-old woman with an extensive history of sexual abuse at the hands of her father and two brothers. Her mother had abandoned the family when Janine was 2 years old. More recently, Janine had been attending college but was expelled as a result of poor grades, not going to classes, and disruptions in classes. The police brought her to the psychiatric emergency room after she called her therapist reporting a suicide plan. While detained at the hospital, Janine made sexual advances to anyone who walked by the room she was in.

In the last three nights, Janine went to bars and picked up strangers to bring back to her apartment, engaging in unprotected, promiscuous, and violent sexual encounters. This hazardous behavior was familiar and soothing, as it connected her, in her vulnerable time, with the only attachment figure that she knew. Additionally, as she saw no hope for herself, suicide was a very real option for Janine. Similarly, she could have died at the hands of any of these strangers she brought to her home.

Janine was psychiatrically hospitalized. Over time, with her therapist, the unconscious meaning of her behavior was interpreted with her. She was kept safe in the hospital and outpatient holding environment. She was joined in her episodes of panic and grief and taught soothing and more adaptive coping skills.

The time spent with Janine was important in allowing her to attain a positive outlook for the future, but this time is not always possible in mainstream mental health facilities that prioritize productivity and billing. Furthermore, society runs at the speed of light, which does not always allow for long relationships with clients to engage with them and perform a comprehensive investigation of early and current stressors and their subjective meaning. This fast pace and focus on productivity and funding diminishes the possibility of engagement, sustainability, meaningful inquiry, and eventual success (Mechanic, 2008; Walsh, 2011). When only limited time is available, we do the best we can at engaging the client, developing trust, collecting necessary information, modulating distress, listening for accurate meaning of expressions, and making swift and necessary interventions. Understanding how to make the best of limited time and what to do with the responses received will still allow for a deeper understanding of a client's psychological expressions.

CLINICAL SKILLS FOR INQUIRING ABOUT TRAUMA HISTORY AND RESPONDING TO DISCLOSURES

Read (2006) suggests that all mental health clinicians in the role of conducting initial assessments/intake should receive training in abuse inquiry and response. Training should include knowledge to motivate and skills, including role-play, for effectiveness. The training program should include local culture and resources, including laws regarding who must engage in mandated reporting and when. Read (2006) constructed a 1-day trauma history training program based on the following principles:

- **All clients must be asked.** This principle removes the opportunity for subjective avoidance of various clients, such as clients who are deemed too psychotic to respond.
- **Ask specific objective and behavioral questions.** For example, "As a child, did an adult ever hurt or punish you in a way that left a bruise, cut, or scratches?" and "As a child, did anyone ever do something sexual that made you feel uncomfortable?" Briere (2004) offers a review of available structured interview tools. Questions should not be asked in the beginning of the interview, before rapport has developed. Trauma assessment questions should be qualified or *funneled* and not presented out of the blue. For example, one might say, "A part of a full assessment is to ask you some personal questions. Is it OK with you if we do that now?" Read suggests that the questions be asked in the context of the appropriate timeline, such as when generally asking about childhood (Read & Fraser, 1998).
- **Ask at initial assessment.** If the client is not asked about trauma history for any reason upon intake (*already too upset*), then they are almost never asked later on (Read & Fraser, 1998). If there are sound reasons why a full assessment is not conducted at intake (client is imminently suicidal or extremely disorganized), then the clinician should make a clear note that the trauma history assessment was not conducted and be specific about when this history will be taken and by whom. "The tendency of some clinicians

to wait for an imagined magic moment when rapport is just right should be challenged, not least with the point that for some clients the act of asking may be crucial in establish[ing] rapport" (Read, 2006, p. 210).

- **Hold awareness of types and prevalence of abuse.** Knowing how commonly different types of abuses occur will likely increase the chance of the clinician asking about trauma history.
- **Hold awareness of the effects of abuse.** When clinicians can see that abuse manifests across all different types of diagnoses, they are less likely to only ask about trauma among clients who manifest classic PTSD symptoms.
- **Hold awareness of current clinical practice.** Offering effective and respectful clinical skills will motivate clinicians to ask.
- **Know how to appropriately respond to disclosures.** Clinicians need training on how to accurately respond, in the moment, to trauma disclosures. Appropriate clinical responses include both clinician skills and mandated reporting practices. Read (2006) offers six clinical skills for disclosure response: (1) Don't be aggressive in collecting all the details; (2) Affirm that disclosing the abuse and experiencing and talking about emotions are all positive; (3) Explore past and future supports; (4) Assess for current safety of client and other potential victims; (5) Check for emotional stability at the end of the session; and (6) Ascertain immediate formal and informal supports.
- **Hold awareness of vicarious traumatization in clinicians.** Clinicians need to be prepared for the traumatic stories they will hear. Clinicians need effective supervision, peer support, and the availability of personal therapy.

Additionally, as the person at the center of concern discusses distressing memories or affairs, the clinician is wise to be cognizant of modulating the associated emotions to avoid becoming overwhelmed (Sullivan, 1955). This supportive and connected relationship allows for emotional safety so that the person will come back to this relationship when he or she is feeling distressed and needs help to understand or mutualize these emotions and perceptions.

I Am a Husband's Wife!

Elizabeth was brought to the psychiatric emergency room by police officers because she was yelling, "I am a husband's wife!" and racial slurs to strangers at a trendy family tourist area. She was unable to calm down or cooperate, scaring people in the neighborhood. The weather was very cold, but she was wearing only a t-shirt and jeans and had lost a shoe.

In Elizabeth's case, the right thing to do was bring her to the hospital where she could be cared for and everyone could be kept safe. In many mainstream treatment settings, this moment would be the endpoint in attempting to gather more information about Elizabeth's current stressors and past experiences that impacted her subjective experience, as managing her psychosis and disturbing behavior would take precedence (Read & Fraser, 1998). At the treatment facility, after making attempts to calm her, Elizabeth was questioned about current stressors; even in her acutely stressed state, asking about early life experiences helped with accurate understanding and effective communication with her.

I could see that Elizabeth was extremely frightened and defensive. I spoke gently but firmly with her. Seeing that she was responding positively to me, I sat very close to her on the gurney. She was quickly able to calm down and rationally speak to me, sharing the following story.

Elizabeth was at the tourist area that day because she was to start a new job. On her way to work and already stressed, she was reminded that this was the place where she was sexually assaulted by a man of color just 2 years prior. She also told me that her husband recently left her and took her children, whom she ever so greatly missed. She said that she had a therapist but had not been able to see her for the last 2 months. She gave me the therapist's name and phone number.

The therapist was able to give even more information about Elizabeth's past life. Elizabeth was the youngest of eight children. Her parents were extremely poor and did not have enough money to feed all the children. Elizabeth and the other two youngest children were placed in an orphanage. Elizabeth did not have contact with anyone in her family ever again. It was her life dream to have a family, which she did with her husband and two children. When he took the children and left, this experience took Elizabeth back to her own early abandonment, which left her devastated.

With all this information about Elizabeth's early life, having a deep appreciation for her current situation was more possible. In fact, because her mental state was so vulnerable and undefended, Elizabeth, herself, was able to connect the psychological dots between her past experiences and her current situation. She agreed that a brief stay in the inpatient psychiatric unit would benefit her. During her short stay in the hospital, she was able to enjoy a period of recompensation, stabilization, and reconnection with her therapist. With the support of the hospital treatment team and reconnecting with her outpatient therapist, Elizabeth was on a path to mourn the losses of these devastating experiences and adjust to creating a self-determined life worth living today. This process can take time, skill, intention, and optimism. It does, indeed, take a lot of effort, but the alternative is *The River* treatment plan, which can produce grim and disabling results.

For some, asking about both current complaints and early life is an obvious assessment method when working with people experiencing symptoms of psychosis. Assessing for content and subjective meaning of these intrapsychic constructs allows people to no longer be haunted and paralyzed by the past or compulsively and unconsciously forced to relive this unbearable trauma and to regain strength to create a self-determined life worth living.

COMMUNICATE CURIOSITY ABOUT WHAT HE OR SHE IS TRYING TO SAY

Many of the communications of people who experience acute symptoms of psychosis can seem mysterious and bizarre because stories are spoken through metaphor and with word association because of altered brain pathways, especially in the Broca's area, Wernicke's area, hippocampus, amygdala, and basal ganglia.

Helping Juan Find His Magic Portal

When Juan stated, "I want to go to Venezuela to find the cave that houses the magic portal," one could ask, "What could this person possibly be meaning?" That is just the attitude to take! What occurs more often than not in mainstream mental health treatment is this person is deemed incompetent to care for himself, and the guiding thought becomes that the most humane and immediate intervention is to increase the dose of his neuroleptic medication. With that action, the person is often physically and socially marginalized (i.e., put in a locked psychiatric hospital unit) until the medications take a sedative effect. Possibly, additional doses of medication are given until the person is cooperative. Subsequently, we just keep going along with the day, conducting the simple survival tasks of eating, bathing, toileting, laundry, and sleeping. The days turn into weeks and everyone goes along as though nothing out of the ordinary ever happened, all the while insisting that the person remain on the prescribed neuroleptic medication for the rest of his life. From the person's perspective, a meaningful opportunity for personal growth is thwarted. He quickly learns to not reveal any conversation or likeness of the magic portal. Sometimes, he can have the will to not talk about the magic portal; sometimes he cannot resist. When he cannot resist and talks about it to people with mental health legal authority, he runs the risk of losing some of his freedoms (i.e., forced neuroleptic medications, locked inpatient psychiatric units, social marginalization, etc.).

If accurate understanding and effective communication are our goals, we orient our interactions in a manner to embrace curiosity about Juan's thoughts and situation. We ask more questions about the magic portal: What does it mean? How long have you been looking for this? What will happen when you find it? We explore the details of the story and their meanings.

Mainstream mental health professionals are summarily socialized to not pursue delusional material, as doing so is considered a waste of time and only enables untrue content. Mainstream mental health clinicians consider delusional material as symptoms that ought to be minimized or, even better, stopped. Sometimes people worry that inquisitive probing of these stories can be perceived as intrusive or making the clinician appear unwise. Ironically, it is the vague therapeutic script of "Uh-huh, tell me more" that is experienced by clients as aloof and patronizing and results in people interpersonally disconnecting and emotionally shutting down for personal preservation.

An authentically curious interaction would engage the client and result in more accurate understanding so that healing becomes more of a realistic possibility. With some warm, committed, and curious interaction with Juan, he was able to reveal the meaning of the magic portal in Venezuela.

When Juan's mother died, he had an opportunity to explore and develop an identity and life of his own. Juan began seeking a far off, exotic, and unimaginable place/situation (Venezuela) where he could develop an identity and life of his own, which before seemed only possible through magic. When this meaning was accurately understood and interpreted back to Juan, the bizarre nature of his delusion softened and his actual dream of developing his own identity and reflective life was nurtured and actualized.

COMMUNICATE COMMITMENT OF AN UNCONDITIONAL AND HELPING ATTITUDE TOWARD THE PERSON

People who are at the mercy of receiving intervention from distressing symptoms of psychosis through the public mental health treatment delivery system are quite used to not being heard, understood, or handled with commitment, respect, and individualized care. With every engaging interaction, you may need to prove your commitment by overtly and repeatedly saying your intentions (i.e., I am here and I want to help you) until the person comes to be familiar and trusts you. This trust must be maintained by being consistent. This process may take an extended amount of time. Where there are losses, or therapeutic hiccups, such as being late for appointments or misunderstanding client intentions, the clinician or loved one must restate his or her commitment to the client. An example of this may be the following: "I am sorry that I did not understand what you were trying to say to me. I am here. I want to understand you. Can you try again to tell me about the magic portal?" When the interpretation is not accurate, the person may respond with frustration, disappointment, anger, anxiety, or even an increase in disorganization. We can easily understand this reaction. As with any intimate relationships, there will be gaps, conflicts, and bumps. The sustainability and strength of the intimacy lies in the committed and sensitive handling of these interpersonal encounters. Continue to express your commitment to listen, understand, and help. We have understood that people who live with psychotic experiences may have a tendency to feel rejected from society and isolate.

> The [mental health clinician's] presence becomes an antidote to the client's alienation, enhances morale, inspires the expectation of help, and creates a setting where constructive confrontation can eventually take place. Within this relationship, the client comes to appreciate the significance of internal and external limits in pursuing goals, improves reality testing, and experiences learning and enhanced self-esteem. (Walsh, 2011, para. 26)

Glide Memorial Church: A Most Unusual Celebration of Life

Glide Memorial Church, on Sundays, offers a most unusual celebration of life. A visit there is a must-do historical and social experience while in the great city of San Francisco.

From 1964 to 2000, Glide Memorial Church was under the direction of the Reverend Cecil Williams. Reverend Williams consistently included the LGBT community in his outreach efforts, advocacy, and spiritual discussions. His outreach efforts were also strongly impactful during the 1980s, when crack cocaine had a devastating impact on the African American community.

Today, Glide Memorial Church offers 87 social service programs to the San Francisco community. During the week, Glide is a social service center where people with trauma, addiction, homelessness, and poverty are brought back to a dignified and intentional self-determined life worth living. Their website reads, "A radically inclusive, just, and loving community mobilized to alleviate suffering and break the cycles of poverty and marginalization" ("Mission and Values"; see Appendix B).

Glide serves three free meals a day and offers mental and physical traditional and nontraditional healthcare, addiction counseling, job training, housing, child care, and parenting classes. At many other religious gatherings, the sanctuary fills to standing-room-only capacity with people from every imaginable and unimaginable walks of life who have at least one thing in common: the need to unburden pain resulting from being mistreated, judged, and marginalized. In passing any of these individuals on a public street, each person might make every effort to disguise the pain and get on with the day. However, in the sanctuary, there is an authentic outpouring of unconditional love, acceptance, and mutualization of emotional pain. Through inspirational songs, connections, and the telling of personal stories of trauma, loss, addiction, abuse, pain, and recovery, people are free to identify with this deep spiritual pain. With all of the magical affiliative dynamics in the room, people are spontaneously moved to bring this hidden pain out of hibernation, thus making opportunities to heal his and her spirits.

TRUST YOUR SOUND AND NATURAL CLINICAL JUDGMENT, ALSO KNOWN AS INTUITION

Fromm-Reichmann asserts that the clinician (and any interested person) who seeks accurate understanding should use her intuition to pay as much attention to what is said as to what is not said (1960). What part of the story is focused on and what is left out? What are the common themes? What is the related affect? What is the quality of the self—true self/false self?

Often, natural intuitive insights are discouraged, categorized as *soft, overly emotional*, or *ridiculous*. However, much of our organic communication is conducted through right-brain, unconscious, and intuitive energy. It is essential that intuitions be trusted and heard. The following story is an example of how intuition may have saved lives.

Get Out Now!

Ed reported auditory hallucinations commanding him to jump in front of a subway train and brought himself to a psychiatric emergency center within a general emergency department in a large teaching hospital. After Ed was medically cleared, he was to be evaluated for legal hold and treatment on an acute inpatient psychiatric unit. I spoke with the medical staff, receiving reports about Ed's needs and capacity for cooperation. They told me that he had been sleeping for hours and was cooperative when needed.

Several medical students and I entered the interview room, where Ed was sitting on the edge of a gurney. Standing across the room from Ed, I introduced myself and explained that the medical students were observing our conversation as a part of their training. Ed did not say anything, did not move a muscle, and did not even blink. However, I experienced an intense assault to my core, like one might feel right before slamming into a car that suddenly stopped ahead on the freeway. This interchange was unconscious, intense, and immediate. Gently and immediately, I herded the students out of the room, politely saying that we needed to check on something and would be in the next room. I secured the door. Each eager student asked, "What just happened? What was that about? We were all ready to observe a clinical interview!" I responded by saying, "I don't know, but it was time to get the Hell out of there! I think he was going to lose it, and someone was going to get hurt." Feeling like these eager students needed more of an explanation, I described my somatic sensation in my core; I felt as though I would vomit. Summarily, I told them that my intuition had saved my life in the past, and I just trust it without question. Operating from a scientifically linear perspective, the students skeptically raised their eyebrows. I have to admit, I felt vulnerable not being able to fully explain why I ended the interview so abruptly, especially when everything seemed to be perfectly arranged for an intake interview.

Ed signed himself in to the psychiatric hospital on the self-reported grounds of being imminently suicidal. I communicated my concerns to the receiving staff. Later that evening, when this patient was admitted to the inpatient acute psychiatric unit, he severely physically assaulted two male patients and three staff members. Somehow and unconsciously, he communicated his severely hostile intentions to me, as we had hardly begun the intake interview. Had I stopped to question the patient or, worse, my own intuitive sensations, that story would likely have ended quite differently than it did.

People can gain a great deal of conscious and unconscious information about a person by simply observing another. I have been known to be quite successful by betting at the horse track. I do not count numbers or follow any horse race statistics. I also do not pick the horse by a cutesy or superstitious name. And, I am not a horse whisperer. Nevertheless, I have enjoyed some small horse-betting success. So, how do I succeed? Before every heat, the horses and their jockeys perform a collection lineup by circling outside the racetrack. I carefully watch each and every horse. I look to see if their hair has been neatly brushed and if their mane is too tightly braided. I assess the relationship between the jockey and the horse: is the intimacy loving, aloof, controlling, distant, or nurturing? I assess the horses' energies and behaviors—is the horse rebelling, compliant, or feisty? Is the energy of the horse eager, lethargic, or distractible? Does the horse naturally walk in line or is his bridle constantly being jerked by his jockey? I pick the top three horses and place my $5 bet as a *trifecta box*, which means that I am guessing, without identifying order, the first three horses that will finish the race. Each day that I have bet, I have won at least one *trifecta box*, with winnings of $250–$850. My horse-betting secret is applying everything I know about conducting an inconspicuous mental status exam on a horse.

Sometimes when speaking with someone, I get a sense of his or her profound loneliness and deep wish for acceptance from someone, anyone. In case consultations, when the clinician is providing the client history and profile, often a huge explanatory chunk of the story is missing. Sometimes, clinicians can just get a sense of what that missing portion entails, such as the person was sexually abused or otherwise mistreated, abandoned, or traumatized by one or multiple people in his or her life. Intuitive revelations originate from immediate and unconscious disclosures of the right brain, and these themes and ideas are communicated through interpersonal connection. Trusting these communications will allow for deeper connection, accurate understanding, and more effective communications with everyone in our lives, including the people with whom we are attempting to help and heal.

REDRAW THE ENVIRONMENT-SYSTEM BOUNDARY TO INCLUDE AT LEAST THE NEXT RING OF PEOPLE AND SITUATIONS IN WHICH THE PERSON MOST INTIMATELY INTERACTS

We tend to extend the concept of *person-in-situation* to people in general. When a person is observed as having a hard time, one imagines what might have just happened to him or her to cause this emotional reaction. This concept of putting the person in his or her real context is borrowed from the classic theorist Harry Stack Sullivan (1968). Fromm-Reichmann asserts that exploring a person's "interpersonal dealings is "mandatory" to understand ego defenses, security operations, and the origins of the underpinning anxieties (Fromm-Reichmann, 1948). Alternatively, she asserts that the clinician must pay attention to the person's historical information to understand the contexts and origins of present-day meaning systems.

However, this same person-in-situation perspective is not extended to people who experience psychotic disorders. Consequentially, inaccurate conclusions are made, assuming that the person is intensely emotional and disorganized all the time.

Since 2006, when intense gentrification accelerated in downtown Los Angeles, the residents of Skid Row have been harassed out of their community. These people took up new homes in the surrounding neighborhoods. I am well acquainted with the homeless individuals who share a neighborhood with me. One day, while riding in the car with my family, we stopped at a red traffic light. In the distance, I noticed a disheveled man carrying many bags, cursing, and flailing his arms. I curiously thought to myself, "Hmmmm. I have not noticed this man around before." I assumed he was hearing persecutory voices and arguing with them, even physically fighting with them to preserve his ideal self. The long red light turned to green, and traffic flowed in a different direction. He dashed across the street, just missing the oncoming traffic. I worried for his safety. Just then, I noticed that he caught the attention of an oncoming bus and hopped on. To my surprise, he had been flailing his arms to catch the attention of the bus driver. The next bus would not come for another 40 minutes.

I made many mistakes in this story. First, I assumed that this disheveled man was hearing persecutory auditory hallucinations with which he was verbally and physically fighting. Furthermore, I had not imagined what he might have been reacting to, redrawing and expanding his environment-system boundary. Had I looked around at the more immediate context, I might have noticed the moving bus he was desperately trying to catch. By including the person in his environment, we have a better chance of a more accurate understanding of his expressions and communications.

People with mental illnesses and psychotic disorders have some of the same situational and interpersonal stressors that we all do and some unique ones, too. Sometimes these situations may have just occurred. Sometimes these historical situations have made deep neurophysiological and psychological imprints. The meanings are real and alive, and the person is actively responding to them. Redrawing the environment system boundary to include the meanings of these past and present situations will contribute to more accurate understandings of expressions.

PLACE THE PERSON IN HIS OR HER CONTEXT BY USING VICARIOUS INTROSPECTION TO LISTEN FOR CHARACTERISTICS, FEELINGS, SITUATIONS, AND DYNAMICS

In addition to imagining the person in his or her context, we also imagine how the person may be reacting to contextual surroundings. As stated, psychotic communications can be difficult to understand because people communicate by way of metaphor and word association, which travels in unexpected brain pathways. Once the context is accurately understandable, next we understand the associated emotions. Alternatively, sometimes, we first understand the emotion and then the context details are more attainable. Nevertheless, there are rich opportunities to accurately understand both context and emotion, and these are the points at which healing can begin.

DECODE THE SYMBOL

The person experiencing psychosis unexpectedly alternates from the concrete to abstract metaphorical thinking and expression (Cullburg, 2006). Alternative brain functioning, discussed in Chapter 7, "The Relationship Between Neurobiology and Psychosis," prevents the person from accurately accessing word choices, so he speaks in close, but not accurate, word associations and metaphor. For accurate understanding, we must *desymbolize* the words (Searles, 1979).

Allow for marginal thoughts, or nonlinear or loosely associated expressions, as their exploration may connect the past to present-day repeated situations and emotions. Allowing a person in acute psychosis to just free associate will make no progress, as these free associations have no meaningful grounding root. These associations will simply be ideas without meaning. To achieve accurate understanding, we put the person in context and use that context to inform the imagination about what the person is attempting to say. By establishing a trusting brief or lengthy relationship with the person at the center of concern, others have the privilege of insight into the common and meaningful contextual life of the person who lives with psychotic experiences. The interpretations are not rushed, but patiently accepted with curiosity, which allows for the empathy that Semrad (1955) asserted was necessary, the prioritizing of relationship over intellectual comprehension that Fromm-Reichmann (1952) emphasized, and Havens's (1996) transmission of acceptance.

In addition to environmental context, to achieve accurate understanding, we pay attention to physical sensations, their origins, and timing. The body often experiences unconscious emotions before they are registered in the conscious mind, called psychosomatization. Exploring these physical sensations can uncover deeply rooted and often conflictual, dissociated, or repressed psychological material that motivates a person in their current interpersonal relationships, situations, and subjective perspectives.

> By interpretation the (mental health clinician) translates into the language of awareness, thereby bringing into the open what the patient communicates to him without being conscious of its contents or of its dynamics, revealing connections with other experiences, or various implications pertaining to its historical or present emotional background. It is frequently not the actual events and happenings in the previous lives of patients to which they have become oblivious, but rather the emotional reactions accompanying these events or engendered by them. Consequently, these connections and concomitant emotional experiences and not the events themselves often need interpretive clarification. (Fromm-Reichmann, 1968, p. 80)

The psychological material has become dissociated and forgotten because the person has deemed these memories to be too painful to have in her consciousness. It is only with the help of another that she is able to bring this into her conscious mind and make conscious choices. Additionally, not all dissociated material needs to be interpreted and made conscious. Just as in the broader population, some people just do not want to consciously know about the content of such painful material.

Choosing to not disturb the distressing memories may be adaptive. What is the saying? Let sleeping dogs lie.

Fromm-Reichmann asserted that the person experiencing psychosis understands what is on his mind (1968). When this private language is communicated in a right-brain, nonlinear manner, it is the listener (clinician, friend/family member) who needs these ideas decoded so the person may be accurately understood. Fromm-Reichmann asserted that it is not necessary that every dream, thought, and situation be interpreted but to understand that each has subjective meaning in the mind of the experiencing person. Patients, like people in general, are largely forgiving when approached with frankness, honesty, and respect. Once we have decoded the ideas and accurately understood, we are in a position to collaboratively discuss what to do, if anything, about these feelings and situations.

The communications of people with psychotic symptoms can and should be understood. Even when the clinician gets the interpretations wrong and the client feels misunderstood or the clinician can convey commitment and a warm willingness to try again, the client's perception of *expert* encourages the client's trust in the effectiveness of the therapeutic relationship (Sullivan, 1947). It is through the work of *Listening with Psychotic Ears* that we have the opportunities to *resymbolize* the contexts and communications of people with psychotic experiences who are asking for help (Searles, 1979).

PEOPLE WITH PSYCHOTIC DISORDERS FEEL THE SAME EMOTIONS AS DO OTHERS

Irena was walking down the street and saw a man who had all the *tellings* of unregulated schizophrenia: jumping about and hollering quotations from the Bible. As she approached him, Irena timidly walked around him, allowing for a wide girth, hoping he would not notice her. She walked further down the street to the busy street corner, where she noticed there had just been a severe collision of several cars. The ambulance had just arrived, and the paramedics were helping the injured onto the gurneys. People were covered in blood and crying. Irena was terribly worried about them. Even though she did not know any of the victims, she began to cry as she was reminded of how quickly severe accidents can occur. Immediately, she thought of her own family members. She said a quick prayer that each injured person would recover. Something told Irena to go back to the man she had just tried to avoid.

As she approached him, she saw that he was talking to an imaginary person. Having just heard about *Listening with Psychotic Ears*, she walked even closer, wanting to hear exactly what he was saying. She was able to *decode* the following story: The man saw the cars collide and one truck lift from the ground and land on its side onto the roof of another car with passengers. He intensely worried about the people in the cars and was praying that God would hold each one safe in His arms. That is not exactly what he was saying as Irena passed him, as he was jumping about and reciting sections of the Bible, but she was able to make this interpretation and accurately understand his seemingly bizarre expressions by using the skills of *Listening with Psychotic Ears*.

Irena and the man were reacting to the same situation with very similar feelings and prayer for the injured. As we ask the person with psychosis to explain his story, we can use vicarious introspection to wonder how we might feel in that person's situation. Surprisingly, or not, people who experience symptoms of psychosis often feel very similar emotions as others. The feelings are just bigger and may get expressed in unexpected directions.

STAY CONNECTED TO THE AFFECT THE SYMBOL AND DYNAMIC REPRESENTS

Consider your primal reactions to snakes. I see them as a sneaky and accurate predator. I am both disgusted by and phobic of snakes. What are your initial reactions about the colors of bright orange or dark olive green? Other random things like limousines? Trees? Whole bodies of literature have been developed to document common associations with people, places, things, and situations. Freud used this information to interpret the dreams of his patients (Freud, 1913). Jung used this information in his work on archetypes, word associations, and symbols with his patients (Jung, 1968).

As we attempt to decode the details of both context and emotions, we entertain common possible experiences of people with mental illness. We consider the possibility that this person has experienced significant stigma, discrimination, and marginalization because of mental illness and iatrogenic trauma as a result of mental healthcare treatment. Older patients tend to have more experiences with neuroleptic medications and frequent, long, and mandated stays in psychiatric hospitals where everything was structured. Being categorized as a *mental* patient, with all the stigmatic myths that accompany it, causes a person to be socially, financially, geographically, and interpersonally marginalized. This marginalization is easily internalized, and, as Goffman (1961) asserted with the term "interactional sociology," alters a person's identity, which, in turn, alters his interactions with the world. As you are making attempts to decode the communications of a person with psychosis, entertain the very real possibility that the person is continuing to express the residual, alive, and strong feelings of past and current traumatic experiences.

TRUST IN THE PERSON'S RATIONAL SIDE, AS WELL AS THEIR SPIRITUAL/EXISTENTIAL SIDE

An erroneous assumption is that children, the elderly, and people with psychotic experiences do not know what is going on around them. Some would argue the opposite. If you want to know the truth about what is going on around you, ask a child, the most elderly person, or a person with psychosis. Children do not always have language to describe (or distract), but intuitively feel interpersonal energy, causing them to naïvely tell the truth. Children are not yet socialized to hold their tongues. Some elderly people are so fed up with conflict and inauthenticity that they seemingly tune out. But, just ask what is going on, and he or she who is not oppressed by the judgments of others will say the truth. The person with psychotic experiences, for better or worse, says what is on his or her mind. This may originate from a thinner repression barrier or because social marginalization is already a reality, so the threat of social rejection is no longer feared.

People with psychosis have similar experiences to those that others have. He or she eats, sleeps, pays bills, watches TV, and is impacted by government politics, time, sickness, joy, dreams, and death. Take seriously the wonderment of explanations of why these experiences might be happening to this person, in this family, in this community, in this point in history.

Just a Hallucination

Billy, a 22-year-old man, was brought to the hospital emergency department by the police because he was talking to himself and agitated. Billy was evaluated by a physician and several interns, who deemed him as medically cleared, asserting that he had no acute medical problems that necessitated treatment.

Then, Billy was brought to the emergency psychiatric center for evaluation, treatment, and placement. Billy could not sit still, scratching his head, arms, and feet. After introducing our purpose and myself, I asked him why he was scratching. He muttered that he did not know why. Seeing that he was terribly uncomfortable and out of sorts, I went back to the medical staff and asked them what they thought this aggressive scratching was about. I was told that it was "a hallucination and there was nothing more to be done." Surprised by this answer, I went back into the room with Billy, who continued to scratch. We tried to begin our assessment, and it was so obvious that Billy was extremely uncomfortable. I asked him to show me where it itched the most. He said all over but especially his head and feet. I went back to the medical staff and requested a physician come to reevaluate Billy. They refused. Seeing that Billy's medical needs were not being taken seriously, I went back to Billy and asked him if I could take a peek at where he was itching. I looked first in his socks. Immediately, I saw tiny lice bugs moving around. I then looked in his hair and saw lice. I went back to the medical staff and reported what I had found. I requested medicine to treat Billy. The chief physician said, "Isn't he going to another hospital? Can't he wait and let them treat him there?" First, this meant Billy would be acutely uncomfortable for another 6–10 hours before he could be treated at the next hospital. Additionally, this meant that Billy would remain contagious to everyone with whom he interacted in this hospital, in the ambulance that would transport him, and everyone in the next hospital. I demanded that he be treated immediately. I was given two bottles of Rid, a de-lice medication. Together, Billy and I treated his lice before transferring him to another psychiatric hospital.

Just a Somatic Hallucination

Sara, a 29-year-old woman, had just begun her mental health treatment by seeing a social work intern at her community mental health center. Each time they met, Sara would complain about her intestines falling out each time she had a bowel movement. She explained how she had to "push the tissue back inside." Sara coped with this embarrassment and physical pain by severely minimizing her food intake so her feces would be infrequent and tinier. She had been to one physician, and before a physical exam was conducted, Sara was categorically dismissed as crazy. Believing Sara, the social work intern escorted her to another physician. The physician took a quick peek but concluded that this was a somatic hallucination because there was no physical evidence. The social work intern persisted, escorted Sara to another physician, and firmly requested a comprehensive evaluation. This physician was able to locate evidence of trauma and diagnosed Sara with a prolapsed bowel. An adult male had sodomized Sara when she was 7. This medical diagnosis rationally and spiritually validated both her physical and psychological pain. Sara was given appropriate medical treatment and relief from this pain.

As much as I am emphasizing that we make every attempt to accurately know what is going on in the life and spirit of the person who experiences psychosis, we must also expand tolerance of not knowing things for certain and let go of controlling others and situations. Asking and probing are necessary to collect all possible information, but there are times in which some or even most of the details will not be known. Still, we proceed with commitment, gentleness, respect, and compassion. We expand our capacity for patience.

Alternatively, do not go overboard in getting accustomed to *Listening with Psychotic Ears*. People who experience psychosis do not always speak in metaphor and will communicate quite linearly and logically. The effective listener needs to be able to listen with both sides of the brain: the left bringing linear and logical conclusions, and the right brining creative, tonal, and holistic conclusions.

TRUST, RESPECT, AND ACCURATELY UNDERSTAND INNATE ATTACHMENT NEEDS IN THERAPEUTIC AND OTHER INTIMATE RELATIONSHIPS

Humans are hardwired for interpersonal relationships. Being in relationship is a vital need like sleep, breathing, eating, and waste elimination that cannot be denied or else the person will perish. Much Fromm-Reichmann's writing addresses the client's dependency needs and fear of destroying the relationship on which the client can depend (1960, 1974). The interpersonal and social marginalization that so frequently occurs among people who experience psychosis can leave a person starving for interpersonal affection, causing an exacerbation of mental and physical symptoms. Upon entering into a therapeutic relationship, he or she brings innate desires for relationship, along with the negative results of all previous meaningful relationships. Wishing for a positive intimate therapeutic relationship with the therapist, his or her wise mind or implicit memory (hippocampus and amygdala) will caution him or her out of fear of, again, being rejected and disappointed.

Sharing a relationship with a person who experiences psychosis should embody the same rules of engagement that a relationship with any person would embody. In her book *The Center Cannot Hold: My Journey Through Madness* (2008), Elyn Saks writes of an experience she had with her analyst, Mrs. Jones, of several years. Elyn was leaving England and Oxford University to return to the United States to attend Yale Law School. The therapeutic relationship with Mrs. Jones that had so accurately held Elyn had come to an end. The following excerpt is a summary of one of Saks's experiences. You can imagine how you might feel and how Elyn might have felt.

ELYN SAKS: You will not leave me. I will kidnap you and keep you in my closet. I will give you nice clothes and good food. You will give me psychoanalysis on demand.

HER (MRS. JONES, ANALYST): You want to deny I am a separate person from you. You want to control me. It is too painful that I have my own life, outside of yours.

ME: You are mine. You have no choice. My every wish is your command.

Most of my refusal to accept the passage of time was talked about, and not acted upon. But the impending loss of Mrs. Jones when I was to leave Oxford and return to the United States to go to the Yale Law School led to behavioral acting out. I could not bear the thought of losing Mrs. Jones. I started locking myself in her bathroom after sessions and not leaving, which led to her analyst-husband, Dr. Brandt, removing the lock on the door. I would stand outside her home office and rock in place. In the evening, I would drive to the end of her block and spend time in the vacant lot thinking how I will get to stay with her. I would deliver gifts through her mail slot—things like twigs.

The very last day I was to see her, I left her consulting room and went straight to her waiting room and wouldn't leave. I began sobbing (I am someone who almost never sheds a tear). She and her husband came in and said I had to leave—that my being there would upset other patients.

ME: I can't leave. I will die if I leave. I must stay, stay. Stay.

HER: The time has come for your sessions to end. You need to go home now.

ME: I'm not leaving. I can't.

THEM: You have to.

ME: No.

HER: We need to call the police.

HIM: They'll just take her to a mental hospital.

Mrs. Jones and Dr. Brandt attempted physically to remove me from their waiting room. I grabbed hold of the pipes along the wall. He was pushing me, she was pulling my hair. I was wailing—indeed, screaming at the top of my lungs.

They then left me to take their next patients. I spent the day in Mrs. Jones' waiting room sobbing. At the end of the day, Dr. Brandt came in and said if I didn't leave now he would have to call the police. Mrs. Jones was downstairs waiting to say good-bye.

I went down and hugged Mrs. Jones, sobbing loudly. She pat patted me on the back and said, "Take courage, Elyn, take courage."

My flight back to the States left the next day. I sobbed the whole way home. From time to time, I considered asking the flight attendant whether she would mind if I jumped out the emergency door. (Saks, 2008, pp. 113–116)

This is an example of a person's extreme reaction to an impending deep and meaningful loss. Time was passing, and an ongoing relationship was passing with it. There was an omnipotent effort to halt the passage of time and prevent the change. Like all defenses, these efforts were bound to fail.

Saks stated that accepting the loss of her analyst and moving on took a year, a five-month hospitalization, medication, and a new therapist to talk this loss through. She did go back to Oxford and was able to say her good-byes to Mrs. Jones in a manner that she was able to express her sadness and this brought her dignity (Saks, 2008).

We see that Elyn felt the same feelings that any person would feel in any situation involving the loss of someone important or special, but her expression of those feelings were more magnified. But, as suggested by Fromm-Reichmann (1974), her feelings came out larger and sometimes from unexpected directions. Fortunately, Mrs. Jones was able to accurately understand Elyn's despair as a reaction to the impending termination of their relationship, respect where those feelings originated, and interpret them to Elyn. Still, Elyn needed to be kept safe in psychiatric hospitalization.

Many times, the clinician or family member is one of very few, if not the only one, who can be trusted and is reliable and dependable. This person is breathing life and exercising all of his or her fragile, fierce, and abundant relationship needs with you.

These relationship dynamics must be trusted as natural, accurately understood, and respected. Because people who experience psychosis often express the same feelings as others, just more flamboyantly (i.e., sobbing for several days) and sometimes sideways (i.e., giving farewell gifts of twigs through the analyst's mail slot), accurate understanding and care will require additional clinical skills, such as those identified in the *Listening with Psychotic Ears* philosophy.

VALIDATE YOUR ASSUMPTIONS WITH THE PERSON

Accurate understanding requires validation with the other person, not just assuming that your interpretation of meaningful connections in the person's story or about his or her behavior is the correct one. Remember Gene, the man who had not had mental health treatment in over 20 years? He brought himself to the psychiatric emergency room because he was experiencing auditory hallucinations commanding him to take his own life. In the beginning of the conversation, his speech was incredibly disorganized and difficult to comprehend. It took him all of 2 hours to fill out an intake form with his name, address, health insurance, and request for help. The following is a transcript from my conversation with Gene:

GENE: I have taken Thorazine, Lithium, Haldol, Stelazine, Cogentin, Depakote, Trilafon, Mellaril. I have tried a lot since the 1980s.

CLINICIAN: Do you take any medications now?

GENE: Not since the 1990s.

CLINICIAN: Why did you stop?

GENE: Doctors are teachers and patients are doctors. I considered the medications to not be appropriate treatment, action, cure, healing.

CLINICIAN: Why was the medication not appropriate treatment for you?

GENE: I took the prescriptions as I was told, every six hours, 12 hours, 18, and 24 hours. I took it for far too long, long as a dog's tail. Are there no other possibilities?

CLINICIAN: Did the medication help you at all, and did you experience side effects?

GENE: Do you know about the Physician's Desk Reference? I am well versed in the Physician's Desk Reference. The Physician's Desk reference lists A–Z side effects. Quickly, you reach a point of no return. There are many and varied side effects, lots and lots of side effects. I was able to tolerate all that I was experiencing for two decades without the medications. Just lately, I was slip sliding away. Doctors ought to be teachers and patients ought to be doctors. I was employed by a rehab center. I worked 11 pm to 7 am. I was lifted by a 6 foot 4 man, a big guy. Is a hospital for osteopathic reasons? He came to me and caught me by the bees knees. I had a dislocated bilateral. It was recurrent. I had one, two, three operations. I couldn't bend my knee. It was black and blue. It was stiff and sore, stiff as a brick, swollen the size of a cantaloupe.

CLINICIAN: Did you get help?

GENE: Yes. I had physical therapy for a year, Mondays and Thursdays—these are my days of the week. I was able to experience an increase in my range of motion. When that was over, at the grocery store where I bought my bread and milk, the black mat at the front door was used to prop open the door. There was a defective sidewalk. Both feet fell. I had muscular trauma bilateral to my knees and elbows. It was the same grocery store where I bought my bread and milk. I almost put my head through the plate glass. There were tests, exams, samples, x-rays, and assessments. There were no firm conclusive evidence, no official diagnosis. I had a lot of symptoms, double vision, nausea, spots, dizziness, stiff, and headaches.

CLINICIAN: So, you tripped on the black mat that was used to prop open the door at the grocery? Sounds like you were severely hurt and had to have lots of tests, surgeries, and physical therapy. Do you still have those symptoms?

GENE: Headaches, lots of headaches still. Yes. I even have migraines in the neck, head, humerus, clavicle, femur, fibula, tibia, foot, and ankle. I have been coming to the doctor for those symptoms. They recommended for me to get psychiatric treatment. I have a stack of business cards this thick [showing 2 inches]. There are a thousand doctors and new $5 billion new hospitals. They say I am a prospective patient for tests, exams, samples, and examples. They give me back and brain procedures. I have an appointment the day after tomorrow.

CLINICIAN: Do you want to come here to this hospital for help?

GENE: What sort of help, assistance, support, aid, or benefits do you have to offer?

CLINICIAN: We could offer you several things. First, we have someone who you could talk to about the things that are on your mind.

GENE: That sounds great, terrific, fantastic, and ecstatic.

CLINICIAN: Another thing you could get here are medications.

GENE: [BURP!!!] After dark, when the sun goes down. He was 6 foot 4 and weighed 280 pounds. I was attacked! I weighed 180 pounds. I was attacked by a doctor, a physician, a psychiatrist by overmedicating, by overmedicating, by overmedicating. They were busy as bees. It was a J-O-B. I looked in the white and yellow pages. There was no criminal liability. They were overworked and underpaid and got lost in the universe. I thought that might have been the case two decades ago. Medications, medications, medications! I am well versed in the Physician's Desk Reference. I am aware!

CLINICIAN: Are you trying to say that you are scared that the hospital staff and doctors will, against your will, inject you with medicines that physically hurt and leave you feeling groggy and confused?

When we make attempts to validate what the person is saying, sometimes, desperate and uncomfortable, he or she will holler out of frustration, "Hell no! That is not what I am saying!" In Gene's case, he loudly burped as if to emphasize a strong emotion. He especially burped when I got wrong a part or all of what he was saying.

Sometimes, the clinician will accurately catch on to a piece of the content. Sometimes, the volatile psychotic person will look you right into your eyes, exhale, and say, "Yes. Yes! That is what I am trying to say." And, with this continuing accurate understanding of the person, you can witness the anxiety deflating and him or her being able to access a linear and logical method of communicating right before your eyes and without neuroleptic medication. Gene's situation was no different.

I listened a lot, verified what he was saying, and offered psychiatric resources. He did not always like what I had to say or thought I got it wrong, to which he always responded with a loud burp. Sometimes, I got it right, and he felt heard, validated, and soothed. To those feelings, he also responded with a loud burp. By the end of our conversation, Gene stopped saying the five synonyms at the end of every sentence and became more linear in his thoughts and speech. However, he did not stop burping, and that was OK with me. I came to rely on his burping as a decoding tool. It takes a long time to overcome 25 years of anger at the mental health treatment delivery system. The healing work with Gene had begun and would be ongoing.

NORMALIZE USUAL FEELINGS, REACTIONS,
AND SITUATIONS WITH VALIDATION AND THOUGHTFUL
AND APPROPRIATE HUMOR

Nonhuman Statue Attempts CPR

Mutual and thoughtful humor can level the interpersonal playing field and allow for a fresh sense of intimacy. Recently, I presented this *Listening with Psychotic Ears* content in a poster setting at a conference called "Tools for Change," aimed at fostering collaboration between professionals and people with mental illness. A woman approached my poster, stopped, and stared at it. As I turned to her, she quickly said, "I have that, psychotic ears." I think what she meant was that she has experienced symptoms of psychosis. We chatted about my material momentarily before she shared the following story:

She had been meeting with a psychiatrist and felt as though she was talking to an unresponsive statue. Needless to say, she was not feeling him or connected to the therapeutic relationship that she so desired. At the beginning of one session, she pulled from her backpack a plush monkey toy she had shaven with a razor. She held it up for the psychiatrist to see.

PSYCHIATRIST (P): What is this?
CLIENT (C): What do you think it is?
P: It looks non-human. It scares me.

This is precisely the reaction that the client wanted. She had been feeling, for duration of her meetings with the psychiatrist, that she had been talking to an unresponsive nonhuman, which left her feeling emotionally and spiritually shut down and nonhuman, as well. She was scared for her well-being. She was looking for some way to emotionally shock the psychiatrist into being present with her.

I asked the woman what happened next. She told me she left the psychiatrist's office that day with an increased dose in her psychiatric medication. I asked her how long she continued with that nonhuman unresponsive statue of a psychiatrist. She said that soon after, she fired him and found someone else. I supported her decision by telling her that it may have saved her life and spirit. We shared a meaningful smile. She went on to say that she had found a different psychiatrist and a therapist with whom she works and feels heard and helped. With this understanding and support, she is now very active in creating a self-determined life worth living for herself and others through her peer-support work.

Maynard Rides with His Friends to a Party in a Limousine

In my university-based courses, I teach about working with people with psychosis, and I make a special effort to bring in guest speakers to tell their personal stories. On one occasion, I invited Maynard. On the day of the class, he did not show up. After the class, we spoke on the phone, in which he informed me that his brother had just committed suicide, and he was traveling to Iowa to be with his family. He all but begged me not to forget about him and promised that he would call when he returned. As promised, 2 weeks later, he called wanting to schedule a time to speak to my class.

Maynard and his friend/assistant arrived 30 minutes before the class. We checked in. As I do with any guest speaker, I welcomed him by asking him if he found the location OK and whether he needed anything. He sat down and explained to me that while driving, he had to pull off the freeway to catch his breath, also explaining that his left arm felt numb. Because my family member had recently experienced a stroke, I was familiar with some of the symptoms. I explained to him that it was urgent that he be evaluated by a medically trained professional. He refused, saying he really wanted to keep his commitment to my class and me. We went back and forth for about 15 minutes. He refused to go to the hospital. Attempting to assess his bilateral facial muscular ability, I asked him to smile. He had calmed down and seemed OK, though I continued to be watchful for any symptoms. He gave a jaw dropping, show-stopping performance, going through a skit about his wish to ride with his friends to a party in a limousine. The audience was left asking, "Is this a real story of Maynard's bizarre life, or was this all a hallucination?" This reaction was precisely what Maynard had hoped for.

After the performance, I checked in with Maynard again, asking him about his physical symptoms. While he reported that he was OK, he finally agreed to allow me to call for an ambulance to take him to a nearby hospital so a medical professional could properly evaluate him. I waited with him and chatted. I stayed close to the paramedics so they would not disrespect Maynard. "On 3, we lift," one paramedic said to his partner; "1, 2, 3," and up went the gurney with Maynard strapped down. His eyes invited me close to him. He thanked me for taking him seriously. It meant a lot to him that he would fulfill his promise to my class and me. I took his hands in mine. I paused for a really long moment and thought before I spoke the next sentence. Feeling a sense of closeness with Maynard, I said, "Now, you finally get that limousine ride with your friend!" Together, we roared with laughter. Later that night, I called Maynard to check on my colleague. He reported that he had gone to the hospital, had a full medical workup, and, since all the physical tests came back stable, was released. Using thoughtful and appropriate humor with Maynard created a balance in our relationship, possibly helping to normalize his circumstances and empower his sense of worth. We can normalize feelings, reactions, and situations with validation and through the use of thoughtful and appropriate humor.

BRAINSTORM ABOUT APPROPRIATE, RELEVANT, AND FEASIBLE SOLUTIONS, INCLUDING NEUROLEPTIC MEDICATION, SOCIAL SUPPORT, FAMILY CONNECTIONS, THE USE OF WORK, AND OTHER RESOURCES

People come in to mental health treatment facilities for help with feelings and situations to which, on their own, they have not been able to find solutions. To avoid the label of "mental patient" and the entire associated stigma, people usually try many things before seeking mental health treatment. Interventions that are initially tried include religious activities (i.e., talking to a pastor, attending church services, reading religious literature, and prayer) and using alcohol or drugs.

Because of the focus on neuroleptic medications as the first solution to psychotic symptoms, many treatment agencies go as far as having and enforcing a policy that states if a person does not take the medication as prescribed, they cannot receive any other services through that facility. Why are neuroleptic medications continually pushed? There are many reasons for this trend.

In the studies that were independent of pharmaceutical company funding and influence, Whitaker (2011) uncovered astounding conclusions about the outcomes of neuroleptic medications on mental health treatment consumers. Some of the main findings of those studies are summarized here.

Before delving into those studies, thought, it should be clearly noted that some people find benefit from the use of neuroleptic medications. The intention of this discussion is not to discourage any treatment that individuals deem effective. In fact, many people (psychiatrists, patients, and families) have reported decreases in psychotic symptoms after taking antipsychotic medications as prescribed. Similarly, some people say the medications have changed their lives for the better and they cannot live without them. Still, others have a different report.

The *long-term* outcome studies of chronic administration of antipsychotic medications are quite grim. Study after study shows the outcomes in schizophrenic samples that have taken antipsychotic medications and those who have not (or taken placebo medications). Among those who have taken the medications, the following outcomes are observed: more likely to have more relapses with greater severity, more frequent hospitalizations, persistent and intensifying psychotic symptoms, nausea, vomiting, diarrhea, agitation, insomnia, headaches, unusual motor tics (tardive dyskinesia), emotional numbness, lethargy, social dependency (including Social Security benefits, Medicare, and Medicaid), lack of motivation, and social disengagement (Bockoven et al., 1975; Gardos & Cole, 1977). Additionally, the higher the dose, the greater the probability and severity of these symptoms and relapse (Prein, 1971). Furthermore, as stated, people who are chronically administered antipsychotic medications experience early death, dying 15 to 25 years earlier than individuals who have not ingested psychotropic medications (Morgan, 2003). People with severe mental illness (SMI) are dying of cardiovascular ailments, respiratory problems, metabolic illness, diabetes, and kidney failure (Whitaker, 2011).

Despite the promising results of neuroleptic medications, the United States has seen a significant increase in the rates of disability consumption, such as Social Supplemental Income (SSI) and Social Supplemental Disability Income (SSDI), because of mental illness. Despite the vast availability and assured effects of neuroleptic medications, one cannot help to question the obvious failure of this mainstream practice when quality of life is not improving.

Most patients with mental illness cannot afford to pay for their neuroleptic treatment on their own and look to insurance reimbursement to cover the rapidly increasing costs. Mental health treatment providers, agencies, and hospitals need to get paid. If services are offered beyond what insurance companies will pay, the treatment provider consumes the cost of the already dispensed treatment and services. Mental health treatments are then organized around the nature and time by which insurance companies will and will not reimburse. Insurance companies want the quickest and cheapest intervention, and to them, neuroleptic medication represents the winning option. All other mainstream mental health treatments are delivered surrounding the consumption of neuroleptic medications.

However, neuroleptic medications have not been the omnipotent magic bullet that everyone, including consumers, hoped they would be. In the process of writing this book, I have had the privilege of speaking to many people who have psychotic experiences and no financial choice but to seek their treatments from mainstream public mental health treatment agencies. The topic of medications always arises early and often in our conversations.

What I have found are that there are typically four categories of responses to medications: (1) "Medications have saved my life and allow me to have a normal life." These reactions are present but few and far between; (2) "I take the medications because they help for the short term, but I do not like the way I feel. I do not take as much as I am prescribed"; (3) "The meds make me emotionally numb, and I feel like a vegetable. They give me really bad side effects that are both temporary and permanent. I want off of them, but I have no one to turn to"; and (4) "I don't take that shit." Most of the people I speak to are recovering from the mental health treatment delivery system as much as recovering from mental illness. Many are active advocates for themselves and others like them.

Many clients report serious side effects from medication use, such as emotional numbing, sexual dysfunction, organ damage, a decreased sense of pleasure, tremors, extreme dry mouth, acute allergic reactions (e.g., extrapyramidal symptoms), and serious weight gain, which causes a host of other serious medical conditions. Clients report that the medications lose their efficacy, especially the longer one takes them. These findings are validated by the empirical studies summarized by Whitaker (2011).

A large portion of people who are prescribed neuroleptic medications wish for an effective alternative to manage the symptoms of mental illness, especially psychosis and mood alterations. Even Gene, in his extremely disabling disorganization, lucidly requested any other treatment alternatives. After a few dramatic acute psychotic decompensations, people sometimes come to the position that neuroleptic medications are a *necessary evil*. Almost everyone I have spoken to wishes for other types of effective and humane interventions and want reduced doses of, if not being taken completely off, the neuroleptic medications prescribed.

LISTENING WITH PSYCHOTIC EARS CAN BE USED AT VARIOUS LEVELS OF CARE, INCLUDING CRISIS INTERVENTION AND LONG-TERM INDIVIDUAL PSYCHOTHERAPY

A great deal of professional literature on the topic of work with people who experience psychosis focuses on experiences after stabilization has been achieved, often with the use of psychotropic medications and traditional communication methods. "Psychotic clients can and should be engaged in working relationships even when the active symptoms are prominent, as they may retain or experience recurrences of psychotic ideation throughout the intervention" (Walsh, 2011, para. 3). As the mental health profession moves toward evidence-based interventions, the value and discussion of therapeutic relationship-building has been pushed aside. Professional literature that specifically deals with the therapeutic relationship shows that considering the tone and quality of the therapeutic relationship is necessary for positive outcomes. Hewitt and Coffey (2005) conducted a literature review of therapeutic working relationships with people who live with schizophrenia and found that when clients experience empathy, positive regard, and facilitative efforts, they have more favorable outcomes.

When a person is in an acute mental decompensation and in more private existential wonderment, the clinical skills of *Listening with Psychotic Ears* can be used. The majority of my revelations have come from my work with clients in psychiatric emergency settings, acute psychiatric hospital units, and extended residential treatment facilities. These skills have been and are widely used in long-term psychotherapy with clients who have psychotic experiences. Psychotherapy can be useful with individuals who experience psychosis in helping to understand their past, expand their present situations and perceptions, and develop future goals (Rhodes & Jakes, 2009).

Fromm-Reichmann offers essential suggestions for long-term clinical work for the purpose of healing from the distress of psychosis (1960, 1974):

Taking the required time is essential in establishing an appropriate conclusion of the person's situation and course of treatment. If there is not enough time, and there often is not in our fast-paced and funded-oriented world, another interview should be scheduled before conclusions are made, as these conclusions have major impact. "He (the mental health treatment provider) cannot take care of the responsibility of deciding the future course of events in another human being's life and the possibilities of bringing forth changes in another person's life if he is pressed for time" (Fromm-Reichmann, 1960, p. 48).

Collaboratively, the client and clinician should agree on the problems (at least one) and the course of action. In the medical model, the mental health clinician does the assessment, decides on what the problems are, prioritizes them, and decides on the course of action. This style is fertile ground for an authoritarian power differential, which is disempowering for the client. Furthermore, Fromm-Reichmann asserts that the intervention method of choice should be explained to, not just conducted on, the patient. Yes, the teaching does take a bit of time, but it is necessary for the client to fully understand what he or she is engaging in and working toward. Having taken the necessary time on the front end will allow for authentic, rapid, and ongoing healing work because trust and style are already established (Fromm-Reichmann, 1960).

Clinicians should be conservative about assigning a diagnosis. Diagnoses have so many associations, often negative and discouraging, for people who receive them. Much of what people know about the treatment of mental illnesses is obtained through movies and other media and is inaccurate, stereotyping, and myth-making. Many people do not know of contemporary and effective treatment methods. Young people will remember an older family member, maybe an uncle or grandmother, who received ECT or neuroleptic medications that carried severe and negative side effects or was hospitalized against his or her will for long periods. When a person receives a psychiatric diagnosis, this new identity becomes everything that has ever been associated with the diagnosis (Fromm-Reichmann, 1960).

A diagnosis should be used to accurately categorize a collection of related symptoms and be liberating to the person and family. Imagine the last time you experienced a new onset of medical symptoms. Finally, you sought medical advice, even if you only *Googled* your symptoms. When a diagnosis was concluded, you may have experienced a bit of relief in knowing what additional symptoms could be expected and the limitations of those expectations; others have experienced these symptoms before, so you are not a medical anomaly. You may also have felt relieved to know there were effective and available treatments. All these consequences are also common in the process of mental illness onset and diagnosis. While a diagnosis may be a relief, the gravity of the prognosis can also be quite overwhelming, worrisome, and hopeless to the point that a person receiving a new diagnosis will contemplate suicide. This reaction is common at the formal diagnosis stage of many chronic and life-threatening physical (i.e., cancer, AIDS, Parkinson's disease, Huntington's disease) or mental (i.e., schizophrenia) conditions (Chochinov, Wilson, Enns, & Lander, 1998). Diagnosis should be accurate. Any medical or mental health clinician should diagnose with caution, giving way to hope and effective and humane interventions (Fromm-Reichmann, 1960).

Length of treatment and amount of sessions should be discussed at the front end of the treatment relationship. The answer to these questions should come from the patient's desires and the clinical wisdom of the mental health worker. Some people who have a lot of emotionally laden material to sort through will need a lengthier amount of time, possibly even years, to allow for sensitivity and comprehensiveness. If the person is eager to enjoy the benefits of treatment or needs more frequent support, he or she may benefit from two or more sessions per week. For the person who may need frequent visits, he or she might not be able to tolerate a traditional 45- to 50-minute therapy session. Collaboratively, the length of each session can be decided on within the therapy session (Fromm-Reichmann, 1960).

Make frequent and brief attempts to reach those who are isolative. Many times, the person is isolative as a way to cope with severe interpersonal rejection and emotional pain. The person needs to feel the authenticity in the therapeutic relationship, which can be expressed by knocking on the person's door each day until he or she decides that coming out is safe and worth it. Consider the following example.

Coming Out of Hibernation

John came to the residential treatment facility after a lifetime of severe physical abuse, severe poverty, an excruciating disconnection from his immediate family members, heroin dependence, homelessness, and depression with psychotic features. John was HIV positive as a result of sharing contaminated needles during intravenous drug use.

John's attendance to the mandatory daily drug recovery group was sporadic. He was often more than 15 minutes late, if he came at all. The mental health worker always knocked on his door to invite him to the group. While in the group, John would fall asleep. The worker would warmly nudge John, greeting him with a soft smile.

After about 3 months of these consistent invitations to the group, John's behavior changed. He began to come 5 minutes early to the group. He knocked on the doors of other late members to invite them to the group. He called out members who were sleeping or otherwise passive in the group. He spoke courageously about his innermost emotional life.

Later on in John's stay, he sought out his primary mental health clinicians to talk about his small but significant accomplishments (i.e., artwork), ask them to read poetry to him, and mutually engage in activities (i.e., walks and watching movies).

As they continued to seek John out and attempt to engage with him positively, John began to feel safe enough to make meaningful interpersonal connections and deal with his emotional pain, and his symptoms of distress significantly subsided. John became a leader in the group, and others greatly benefited from his presence.

THERE IS NO ROOM FOR JUDGMENT IN THIS WORK
WITH PEOPLE WHO EXPERIENCE PSYCHOSIS

Judgment will quickly turn a person off, sending him or her into social isolation and paranoia. Because of the nature of psychosis and potentially few coping resources, you may see some behaviors, speech, and situations that are out of the ordinary, to say the least. Addressing these situations may be necessary, but judgment will cause an increase in symptoms and regression.

Strongly hold the intention of "I am here. Let's keep trying." The professional literature terms this "sustainment" (Goldstein, 1995; Walsh, 2011). As the listener focuses on engagement, trust, and a nonjudgmental and accepting environment of making sense of threads of meaning in fragmented or bizarre expressions, the person at the center of concern will naturally not need psychotic defenses and will manifest a natural "trusting response to being understood that facilitates his or her movement in the direction of personal integration and more adaptive functioning"

(Walsh, 2011, para. 26). Remember, most people experiencing psychotic symptoms have experienced major rejection from the people they value most. They will be extraordinarily sensitive to rejection, sensing it even before others act on it. There will be many misunderstandings and other therapeutic hiccups. When these occur, communicating commitment and intentions of moving forward are necessary.

MAINTAIN AND LEAD WITH AN INTERPERSONAL FEELING OF RESPECTFUL WARMTH

Mental health professionals often receive overt education about being *the blank slate*, attempting to withhold self-disclosure to an extreme degree. This coldness can be experienced as aloof and sullen and has the potential of causing disconnection with a person who experiences symptoms of psychosis. Without any interpersonal cues to connect with, the person who is vulnerable to psychosis will often fill in the blank with his own ideas, such as you do not like him or, worse, you are angry or negatively judging him. Alternatively, Semrad (1955) uses his charismatic self, curiosity, animation, empathy, and humor, toward establishing and maintaining an authentic connection that helps clients to take on what has previously felt unbearable and understanding, problem-solving, and creating an existence that feels more comfortable and rewarding.

DO SOMETHING WITH THE PERSON THAT HE OR SHE ENJOYS

Playing cards, listening to or playing music together, looking at magazines, playing basketball, or going to the library or park with a client can be beneficial in forming a positive and trusting relationship. Many times, in the beginning of a therapeutic relationship, the person may not be open to the spontaneous and delightful feelings that come up because of previous negative experiences when engaging with someone for the first time. Doing things that people enjoy relaxes anxieties and brings about authentic connections.

HAVE EXTRAORDINARY PATIENCE. THIS WORK CAN BE SLOW

Results of this work can be immediately witnessed or occur at a glacial pace—in other words, extraordinarily slowly. We may find ourselves working with the same person for long periods without seeing much progress. We should generously receive consultation about our intentions and be consistent, warm, and gentle in our approach. Fromm-Reichmann (1960) said to give the person the ripe environment and a reason to come out of psychic hibernation. We appreciate every small movement. These movements add up and can heal the spirit in time. Consider the following example of extremely slow and important work.

No Liquids for Me

James, a 54-year-old man and a Vietnam veteran, was trained as a registered nurse in the Army. After coming home from Vietnam, where he cared for the acutely wounded from combat, he began experiencing delusions about poisonous chemicals in his food. Well, like most delusional thoughts, there may be a grain of truth. We remember Operation Ranch Hand during 1962–1971, in which the US military sprayed approximately 20 million gallons of chemical herbicides and defoliants over rural areas of South Vietnam from the sky, leaving approximately 400,000 dead or seriously marred. As a result, approximately 500,000 children were born with birth defects. Women and livestock experienced an unthinkable increase in miscarriages and stillbirth. Many veterans were left with cancer, respiratory failure, and digestive symptom disorders. James believed he ingested these chemicals.

James now lives his life as a strict vegetarian and will not eat anything that does not come from a seed. He drinks no liquid, obtaining his only liquids from fruits and vegetables. He lived under a bridge for 4 years but, on the consistent, gentle, and encouraging care of his caseworker, agreed to live on his sister's porch. He never goes inside and has not bathed in 36 years. James's clothes are only removed as the clothes that touch his skin rot off. He wears layers of garbage bags in an attempt to protect himself from being further contaminated. For 7 years, he was mute.

With his caseworker, we approached James's porch home, where he sat waiting. With urgency, James said he wanted a driver's license and said, "Let's go now and get one." Gently, assuredly, and quietly, almost muttering so no one else could hear, the worker explained, "The world does not work that way. You need identification and to pass a written and driving test. We can work toward getting you those things." After they spoke for a few more minutes about making a plan, the caseworker warmly said, "See you next time, Buddy." As a premeditated afterthought, the caseworker reached into his jacket and offered James some garbage bags, saying, "You never know when you might need these."

On the drive away from James and his porch home, the worker said, "He doesn't ever come with me, but one day he will. In the meantime, I keep meeting with him. He has made some little and substantial changes over the time I have known him."

We appreciate all sizes of progress, including taking intermittent showers, wearing clean clothes, ironing one's clothes, wearing a piece of jewelry that reflects personal style, reducing substance use, making attempts to connect, making and reaching goals, and walking with dignity.

BE AS CONSISTENT AS POSSIBLE, CHOOSING THE SAME TIME, SAME MEETING PLACE, AND SAME LENGTH OF TIME SPENT TOGETHER

People build trust and a sense of safety through consistency and predictability.

These principles can be used by families or mental health professionals who either prescribe medications (such as psychiatrists and nurse practitioners) or do not prescribe medications (such as peer workers, social workers, psychologists, art therapists, occupational therapists, and marriage and family therapists). Additionally, narrative therapy is a therapeutic model that is formally and informally used in healing the distress of psychotic experiences.

NARRATIVE THERAPY

Narrative therapy, developed by Michael White and David Epston in the 1970s, is a widely used method to construct a cohesive and comprehensive story that explains the past and introduces hopeful and feasible intentions for the future, fostering a self-determined life worth living with symptoms of mental illness (White, 2007; White & Epston, 1990). Narrative therapy can be practiced in groups and with individuals and can be used in both brief and long-term situations. The story can be created around a portion of the person's life that he or she is trying to understand (such as a mother leaving the family or an automobile accident) or the entire collection of life stories up to current times. People who work toward sobriety practice constructing and telling their story in 12-step communities, such as Alcoholics Anonymous. The first time the person tells his or her story, it is either overlaid with overwhelming emotion or absent of emotion and often chaotic, incomplete, and peppered with searching pauses. On the other side of exploratory emotional work, the story is told linearly and with confidence, as he or she has discovered many accurate truths, including the aspects of his or her current hopeful self-determined life worth living. Consider the following example.

The Truth, the Whole Truth, and Nothing but the Truth

Jessica grew up in a family who struggled with addiction. She was the youngest of seven children. For many of her young years, there was little to no adult supervision, and the children did what they could to find food and get themselves to school. Between the ages of 5 and 12, Jessica was sexually molested by a friend of the family. She did not tell anyone because he threatened to kill her family if she told. She wondered how her parents, brothers, and sisters could not know that this was happening. She came to believe that everyone did know and was allowing this to happen. From that misperception, she felt that no one loved her and felt undeserving of any good things or love. She was isolated from her family and opportunities for close friendships. She began to use marijuana and other drugs to dissociate from her unbearable emotional experiences. She experienced hallucinations, including smells and sounds from the perpetrator, nightmares, and delusions that someone was trying to kill her and her family.

Finally, Jessica was able to tell her cousin about what had happened to her. Her cousin was able to rally the family so everyone would know. Still, her family refused to talk about it. Jessica perceived this refusal as them being angry with her for allowing the abuse to occur.

Jessica began working with a gentle and patient therapist, who saw that Jessica had been mistreated and the family members did not have the coping skills with which to recover from this trauma. She also recognized that Jessica had developed some misperceptions about herself and her family that led to disconnection, oppression, substance misuse, and severe depression.

Together, over a period of 3 years, Jessica and her therapist were able to construct a comprehensive story that explained the family dynamics with regard to addiction, neglect, and abuse. Their work also included clearing up the inaccurate beliefs that Jessica had concluded. She was able to see that in the process of her father's addiction, he and other family members were dissociated, disconnected, and truly not aware of Jessica being sexually molested. Also, Jessica was able to understand that the family's refusal to talk about this time was because they lacked the necessary communication skills to do so. Additionally, each person had so much guilt and anger that refusal and denial were the only methods with which to cope with such strong and uncomfortable feelings.

Jessica's father had since attended Narcotics Anonymous and had been on his personal recovery path for 7 years. While he did not know how to approach this difficult conversation with his traumatized daughter, he had found personal ways to express his sincere apology and care for Jessica that felt authentic and forgiving to her.

The therapist was able to conduct several family therapy sessions, during which she taught and modeled effective communication skills to Jessica's family. Over a period of a year, most of the family members had been able to have a few important conversations about the volatile time, describing their own personal coping styles, clearing up misperceptions, and expressing wishes and plans for future closeness in the family. As a comprehensive and accurate story was constructed and family relationships became more supportive, Jessica's hallucinations, delusions, substance misuse, and depression were significantly reduced. She began pursuing an intentionally healthy lifestyle, including her own therapy, good nutrition, education, and mutually rewarding interpersonal relationships, all creating a self-determined life worth living.

FINAL THOUGHTS

Many individuals and treatment programs throughout the United States and the world have exercised parts of the philosophy of *Listening with Psychotic Ears*. People with mental illness and psychotic experiences have opportunities to increase quality of life and live a meaningful self-determined life worth living. The philosophy and skills of *Listening with Psychotic Ears* facilitate a therapeutic relationship that is experienced as a sanctuary embodied with accurate understanding and effective communications with people who are vulnerable to experiencing symptoms of psychosis, thus empowering people and improving their sense of worth. We have no idea about the potential of people who have experienced psychosis because we have not had accurate and effective treatment methods.

Listening with Psychotic Ears takes everything out of us to give all of ourselves for the betterment of another. Self-care techniques in the presence of working with a person with psychosis are elaborated on in Chapter 12, "Survivor and Self-Care for Good and Noble Families and Clinicians Who Work with People Living with Symptoms of Mental Illness."

11

Practice-Based Interventions for Engaging

the Most Difficult/Impaired

WHEN CHRIS WAS in his senior year of high school, he became obsessively interested in public transportation systems in large cities. He reported being "called" to various cities, and would spontaneously travel to these cities to ride their trains and buses. On several occasions, while in a strange town, using alcohol, and speaking back to the voices he heard, he was detained by the police and hospitalized in psychiatric hospitals. Now, at 34 years old, diagnosed with schizophrenia, no job, and off and on neuroleptic medications for years, Chris has been in and out of psychiatric hospitals and jails for minor offenses. Chris's family worries for his future well-being.

Clients come with all kinds of needs and challenges, and not every person who is seeking mental health treatment is easily approachable or entering treatment willingly. Many people exhibit behaviors that make therapeutic engagement quite difficult, seemingly impossible, alienating, and hopeless at times. Words that unprepared or unknowing clinicians often use to describe these behaviors include resistant, angry, help-rejecting, noncompliant, untrusting, irritable, conflictual, moody, selfish, and inconsiderate of others, just to name a few.

Jeff had experienced a lifetime of depression, PTSD, alcohol and other drug misuse, and physical assault from others. One night, his wife started an altercation because he would not agree to pay her mother's bills. She cut him with a broken beer bottle in several places (requiring surgery). When he called the police, she reported that he was the one who assaulted her. In addition to this fabrication, she told the police that he was at risk for suicide. After being roughed up by the police,

Jeff was taken to jail, where he was put on suicide watch for the weekend. He was left naked and without a mattress. Upon his release from jail, Jeff was so filled with shame that he did not pursue these civil rights violations. After 3 weeks, he reunited with his wife.

A 56-year-old man came to the hospital emergency department requesting a sandwich. When refused, he reported that he had chest pains and needed to see a physician. After a $75,000 cardiac workup that was unfounded, he was discharged from the emergency department. On his way out, purposefully, he defecated on the paramedics' walkway.

Neil, a well-known patient, presented to the emergency department requesting admission to the psychiatric unit. It was an extremely cold February night in downtown Chicago. The emergency department physician was notably angered by Neil's request. The physician hollered to Neil, "Get up! Get dressed! And get out!" Neil did just that and walked to nearby store, purchased a gallon of antifreeze, and drank it. He came back to the hospital, with the bottle of antifreeze, stating that he felt hopeless, suicidal, and had drunk half of the bottle of antifreeze.

Kevin was a young man who spent his days going from one hospital emergency department to the next. Kevin made a habit of finding new workers and telling a story that he was hearing voices of monsters and demons. With these details, the worker would initiate a complete mental status exam. Kevin always insisted that the interview be conducted in private. At this point, Kevin would corner the new worker in a private room, unzip his pants, and proceed to masturbate. Sometimes, when Kevin did present to the emergency department, he really did seem to be hearing command distressing voices and needed psychiatric hospitalization. During these visits, Kevin would go through the half-hearted motions of attempting to corner the mental health clinician, just out of habit. Redirecting him seemed easier during these visits, as Kevin really seemed to be in distress and needed supportive help.

What do all these people have in common? Each one employed extremely desperate measures to get their needs met. Addiction, mental illness, poor judgment, little to no support, few resources, and big and overwhelming feelings cause people to resort to unimaginable strategies to meet their natural needs. These kinds of behaviors result in furthering negative consequences and alienating family, friends, and caregivers.

Let's stop and explore how the person got this way in the first place. A large majority of people who find themselves seeking social services in the mental health treatment system have experienced extraordinarily high rates of early, ongoing, and increasingly severe trauma. Some of these traumatic experiences include various types of physical, sexual, and emotional abuse and torture; repeated parental abandonment; addiction in parents, siblings, and extended family members; physical illnesses and disabilities; and early and ongoing involvement in the criminal justice system. These experiences cause significant distress and permanently imprint the mind, subjective meaning system, brain tissue, and neurotransmitter functioning. *People with these types of experiences learn to tolerate great deals of intrapsychic and physical pain.*

Consequently, this quality of distress and impact results in some of the behaviors that clinicians describe as *difficult to reach*. The traumatized mind will naturally construct defense and coping mechanisms in an attempt to avoid future similar emotional traumatic experiences. Unfortunately, these desperate defense and coping styles further sideline the person and lead to more severely distressing and marginalizing experiences, such as rage, addiction, and homelessness.

At this point, these people often receive pejorative labels such as hopeless, thug, and sociopath, and with that, the countertransference reactions from clinicians and others include irritability, annoyance, avoidance, loss of empathy, and disrespect. These reactions make everyone (the individual, family, and clinicians) feel miserable. How, in a timely manner, can these people, their behaviors, and their situations be more accurately understood and humanely and effectively responded to? How can we cause a paradigm shift from *a problem with the person*, to *a person with a problem*? We are dealing with a unique individual with a unique story that deserves accurate understanding and effective responses.

Jackie was a 37-year-old woman who was well known for her frequent visits to the hospital emergency room. Jackie usually presented with a similar story that included her intense and dysregulated emotions that resulted in her physical injury. For example, she often would experience a loss, such as another person took her marijuana supply. Jackie would verbally attack the person, ferociously calling him every name in the book. That person would physically assault Jackie, sending her to the hospital to tend to her injuries. Jackie also would prostitute herself for even a small portion of drugs or food. Her extremely poor judgment would take her to unsafe people and situations, during which she would often experience brutal sexual assault. As a result, everything in her life was extremely unstable, including housing, relationships, social support, physical health, mental health, and finances.

On one occasion, Jackie was evicted from a residential addiction treatment facility for using drugs. She had nowhere else to go and was now homeless. Like many people, she did not want to go to a shelter. Feeling rejected and abandoned and with nowhere to turn to for help, she reported an impulse to kill herself. The emergency department physician told her that she was "a lazy, manipulative drug addict" and she would not be admitted to the psychiatric hospital. With this news, Jackie, whose resources were bankrupt, went outside to a bench that was situated just outside a large window. She sobbed and rocked herself.

She desperately looked around and found a beer bottle. She looked back at the window. Holding the bottle by its neck, she smacked the bottle on the bench. Then, she held the broken bottle edge up to her wrist, which she held high in the air, pausing a moment to make sure people could see her through the window. Jackie purposefully slashed her forearm with jagged beer bottle. With that, she *bought* herself an admission to the psychiatric hospital, despite what the emergency department physician had said.

When crises like these occur, it is natural to have strong emotional responses that derail therapeutic intentions and goals. It is crucial to get a grip on an accurate understanding of the client and his or her situation, else *the wheels will fall off the bus*, and destructive emotional interactions will ensue. With accurate understanding, we are more able to offer effective interventions and minimize destructive emotional reactions.

CLINICAL SKILLS

The use of clinical skills are required for working with people toward therapeutic healing. Below you will find several skills that have been used with this population with whom are the most challenging to work.

Enlisting Objectivity Puts Necessary Emotional Distance Between Client and Clinician or Family Member

Keep your personal distance from the content of the dynamics that occur. Life is often like playing chess. One person makes a move, and then the other person makes their move. It is not personal. Often, a supervisor, consultant, or friendly interested person, upon hearing the story, can sometimes share insight that might otherwise seem so obvious. Enlisting objectivity helps the clinician to not take personally the client's offensive behaviors, such as calculatedly and violently cutting herself or defecating in the paramedic's walkway. Since this happened, now another move is necessary. The clinician can understand that this desperate person, who has very little resources and adaptive coping skills, did the best she could do to elicit help or express frustration. We understand that this anger could be directed at anyone, everyone, himself or herself, or no one.

Once some emotional distance and objectivity has been established, it is much easier to allow for an *empathic view* of the isolated person. It is easier to imagine what the person might be feeling and reacting to. Then, we can normalize these emotional reactions in desperate situations. So, how do we access this emotional distance, especially when the emotions are so very strong and consuming?

A famous Buddhist story, "The Spider's Thread," by Akutagawa Ryūnosuke comes to mind:

> The Buddha Shakyamuni is meandering around Paradise one morning when he stops at a lotus-filled pond. Between the lilies, he can see to the depths of Hell through the crystal-clear waters. His eyes come to rest on one sinner in particular by the name of Kandata. Kandata was a cold-hearted criminal but had one good deed to his name: while walking through the forest one day, he decided not to kill a spider he was about to crush with his foot. Moved by this single act of compassion, the Buddha takes the silvery thread of a spider in Paradise and lowers it down into Hell.
>
> Down in Hell, the myriad of sinners is struggling in the Pool of Blood in total darkness except for the light glinting off the Mountain of Spikes and total silence except for the sighs of the damned. Kandata, looking up by chance at the sky above the pool, sees the spider's thread descending toward him and grabs hold with all the might of a seasoned criminal. The climb from Hell to Paradise is not a short one, however, and Kandata quickly tires. Dangling from the middle of the thread, he glances downward and sees how far he has come. Realizing that he may actually escape from Hell, he is overcome by joy and laughs giddily. His elation is short-lived, however, as he realizes that others have started climbing the thread behind him, stretching down into the murky depths below. Fearing that the thread will break from the weight of the others, he shouts that the spider's thread is his and his alone. It is at this moment that the thread breaks, and he and all the other sinners are cast back down into the Pool of Blood.
>
> Shakyamuni witnesses this with a slightly sad air. In the end, Kandata condemned himself by being concerned only with his own salvation and not that of others. But, Paradise continues on as it has, and it is nearly noontime there. Thus, the Buddha continues his meanderings. (Kelly, 2012)

This story was first told to me on a Thursday night by a Buddhist reverend. On Monday morning, I entered my job site, an urban general hospital emergency department about 2 miles from Skid Row in downtown Los Angeles. By 7:30 am, a 73-year-old homeless woman had been to every administrative office in the hospital seeking acquiescence. She was viciously demanding prescription opiate pain medication for her intellectually challenged and silent 54-year-old daughter, whom she had in tow. She had aggressively addressed her demands with the nurse manager of the emergency department, security department supervisor, patient advocate, and CEO of the hospital and even called 911 from the hospital emergency department. Each department directed her back to the emergency department physician, who refused to give her the requested and unwarranted opiate prescription. The woman viciously cursed out everyone in her blazing path.

At that point, given that her evaluation and treatment had been fulfilled, with a firm united team of hospital representatives, she was directed to vacate the hospital. After bitterly and unforgivingly using every curse word in the book, she departed with her silent daughter still in tow.

In my previous days, this woman's unbridled rage and shrieking demands for addictive and dissociative medications would have left me with an abundance of negative countertransference reactions, including feeling emotionally rattled and increasingly frustrated. Her entitlement would have left me offended and alienated from her. I would have felt that she was wasting my time and snatching the hospital's and my integrity. Given these perceived threats, my amygdala would have responded in kind, causing me to feel threatened, increasing my adrenaline, heartbeat, and the volume of my voice, resulting in decreased whole brain activity and impeding my capacity to think about effective interventions. These emotional reactions are what leads a person straight to professional burnout.

But this Monday, I had the enlightenment of "The Spider's Thread" and was able to see this *rageful, cold-hearted* woman's desperate actions through the objective and empathic lens of "The Spider's Thread." I saw her as likely having a very long history of traumatic experiences, including the daily stressors of now being an elderly woman with an adult dependent daughter, being homeless and living in extreme poverty, and being addicted to opiate medications. Clearly, she and her daughter have very few resources to which to turn to meet their daily needs. The mother was desperate in her need to get the pain meds to use herself, sell, or both, to meet or avoid her/their needs being adequately met. The daughter responded by emotionally shutting down, likely to avoid her mother's rage. With no viable choices, the adult daughter experiences psychogenic death: a death of the spirit or sense of agency.

This raging mother was not ready for enlightenment; furthermore, in this moment, she completely lacked the insight necessary for the beginnings of a stable life. While maladaptive, the drama and instability served her needs at this point in her life. Her destructively rageful, desperate, and self-serving actions left her both empty handed and falling back down into "The Spider's Thread" realm of Hell.

On this special Monday, I felt no attachment to her rage; I had no impulse to rescue her. This mindframe was where she existentially needed to be, and I had respect for that. I did feel the need to protect the safety and morale of the other patients and hospital workers and the integrity of hospital patient care. This need allowed me to be the leader of the hospital representation and stay emotionally neutral. I informed her that she would not be given any medication and she had to vacate the hospital, as her evaluation and treatment were complete. Her fragility left me seeing her desperate attempts to get her needs met as simply so sad.

The following tools are both evidence-based practices and things I have discovered to be true for effective engagement and intervention during challenging situations with people who experience symptoms of severe mental illness (SMI).

Kenneth Minkoff, MD, asserts that *an empathic, hopeful, continuous treatment relationship* is necessary for recovery from SMI and addiction (Minkoff, video). All too often, our overloaded mainstream mental health treatment system does not allow for this type of relationship. Clinicians are often overloaded with too many clients with an abundance of complex needs. Whereas the majority of clinicians entered into the mental health treatment field with passion to deeply help people, this passion is quickly and persistently eroded by (1) a never-ending workload, (2) inconsistent resources and structure, and (3) unprepared supervision and administration, causing burnout and *zombie-like* job performance. In this environment, there is little energy left for empathy for clients in desperate situations. Without empathy, consistency, and resources, clients also become zombie-like in the treatment relationship, causing them to simply go through the motions, act out by engaging in risky drama and drug use, or drop out of treatment. These unfortunate consequences cause the clinician to see many people not doing well. The belief that people can and do recover becomes a fantasy, not a reality, which can quickly and severely erode hope.

A very similar dynamic can occur among families. Generally speaking, families simply wish for health and well-being for the family member with symptoms of mental illness. Family members often sacrifice a lot of emotion, money, time, and energy toward these goals but may not accurately understand the symptoms of mental illness. The emotional, financial, temporal, and energetic drain may be too much, so resources become withdrawn from the symptomatic person to use for the family member's own survival preservation; as a result, family members and friends may withdraw their support. These dynamics explain why a significant number of adults with SMI do not have family support.

How do mental health treatment centers and family members maintain an empathic, hopeful, and continuous treatment relationship with the person with symptoms of mental illness? This is the million-dollar question!

As previously mentioned in this book and by the abundance of psychiatric survivors, much of our public mental health treatment system is broken. That said, there are feasible efforts that can be implemented by clinicians to allow for empathic, hopeful, and continuous relationships with clients.

Mental Health America's Village of Long Beach (see Appendix B for website) teaches and operates on many of the concepts mentioned here. Mental health treatment delivery clinicians and administrators come from all over the world to

Mental Health America's Village of Long Beach to study and witness how comprehensive, integrated service treatment delivery principles work effectively in increasing quality of life for people who live with SMI.

Recovery Aspects

- **Hope**—People need hope that recovery and a better life are real possibilities.
- **Empowerment**—People need to experience authorization to pursue personal choices.
- **Self-responsibility**—People need to be accountable for the choices that are made. While mistakes are expected from anyone, individuals need to be responsible for trying new behaviors and correcting situations as needed.
- **Meaningful roles**—People need normalized and rewarding aspects of their lives with real consequences that are separate from their mental illness.

Recovery Philosophy and Principles

- **Client choice**—People get to work on the issues of their choice with the staff of their choice.
- **Quality of life**—Recovery is focused on life areas that immerse the person in the fabric of the community and will increase life's comforts, including employment, education, housing, healthcare, finances, and social network.
- **Community choice**—Clients are met within natural community locations, not in an unnatural office setting.
- **Whatever it takes**—Staff members are available for crisis support 24/7. Staff members have a *no fail* philosophy, and there are a range of resources and supportive services to meet clients *where they are*. Staff members are highly committed to clients and their goals.

Services

- Personal service plans
- Psychiatric care
- Employment
- Substance abuse recovery
- Housing assistance
- Financial assistance
- Community involvement

In addition to these effective, life-sustaining, and award-winning practice principles, Mental Health America's Village of Long Beach makes a practice of teaching their mental health workers how to chart service delivery in a way that is both truthful and meets funding requirements (Personal communication, Anonymous). This practice allows for flexibility in meeting places and timing. For example, members do not come to a mental health treatment agency for a social skills group. Instead, they might go to a baseball game and practice social skills in a naturally occurring environment. This setting allows for naturally occurring situations with more sustainable learning.

Many strong evidence-based mental health treatment interventions begin authentic engagement with the principle of genuinely *validating and joining the person in their desperate feelings.* Having a mental illness can be excruciatingly difficult to cope with. In the following example, Minkoff offers the spirit of validating the person's illness.

It must be so very difficult for you to cope with your mental illness. You have tried so many different things and so many times to make things better for yourself. I wish you could accept as much help and support as you deserve. You deserve a lot more help and support than you are receiving. (Minkoff video)

MOTIVATIONAL INTERVIEWING

Motivational interviewing is an intervention philosophy for working with any person through the change process (Miller & Rollnick, 2012). We all know that telling people what to do rarely works. We know that when an individual decides to make a change, it is much more likely to be sustainable when he or she decides a change is necessary. The purpose of motivational interviewing principles is to internally enlighten the individual that a change is necessary and highlight the reasons for that change. Motivational interviewing involves several main principles:

- Use empathy.
  - "Things must be really hard for you these days."
- Ask for permission to engage in a conversation about necessary changes.
  - "Do you mind if we talk about your drug use and how it is impacting your goals?"
- Engage in change talk.
  - "What do you think would happen if you continued to use at the pace you are now going?"
  - "What do you think would be different if you were able to stop using?"
  - "If you did decide that you would stop using, what would you need to make that happen? How could I help you in that process?"

- Help the person imagine extreme situations.
  - "How do you imagine your life if you do not make this change? What is the worst thing that could happen?"
  - "If you do make this change, what is the best thing you can imagine that would be different in your life than it is today?"
  - "If you do not stop or slow down, what can you imagine your life will be like in four years?"
  - "What was your life like before this all started?"
- Explore confidence in capacity to change.
  - "What is your rating from 1 to 5 of your ability to make this change?"
  - "Why do you score a 3 and not higher? A 3 and not lower?"
  - "What would you need to happen to be able to score your confidence higher to make this change?"
- Ask open-ended questions.
  - "What has happened since we last met?"
  - "What is it like for you when you get loaded?"
- Use reflective listening.
  - "What you are saying is . . ."
  - "It sounds like part of you is wanting to . . . and the other part is wanting to . . . and you are concerned about . . . ."
- Normalize usual feelings.
  - "A lot of people in your shoes would be concerned about that."
  - "It is common to try to stop many times before a change really sticks. This is a major lifestyle change!"
- Use a decision-balance (pros/cons) exercise (Miller, 2004).
  - The Internet can provide many more elaborate decision-balance worksheets.

	Pros	Cons
Make the change		
Do not make the change		

- Develop discrepancies.
  - "On the one hand, you are saying that you have no money to contribute to the family and that you hate your job. On the other hand, you are saying that it is important to you to be able to contribute to the family. How is it working for you to work this job that you say you do not like and in which you are not making enough money?"
  - "Help me understand. You are saying that having an active relationship with family is the most important thing to you. You also are reporting that

your sister said you are not welcome in her house and around her children when you are using, yet you continue to use. How is this meth use getting in the way of your value of having an active relationship with your family?"

- Support self-efficacy and self-confidence.
  - "When we spoke last summer, you were sure that you could not go a day without talking to your abusive boyfriend. You now say you have not had contact with him in two months. How were you able to do that?" "How do you feel about making this change?"
- Use affirmations.
  - "In spite of what happened two weeks ago, you are still coming here to try to help yourself. I can see that you really want to make this change!"
- Summary feedback.
  - "I have calculated our assessment and compared you to other people who are in this process. Can we talk about these results?"
- Therapeutic paradox.
  - "You have been coming to meet with me for six months now and have not lost one pound. Maybe now is not the time for you to be making this change."
- Stages of change.
  - Prochaska and DiClimente (1986) have identified common stages that a person goes through when attempting to make a change. A person can move through these changes rapidly or slowly, even getting stuck in one stage or another. The following paragraphs present the stages of change, a description of them, examples of what a person in this stage might think or say, and therapeutic interventions at each stage. The purpose of therapeutic interventions is to cause a person to choose to move to the next stage of the change process.

Denial—Precontemplation

In this stage, the person is unaware of the cost/impact of his or her behaviors. Change is not being considered. This person may say something like "I do not have a problem!" What possible interventions can help someone in this change stage of denial?

- *Offer honest feedback.* "The decision to make a change is yours. You are not interested in making a change at this time. When you are ready to make that change, then you can return here."
- *Give real consequences.* Do not rescue. If a person with a pattern of impairment shows up late for work and gets fired, family members and clinicians

often experience big feelings, including not wanting things to get worse or feeling sorry for the person, and jump in to relieve any hardships. Telling yourself "Oh, just this once" is common; however, these behaviors are considered rescuing, and if this happens, the individual does not have an opportunity to learn from the consequences of his or her behavior. Whereas it might be uncomfortable to see someone you care about facing hardships, we can look beyond the hardships and focus on the learning opportunity available to not repeat a dysfunctional behavior.

- *Have the person hear stories of people who were once gripped by the issue and are now successful in making the change.* This solution is why judges often mandate/sentence people to go to voluntary Alcoholics Anonymous meetings. The person may hear someone tell a story that he or she can identify with. Now, the speaker is stable and feeling the benefits of making the lifestyle change.

Ambivalence—Contemplation

In this stage, the person is aware of the cost/impact of his or her behavior but is unwilling or unable to make a change in the near future. This person might say, "I realize that meth has destroyed my marriage, but I am not ready or willing to stop using." What can be done to help a person in the ambivalent stage of change?

- *Encourage self-exploration.* "What will become of you in four years if you continue to use?" "What would be the worst thing that might happen if you stop?"
- *Develop discrepancies.* "You are saying you want to feel comfortable in your clothes, yet you are eating a quart of ice cream daily." "Is this the right time for you to be making this change?"
- *Continue to give real consequences.*

Preparation—Determination

In this stage, the person knows that a change is necessary. He or she is exploring and considering options. This person might say, "I know I need to make a change and am thinking about the most feasible way of going about it." How can a person be helped in the preparation stage of change?

- *Help to identify feasible options.* As a treatment, or intervention, option is considered, there are several points to keep in mind: if the change is to seek treatment, consider what options the person has available including payment, time, location, and transportation and which theoretical modality may be appropriate, such as self-help groups, artistic expression, Eastern practices, medication, psychoanalysis, or a structured work environment.

- *Continue to nurture self-reflection/self-exploration.* Nurturing can be done with the help of a professional, a mentor, or a peer, and personal exploration can be done via reading and personal practice.
- *Allow time for exploration and consideration; then, create urgency.* Many people will look to make a change or even say they are in recovery of one type or another, but their behavior is not congruent with those ideas. Fear of change is common. In this situation, a direct and caring conversation is necessary, often causing a person to reevaluate choices, and urgency is stimulated.

Action

In the action stage of change, the person is actively practicing change behaviors. We will often witness a sharp learning curve as choices are tried and reward occurs. If the changes are not rewarding enough, relapse is inevitable. While the action phase is much smoother to witness, the person continues to need a lot of support. This person might say, "I have a problem, and I am doing something about it." What can we do to help a person in the action stage?

- *Give lots of authentic affirmations.* "Your courage to try new ways of feeling better is admirable. How are you feeling about these changes?"
- *Keep an eye for the need for reevaluation and change in action plan.* It may take many tries to get a change plan with the correct details that make it sustainable. Do not give up until the miracle happens.

Maintenance

The maintenance stage of change involves the person actively participating in the behavioral and cognitive lifestyle changes necessary to successfully make change possible. This person might say, "I have a problem, and I am doing what it takes to overcome this problem. I am stable and reaping the rewards of my lifestyle changes." In the maintenance stage of change, far less clinical intervention is necessary. The person is independently sustained and may not need much, if any, formal help. However, given that we are considering that people with SMI may need lifelong support, here are some considerations for people with symptoms of mental illness in the maintenance stage of change.

- *Support from a distance.* Micromanagement is not necessary, but we are all in need of support. As the person has life span stressors, such as illness, housing moves, cue precipitants (anniversaries, birthdays, weather changes, etc.), or loss or death of significant persons, make an effort to directly and sensitively check in with the person. "Given this change, how is your recovery going?" "Do you need anything?"
- *Be sure to check in about specific things you know to have been working for the person.* "How is it going with your therapist?" "Are you still drinking your morning smoothies?" Life happens. The therapist may have taken another job. The blender may have conked out. During these naturally stressful times is when the person needs his or her maintenance plan the most to sustain this positive change. If the blender conked out, brainstorm with the person about how he or she might finance a new one. If the therapist went on maternity leave, brainstorm about a new connection. Follow up with the person about making the plan a reality.
- *Discuss that relapse is a process, not an event.* Discuss early warning signs and effective interventions.

Relapse

Relapse occurs after a person has known a period of stability and returns to a maladaptive coping style. Relapse is a process, not an event. Relapse occurs to the majority of people in the process of change. If the person is in continuous connection with empathic, hopeful people, the relapse will be less severe and shorter. With this empathic, hopeful, and nonjudgmental relationship, the person has more of a chance to return to this relationship during or after relapse. The person will likely be feeling a dose of shame, as he or she will experience the perception that he or she has disappointed you. When the person is ready, your authentic connection will invite them back. The person in relapse says, "Oops, I did it again!" If you have not seen the person in a while or you notice some relapse warnings (disconnection, irritability, sleepiness, change in energy: high or low, unexplainable absence or presence of money, change in self-care, unexplainable physical absence, etc.), directly and sensitively check in with the person. Be prepared for a range of stories, including a flooding of honest sharing of shocking details to a wild menagerie of unthinkable drama.

- *As the person shares his relapse experience, use a supportive, nonjudgmental tone.* Listen for and directly ask, "What do you need now to get back on your plan?"

- *Assess for risk of physical, medical, and social harm through direction questioning and your strong observational skills.* Call in collaborative professionals, as needed, for secondary and tertiary care, such as medical professionals, housing, and food banks, to name a few.

Remember, the point of motivational interviewing is to cause the individual to decide for himself or herself that a change is necessary. With your support, the person has an increased chance of becoming ready, willing, and able to make these necessary and life-giving changes.

HARM REDUCTION

There are some people who will not, in any near future, make the necessary changes for a more positive, sustainable, and healthy life and lifestyle. At this time, abstinence is not a goal. These people are not to be ignored or avoided by mental health treatment providers just because they are participating in these lifestyle choices. For these people, who regularly engage in risky substances or behaviors and cannot stop in the near future, we exercise the principles of harm reduction.

The intention of harm reduction is just as it sounds: to reduce the inevitable harm that is a result of risky behaviors. We teach people who cannot stop how to do these behaviors so that the most serious harm does not occur. If a person chooses to ride a bike, harm reduction indicates that the person wear a helmet and take an unpopulated route with a clearly marked bike path, not the freeway. If he or she is going to binge eat, harm reduction indicates that he or she eat a large bowl of strawberries instead of an entire cake. If a person is going to use drugs by way of an intravenous needle, harm reduction indicates that he or she use a sharp and sterile needle with sterilized water, not a needle that has been used 50 times and shared with other users. If a person is going to have sex with strangers, teach him or her to choose safer people to go with, which persons to avoid, and to always use condoms and dental dams.

Keep in mind, there is a difference between *use reduction* and *harm reduction*. use reduction, a practice that may or may not be within harm reduction, suggests that the person slow down the frequency and amount of use in an attempt to reduce potential harm. Use reduction principles include practices that break the unconscious habit of overindulgence. One example is when trying to quit smoking, one might put away/throw out all paraphernalia, such as ashtrays, lighters, or fancy and glamorizing cigarette cases. The effort to reattain the paraphernalia will cause the act of using to be conscious and intentional. Another example is to find a specific and inconvenient place to smoke, such as outside, rather than on the couch. The effort of going and using outside will cause the person to make a conscious choice, rather than an unconscious habit. Use reduction is one effective practice to reduce the harm of risky behaviors.

Now, some readers might be offended by all this harm reduction discussion. The philosophy of harm reduction is often misunderstood as a delicate way of rationalizing the enabling of risky behaviors. This belief is a common mistake. Harm reduction is not the first line of intervention for dealing with risky behaviors. It is intended for those who are participating in very risky behaviors and *cannot stop*. These risky behaviors can and do result in very severe consequences, such as getting fired from employment, contracting life-altering illnesses, participating in activities that land a person in jail or prison, and death. Harm reduction practices are intended to teach those who cannot stop to divert some of these stark risks.

Harm reduction is an international philosophy that emerged in Liverpool, England, in the 1980s. Its ideas are adapted from the *responsible use* philosophy of the 1970s. While prevalent in the United States, it is even more strongly active in Canada, Europe, and Australia. In Vancouver, Canada, there is a safe and supervised injection clinic called *Insite*. You can watch a CNN documentary about *Insite* at the link listed in Appendix B. No drugs are provided here, and medical staff members are present. People come to this facility to safely intravenously inject drugs, primarily heroin, cocaine, and morphine. As a result, potential harm, such as the contraction of illness, spreading of disease, and overdose are avoided.

The principles of harm reduction are borrowed from The Harm Reduction Coalition (see Appendix B for website information):

- Accepts, for better or worse, that licit and illicit drug use is part of our world and chooses to work to minimize its harmful effects rather than simply ignore or condemn them.
- Understands drug use as a complex, multifaceted phenomenon that encompasses a continuum of behaviors, from severe abuse to total abstinence, and acknowledges that some ways of using drugs are clearly safer than others.
- Establishes quality of individual and community life and well-being— not necessarily cessation of all drug use—as the criteria for successful interventions and policies.
- Calls for the nonjudgmental, noncoercive provision of services and resources to people who use drugs and the communities in which they live to assist them in reducing attendant harm.
- Ensures that drug users and those with a history of drug use routinely have a real voice in the creation of programs and policies designed to serve them.

- Affirms drugs users, themselves, as the primary agents of reducing the harms of their drug use and seeks to empower users to share information and support each other in strategies that meet their actual conditions of use.
- Recognizes that the realities of poverty, class, racism, social isolation, past trauma, sex-based discrimination, and other social inequalities affect both people's vulnerabilities to and capacity for effectively dealing with drug-related harm.
- Does not attempt to minimize or ignore the real and tragic harm and danger associated with licit and illicit drug use. (Harm Reduction Coalition, n.d.)

Some common harm reduction practices include methadone maintenance, distribution of free condoms, homeless shelters, free taxi service on New Year's Eve, and education for heroin users about Nalaxone to counter an opiate (especially intravenous heroin) overdose. While many of these might evoke passionate controversy, when we get right down to it, there is harm all around us, and everyone participates in reducing harm. Shoes. Smoke detectors. Traffic lights. Seat belts. Handicap rails. Look around your current environment and notice harm reduction practices in action.

Adaptive Coping Skills

Another concept to use when working with people with mental illness who are difficult to reach is to teach adaptive coping skills to manage inevitable life stressors and personal challenging situations. Without adaptive coping skills, people find maladaptive coping skills, such as overindulgence of drugs or food, social withdrawal, avoidance, rumination, self-harm behaviors, psychosis, anger and violence, and denial, to name a few.

Recovery Is Real

Lily, a 27-year-old Latina woman with a substantial trauma history, heard voices daily that would call her derogatory names and tell her she was worthless and useless and should do the world a favor and kill herself. Often, she was able to differentiate her voices from reality, but occasionally, she would accuse a family member, usually male, of saying derogatory things toward her, which led to tension in the family. The client's sister, who also acted as her caregiver, once came to a session asking, "When will she get better?" When asked what she meant by *better*, the sister reported that she thought the medications would *fix* her sister and she could get a job and be normal. Lily's sister became tearful when reporting that Lily would often slam doors, scream at her voices to "Shut up!," and then breakdown crying. "She is tormented! I just want my sister back!"

The treatment team (psychiatrist and social worker) provided psychoeducation to the family, referred the sister (and interested family members) to the family-to-family course at the National Alliance on Mental Illness (NAMI), and increased the frequency of Lily's one-on-one sessions. The psychiatrist suggested Clozaril, a psychotropic medication, but Lily reported she was afraid of needles and did not want to take weekly blood tests. Lily's individual sessions with the therapist focused on reality testing, identifying the triggers and stressors of her voices, and determining ways to distract and reduce her voices. Lily was able to identify ways to reduce her stressors, such as opposite action (e.g., watching a comedy when she started to feel down or going for a walk when she wanted to isolate) and reality testing (e.g., weighing the evidence for and against whether she heard her voices or someone near her make comments). Lily and her sister gradually accepted the reality of Lily's mental illness and what long-term recovery would look like. Lily reported her long-term goal was to return to school. After a few years of increased treatment, she started attending an adult school and taking computer classes. Lily reported that the classes and homework distracted her from the voices. Lily's sister bought her a computer so she could practice her new skills. Lily still hears voices daily, but the intensity has gone down considerably, and she reports reduced depression, anxiety, and a higher quality of life.

Teaching and using adaptive coping skills requires a conscious and active process within a safe relationship. We want to, first, be able to identify the stressor and, then, the maladaptive coping skill. Then, we want to identify a healthier, more adaptive, and more desired response to this stressor. Teaching the desired response can be done through role-play.

Role-play is an effective tool for teaching adaptive coping responses and skills because it allows the person to consciously and actively choose a new behavior when he or she does not feel threatened or stressed. The nuances of the situation can be identified, discussed, and incorporated into the practice. Then, when the person is in the stressful situation, that behavior is readily available to him. Getting the response to be immediate and accurate may take a lot of practice over time.

When role-play practice is done in safe and quiet times, this process is actually creating new pathways in the brain. When the stressful situation occurs, the brain is in survival mode, using more lower-brain activity. The pathway to the higher brain will have already been created, allowing for more adaptive coping skills to be used during stressful situations.

Here is a short list of adaptive coping skills that can be used in stressful situations. It is a good idea to keep a running list of skills and activities to turn to when needed.

- Deep breathing
- Writing a letter or in a journal.

- Taking a walk or engaging in another favorite physical exercise activity.
- Taking a warm bath.
- Listening to music or playing a musical instrument.
- Sitting quietly and hearing the natural sounds around you.
- Cooking a meal.
- Calling a friend.
- Altruism or helping someone else with no expectation for them to return the favor.
- Making a pro/con list.
- Brainstorming about ways to solve the problem. Focusing on ways/methods in which you are in control.
- Laughing.

DIALECTICAL BEHAVIORAL THERAPY

Dialectical Behavioral Therapy (DBT) is a detailed evidence-based intervention method used with people who have severe life-threatening behaviors and difficulty coping when emotions become dysregulated. Dialectical Behavioral Therapy focuses on teaching skills to cope with emotions that are difficult to tolerate or regulate. Dialectical Behavioral Therapy teaches four sets of skills: mindfulness, distress tolerance, interpersonal effectiveness, and emotion regulation. Skills are taught in a class-type group setting that meets for 2.5 hours per week, taking 24 weeks to get through the curriculum. The *DBT Skills Training Manual* is available for purchase (Linehan, 2014). Also, a variety of trainings are available around United States and online at the Linehan Institute (see Appendix B).

People who have symptoms of SMI especially need help with learning adaptive coping skills in crisis situations, such as during interpersonal conflict. Additionally, learning and using adaptive coping skills includes accessing needed resources, such as suicide and coping resource hotlines, therapists, trusted social relationships, hospital emergency departments, and respite care centers.

The practice of appropriately accessing these needed resources is especially necessary for people with symptoms of mental illness. Many people have learned not to trust others, ask for help, or talk about what is going on or manage crisis situations alone. That said, one of the first things to point out with this person is that they have permission to access these resources and ask and receive help. Crisis resources may have to be clearly identified, written down, and kept in accessible places. You may find that the person will have many crisis situations and will not readily access these resources. Calmly and patiently, revisit these resources as options. Inquire about the reasons why the person did not turn to these resources. It may take a lot of practice for the person to internalize that these resources are options and it is OK to access them.

Is This Real?

Ann was a 50-year-old female who had been engaged in mental health treatment for 5 years. Her psychotic experiences started when she was in her early 20s and led to several involuntary hospitalizations, a divorce, the loss of her children to their father, and eventually homelessness. The client lived in temporary shelters. Ann was completely immersed in delusions and hallucinations for a decade. She believed her food was being poisoned. In a life-preserving effort, she had been severely limiting her food intake, resulting in body weight of 97 lbs. (She was 5'5".) One day, in the shelter, she saw a movie in which the protagonist sought mental health treatment and got better. Ann concluded that she had nothing to lose and voluntarily entered the psychiatric hospital. She reported that her auditory hallucinations were reduced by Zyprexa, a psychotropic medication, but she still felt anxious and paranoid. She reported that she would spend a lot of mental energy on trying to differentiate reality from her illness. For example, Ann would bring in a copy of an e-mail from one of her adult children (whom she had reconnected with after she started making progress) and ask her therapist if she saw any hidden meaning or accusations. Ann met with her therapist twice a month for an adapted cognitive-behavioral therapy (CBT) for psychosis. Most of the skills focused on reality testing and looking at evidence for and against automatic thoughts. The therapist also included mindfulness for times when Ann felt overwhelmed. Ann enjoyed her CBT handouts so much that she made copies for her adult children. On weekly calls with her daughter, they would go over mindfulness techniques and different CBT interventions.

Ann was able to get to a much more adaptive quality of life. She would come to the session and share how she had a distressing automatic thought over the weekend and was able to work through it or refocus with mindfulness techniques and get through the process without too much stress or mental energy. Ann continued to work through the distressing guilt she felt for having abandoned her family because of her mental illness. Ann's father bought several copies of *The Center Cannot Hold: My Journey Through Madness*, written by Elyn Saks (2008), for family members to help them all understand schizophrenia. Reading and discussing this book has helped to mend their relationships.

The idea of a recovery lifestyle must be clearly envisioned and strongly embodied. Mainstream mental health treatment delivery does not envision recovery as a real possibility. Low expectations are pervasively communicated. People with symptoms of SMI are often told not to work to avoid stress and future decompensations, to seek supervised housing, and to take the medication for the rest of their lives, which, as noted, may leave them lethargic, emotionally numb, and with impediments in brain functioning. While all this is told to a person with protective intentions, low expectations result in comprehensively shutting down the individual's capabilities. Without dreams, a person is spiritually bankrupt. Without his own living space and source of money, a person is forever dependent. Without experiencing a range of emotions, including the pain of loss and the bliss of enthusiasm, a person is living life going through the motions without an authentic connection.

WELLNESS AS A REALISTIC GOAL

We look to the literature and practices on wellness, the recovery model, and spirituality to guide visions and embodiment of a *recovery lifestyle*, which also must be extended to people with symptoms of SMI who are categorized as *difficult to reach*.

First, we must recognize, accept, and identify specific symptoms of mental illness. We should not be naïve and dismiss the symptoms of mental illness and the subsequent impact of them on subjective experience and quality of life in search of a cure. Auditory hallucinations and delusions can be terribly distracting. Word-finding difficulties can be limiting. Low energy can be paralyzing. The symptoms are real and must be appropriately dealt with by means of psychotherapy, cognitive-behavioral skill-building interventions, appropriate dosages and types of neuroleptic medications, nutrition, artistic expression, and exercise. With these types of appropriate interventions, even the most distressing symptoms of mental illness can be minimized or accepted and held in a safe place internally, where they do not haunt and paralyze the person.

The construction of a successful recovery lifestyle begins with a visionary foundation. We must explore and discover the person's individual interests, strengths, and dreams. Would he like to pursue digital animation? Would she like to care for animals? Is he good at poetry and imitations? Does she have a knack for computer work? Searching, pursuing, and nurturing these interests and strengths give motivation, enthusiasm, and confidence to any person, including people with symptoms of mental illness.

Identifying and working toward specific goals builds structure, motivation, and confidence. Goals must be hopeful, flexible, productive, and realistic. However, some common mainstream mental health treatment goals are as follows: "Patient must attend two groups a week" or "Patient must be compliant with medication." Where is the motivation here? Instead, we can construct a hopeful, flexible, productive, and realistic goal, such as "In one year, Carlos will be employed as a digital animator."

Then, we work backward. Collaboratively, we work with Carlos to explore and discover what he needs to realize this dream. Consider the following examples of how recommendations for Carlos might proceed:

- Carlos needs regular and frequent access to a computer, preferably his own.
  - Does he have money to purchase a new/used computer?
    - Options include Craig's List, Goodwill, yard sales, and donations.
  - Does a friend/family member have a computer that Carlos can have?
  - Contact local businesses for a donated computer.
  - At the very least, Carlos has access to computers at the public library.
- When Carlos gets his own computer, computer care/maintenance knowledge is necessary, including keeping it in a secure place and not loaning it out.
- Carlos needs to know how to work the computer and the necessary software.
  - Take a class online or in person.
  - Connect with a friend who has computer skills.
  - Access free online instructional videos.
- Carlos needs to enter the digital animation world.
  - Talk to successful digital animators.
  - Explore and discover digital animation media: websites, magazines, etc.
  - Connect with one or more mentors.
- Carlos will need focused attention and cognitive clarity.
  - Assess for symptoms of mental illness that may be barriers to learning and focus.
  - Are medications needed?
  - Does Carlos experience self-induced barriers, including a low capacity for feeling deserving? If so, support through working these feelings with narrative therapy and CBT.

EMPLOYMENT AND RECOVERY

Employment is an evidence-based intervention toward recovery from SMI. There is a pervasive and erroneous myth regarding employment and individuals who live with SMI. Lots of frontline clinicians communicate this mantra: "Employment causes stress. Stress causes an exacerbation of psychiatric symptoms. Individuals who experience symptoms of mental illness should not work." Much is lost in this erroneous conclusion.

A working definition of *institutionalization syndrome* is when people's natural independence and developmental needs are oppressed and go into hibernation because the institution, family, or society provides for these needs. One well-known example of the institutionalization syndrome is from the 1994 movie *The Shawshank Redemption* (Darabont, 1994). Brooks had been imprisoned for most of his adult life. When the parole board decided he should be released, Brooks panicked for fear that he could not survive outside the prison. When released, he could not adjust to civilian life and meeting his own needs, especially developing a social network. Ultimately, Brooks took his own life out of abject loneliness and helplessness. This spiritual death is what can occur among individuals who live with social stigma and marginalization from mental illness. This impact is another form of iatrogenic trauma from the mental health system.

Among individuals who live with SMI, unemployment is upward of 85% (Lehman, 1995; Ridgeway & Rapp, 1998). The annual cost of this unemployment to society is greater than $78 billion. Approximately 90% of individuals who live with SMI want to work (Hatfield, Huxley, & Mohamad, 1992; Shepherd, Murray, & Muijen, 1994). Recovery-oriented work suggests creating a complex identity that is not defined by mental illness and should, if possible, include employment.

We are reminded of the empirical and consistent findings of the World Health Organization (WHO) that show that, in the long run, individuals who live with schizophrenia and related disorders in the industrialized West (chiefly Europe and the United States) have less favorable outcomes than their counterparts in developing countries (countries in Africa, Asia, and Latin America) (Hopper & Wanderling, 2000; WHO, 1973). Why is this? Many developing countries encompass a culture that endorses a competent work philosophy, meaning most people maintain a *can do* work ethic, but combined with extreme poverty rates, many live by a *must do* work philosophy, even those experiencing symptoms of physical or mental illness. For example, in many of these cultures, a psychotic episode is just that—an episode that disrupts daily living momentarily. The person experiencing this episode, rather than being sedated or institutionalized, will rejoin his or her daily work duties as soon as the episode passes and he or she is able. This dynamic creates competency and strengthens complex identity, which the previously mentioned research suggests leads to the more favorable outcomes for people who live with psychotic experiences in these countries.

Employment provides rewards in personal meaning, mastery, a needed role with responsibility, socialization, a creative outlet, and, sometimes, financial rewards, which bring additional power and a strong sense of agency. There are additional factors that contribute to these positive findings in developing countries. These countries enjoy unconditional and extended family support, especially when one is vulnerable as a result of symptoms of episodic mental illness. For better or worse, these countries do not have the presence of pharmaceutical companies and their psychotropic medications and forced psychiatric treatment in which people experience iatrogenic results. Supported or independent employment (paid and unpaid alike) can provide individuals who live with SMI purpose, personal meaning, socialization, and mastery. Employment helps to reduce physical and mental symptoms. Employment increases medication compliance, as individuals have the idea, "I will do whatever is in my power to be and stay well so I can receive the benefits of my job." In doing so, employment decreases the frequency and length of psychiatric hospitalizations. As one begins to enjoy these personal benefits, self-esteem and self-efficacy increase. Employment helps to add another dimension to one's personal identity and integrates the individual into the community. For example, one can be known for his or her knowledge, assistance, and presence in the paint department at the hardware store. As the individual enjoys increased positive socialization, he also experiences an increased perception of quality of life, and all this is what recovery-oriented work is all about.

It is not uncommon for any individual to experience errors on the job. Many of these errors occur as a result of being socially naïve or not understanding the culture of having/maintaining a job, such as showing up to work on time. The philosophy of supported employment asserts that putting a person in a job and supporting any limitations, including lack of understanding of tasks and culture, is a more recovery-oriented way to success. There are many kinds of employment situations, such as seasonal work, day labor, agency placement, temporary job placements, part-time and full-time work schedules, and volunteer work, all of which can allow a person to enjoy the various benefits of employment.

There are many reinforcers for individuals with mental illness to NOT work. Many people have peers who do not work. Family members and mental health providers discourage work because of the fear that work stress will cause an increase in psychiatric symptoms, causing the individual to lose the job and decrease self-esteem, furthering a psychiatric disability. Many individuals who live with symptoms of SMI receive monetary federal (SSI and SSDI) and state (General Relief) benefits and worry that employment payments will interfere with these benefits. Each of these concerns has its pros, cons, and limitations. Exploring the right balance and the optimal situation will allow individuals who live with symptoms of SMI to enjoy the various benefits of employment, which all goes toward increased quality of life.

WELLNESS AND A SELF-DIRECTED LIFE WORTH LIVING

Truly effective and humane mental health treatment has taken on a new face called *wellness*. Wellness has to do with achieving mental health stability and realizing personal goals, creating a self-determined life worth living. Wellness-based mental health services begin with realistic recovery attitudes among mental health professionals, including psychiatrists. These attitudes include first realizing and then assisting clients to lead a self-directed, affirming life and realizing related goals. Wellness and recovery requires discovering new resources. Wellness incorporates peers (people with lived experiences) on boards of directors, leading groups, designing programs, and as direct service providers. Peers as mental health workers can offer pervasive integrity and uncomplicated, trusted communication with clients that have a different qualitative tone than conversations with clinicians. Wellness includes everything necessary for symptom management, including social supports and neuroleptic medications. Wellness services are necessary supportive and stabilizing services of all kinds that extend beyond traditional mental health services, taking mental health services out of the community mental health center and into the normalized community, creating a self-determined life worth living (Pandya & Jän Myrick, 2013; Ursuliak, Milliken, & Morgan, 2015; Jacobson & Greenley, 2001).

When working with people who experience symptoms of SMI, we continue to evaluate the feasibility of hopeful, flexible, and realistic goals. The following questions should be considered. Is the person enjoying or finding reward in working toward or maintaining the goal? Are additional resources or supports needed? Are the expectations realistic, or should parts of the goal be revised? It is important to keep the expectations as high as possible to preserve a challenge and integrity and allow a person to reach his highest potential.

The following is a list of mental health service providers' characteristics by which clients say they most feel engaged and inspired:

- Energetic/enthusiastic
- Not burnt out
- Focusing on me, not focusing on paperwork
- Being conscious and respectful of the person in situation
- Positive, honest, and open communication
- Remembering the details of a person's stories
- Thinking of the client as a person, not a statistic
- Giving the client individual care that is personal and friendly
- Familiar rapport
- Recognizing symptoms of real mental illness. Being able to identify people who fake mental illness (malingering and other sociopathic behaviors) so they can qualify and receive services, such as housing, SSI, and mind-altering medications.

SHARED (SELF-DIRECTED) DECISION-MAKING

Shared (self-directed) decision-making is an additional effective and humane method of working collaboratively toward recovery goals.

Shared decision-making has a foundation that considers that two or more parties who have important information to offer about healthcare and other important aspects of life, such as nutrition, housing, and legal decisions, to name a few. Expert practitioners have current and accurate information on the situation, including diagnosis, expected course, and possible interventions and their potential risks. Clients or, using recovery language, "the person of the center of concern," are experts in their own lives and offer their values, intervention preferences, treatment goals, and moderating factors, including quality of life inclinations (Charles, Gafni, & Whelan, 1997; Hamann & Heres, 2014; Adams & Drake, 2006; Stewart & Brown, 2001; Noble & Douglas, 2004; Shumway et al., 2003).

Shared decision-making is a divergence from traditional unilateral decision-making, whereby practitioners make their own assessments and then prioritize problem areas and give intervention direction to the "subordinate patient." Some subgroups in NAMI, for example, have advocated for complete control over the family member with mental illness, by way of conservatorship. Furthermore, even when conservatorship is indicated, the person at the center of concern can be fully included in the shared decision-making process. Shared decision-making is more congruent with recovery model values that include autonomy, choice, accountability, and empowerment (Nelson, Lord, & Ochocka, 2001).

There are many benefits of using shared decision-making. This model includes the person at the center of concern and her values, lifestyle trade-offs, and needs. While these are pragmatic concerns, including these factors is congruent with ethical considerations that assert that people have a right to choose influences on their own lives and bodies. Additionally, including the values of the person at the center of concern increases the likelihood of success, as there will be fewer barriers to implementation (Charles & DeMaio, 1993; Nelson et al., 2001). And given that there are fewer barriers and more likelihood of the implementation of intervention recommendations, successful outcomes are more likely, which translates into fewer dollars being spent on expensive and repeated secondary and tertiary care (Polsky et al., 2003). Shared decision-making has benefits in the areas of client satisfaction, ethical congruency, therapeutic relationships, economics, and epidemiology of healthcare outcomes.

Some have suggested that shared decision-making with individuals with SMI results in negative outcomes. One proposed idea is that including the person at the center of concern offers yet another choice point and too many choices can overwhelm the individual (Kahneman & Tyersky, 1979). Others suggest that the experience of making the wrong choice may instill a feeling of lost opportunity and regret and the individual may make decisions based on avoiding this feeling. Additionally, the individual may have goals that are unrealistic in the actualities of healthcare and other contemporary systems (Loomes & Sugden, 1982). These ideas are a manifestation of patronizing and oppressive low expectations for individuals who live with mental illness. The professional should be educating the individual about the complete parameters of the situation and doing so in evidenced-based communication styles, such as motivational interviewing. Where individuals are overwhelmed and defer necessary decisions to professionals or others, this in itself is considering the individual's wishes.

Another concern about shared decision-making is that the individual may have difficulty fully anticipating and appreciating the manifestations of illness and as a result make wrong decisions (Kievit, Nooij, & Stiggelbout, 2001). This suggests that once decisions are made, reevaluation is not possible and decisions made are irrevocable, which could not be further from the truth. Individuals and professionals are forever able to reevaluate and revise necessary choice points. Another concern is the time (i.e., money) it takes to include, hear, and discuss the wishes of the person at the center of concern. It is well known in many professional industries that spending time on the front end in developing a relationship often accelerates efficiency in the future, through using empathy, appreciating values, developing trust, and agreeing on a foreseeable plan and outcomes. While there can be barriers to fully incorporating this shared decision-making model, this philosophy should be regularly incorporated into discussions of care.

In all choice points in life, we are forever weighing the benefits and risks. Shared decision-making is congruent with recovery model ethical values, including autonomy, choice, empowerment, accountability, client as expert of her own life, and reaching self-potential. Shared decision-making has shown positive outcomes in healthcare and other aspects of life. This model is not a guarantee of perfection, but no existing model promises perfection. Where professionals can provide current and relevant information and work collaboratively, people who are at the center of concern should be allowed to articulate their values and concerns, and influence and make decisions that impact their own lives.

UNCONVENTIONAL STRATEGIES FOR THOSE
DIFFICULT TO REACH

Finally, as one realizes that the person is really not aware of the cost of their toxic and destructive behavior and not at all interested in making a change, we use unconventional strategies to preserve integrity and safety of all in a peaceful community.

These strategies are organized, intentional, and firm efforts that, at all costs, hold authority with the rare person who is toxic to a therapeutic environment.

The Opiate Retreat

It was a Friday afternoon at 4 pm in a general medical hospital in downtown Los Angeles. I received a consultation request from a general medical/surgical unit. There was a 27-year-old woman, Jada, who was admitted and now discharged from the hospital and would not leave. She was a registered patient who had been discharged 30 hours before. The consultation was a request to have her removed from the hospital.

First, I spoke with the medical staff to gather the necessary client information and what had been done thus far. Jada had presented to the emergency department 4 days prior seeking relief for back pain. Many medical tests had been conducted, and all were inconclusive, meaning the origin and location of Jada's back pain could not be detected. Jada continued to demand high doses of Percocet, Dilaudid, Demerol, and Fentanyl—prescription opiate medications intended for severe pain and inpatient use only. In the room was her boyfriend, who had stayed with her for the entire time of her 4-day inpatient hospitalization. The medical staff determined that Jada did not need any further medical tests and there was nothing more that could be done for her. It was determined that she was malingering (faking) the back pain symptoms to receive the powerful prescription opiate medications.

With permission, I entered Jada's room. There, I found Jada dressed in a hospital gown, laying in bed, and talking on the phone to her auntie. Her boyfriend was at her bedside. There were empty food trays around the room. Jada was furious, as the medical staff had been trying to get her to leave and she reported that her back pain was not being treated. After introducing myself, I asked her about her specific plans. She simply wanted more prescription opiate pain medication.

I could see that Jada and her boyfriend were homeless. Coming to the hospital, while sterile and seemingly quite boring to me, it was a comfortable respite for the couple. It was safe, clean, and warm. Jada and her boyfriend had their own restroom with a shower. There was a steady stream of food being delivered to her bedside. Furthermore, there was enough food for Jada *and* her boyfriend. Hospital staff spoke to Jada in a friendly or interpersonally neutral tone, at the worst. But, most of all, on her inpatient retreat, Jada had a steady stream of free, sterile, and extremely high potent prescription opiate medication being regularly delivered to her bedside. With her boyfriend also at her bedside, what more could she ask for?

This situation was ripe with rapidly sinking integrity and morale among hospital staff. It was costing taxpayers approximately $3,000 a day and approximately

$50,000 in diagnostic medical exams (MRI, blood work, x-ray, etc.) to fund Jada's opiate retreat. Jada should have been discharged 3 days prior and quite possibly never admitted to the inpatient unit of the hospital. But, she was there now and refused to leave.

In a firm and warm tone, I explained to Jada that the medical staff was saying that there would be nothing more they could do for her. Jada furiously requested a second physician opinion. That had already taken place, and the second physician agreed that there was nothing more that could be done than had already been done for Jada.

I saw Jada with "The Spider's Thread" perspective. She saw no cost to her choices and behaviors. She was destructive to herself and others in her path. Integrity and safety needed to be asserted and maintained. My tone was firm, warm, and unattached to her desperate demands. Jada and her boyfriend vacating hospital property was my goal. Seeing that she had a large range of social and mental health needs, I asked Jada if I could help her find a place to stay and link her with some resources. She refused. I told her that I could see that she was risking everything so that she could get more prescription opiate pain medication and that we could arrange for her to get residential treatment for her drug dependence. She was inflamed and denied being drug-dependent, reasserting that her severe back pain was the only reason for her request for the medications. Again, she refused to leave the hospital. Gently, firmly, and neutrally, I explained the imminent consequences to her. If she did not leave the hospital, the staff would call the police and have her arrested. I told her that I did not want that for her and reiterated that I could connect her with more useful resources.

Jada was repeating everything to her auntie, who remained on the phone. Jada shoved the phone toward me and said that her auntie wanted to talk to me. Neutrally, I denied this request. It was important to keep the conversation between Jada and me to minimize stimulation. Additionally, I made respectful eye contact and spoke to Jada's boyfriend, but I did not ask him for any input.

Impulsively and desperately, Jada claimed that she was going to call the local news to have them do an exposé on the discriminatory hospital practices. I explained to Jada that she was welcome to do that and that there was a payphone outside the hospital on the corner. Jada blurted out that she would go to another hospital for further back pain evaluation and asked me to call an ambulance for her. I explained that because of EMTALA laws (Emergency Treatment and Labor Act, aka, "hospital antidumping laws"), transferring her to another hospital under her circumstances was not possible. She asked me then to arrange a taxi for her to be taken to another hospital. Remaining neutral, I explained to her that this would be considered hospital dumping and the laws prevented me from doing that. Again, I explained to

Jada that the medical staff had concluded that there was nothing medical that they could do for her. I told her that she seemed desperate for the prescription opiate pain medications and that I could help her go to a residential detox program. Aside from that, I explained to Jada that it was time to collect her belongings and vacate the hospital. Moving closer to Jada, almost energetically and sympathetically holding her hand (but not in reality), I added new important prompts for her. I said that if she was not out of the hospital in 10 minutes, the police would be called, and she would be arrested for trespassing on hospital property. I asked her if there was anything I could do to help her collect her belongings. Jada resolved, "I see what is happening here. They have sent the nice lady to come here and kick me out." I said, "Yes, Jada. That is what is happening." Cursing to herself and throwing her things in her duffle bag, she and her boyfriend were out of the room in 5 minutes.

Additionally, seeing how desperate Jada was, I contacted the hospital transportation department and arranged for a wheelchair to safely help her out of the hospital. Funny how elevators sometimes do not close properly or steps may be especially slippery when one is being asked to leave a facility.

That day, I was a hero with hospital staff because integrity and safety were preserved, which was acutely necessary. However, my heart did not feel like a hero for Jada. There she was, a homeless young woman addicted to opiates, with passive boyfriend in tow, on her endless way to the next hospital emergency department, seeking high-strength prescription opiate medications and spewing destruction in her path.

Many unconventional strategies were used in this situation with Jada. At every turn, it was important to treat Jada with respect, honesty, and potency. If she ever had a wink of desire for help, I hoped that our 15 minutes together would have made a strong imprint on her capacity to trust, and she would allow another worker to help her. Recovery is a process of creating a personal self-determined life worth living. Sometimes these steps toward recovery are microscopic steps not immediately known or witnessed. Setting clear and strong limits with neutral emotion was essential. *Love* and *firmness* are my mantras when preserving integrity and safety in situations like this with Jada.

No one wishes to be in the custody of police or child protective services (CPS) or held against her will in a mental institution. Few family members and social service workers look forward to making those calls. That said, sometimes making calls to protective services is exactly what is needed to preserve safety and integrity when a person has consciously or unknowingly crossed boundaries. You are encouraged to do what you have to do. Acting respectfully, ethically, and swiftly will most importantly preserve safety and security in the present moment and, quite possibly, impact a new internal meaning association for the individual in question. That Friday night,

I went home emotionally exhausted, as I often do. All that was done with Jada was necessary but not enjoyable.

FINAL THOUGHTS

Readers are challenged to persistently and consistently assert conscious intentions to practice this commitment of reaching the most difficult paradigm shift. This type of selfless, ethical therapeutic work can be incredibly emotionally taxing on the clinician or family member. It takes everything out of us, sometimes, to give all of our selves with the intent to help another. This work is both rewarding and exhausting. Sometimes the work is intense, and sometimes it is extremely slow moving. In the following chapter, these types of emotionally demanding experiences are validated Additionally, essential self-care techniques are explored for the clinician and loved ones who are *Listening with Psychotic Ears.*

12

Survivor and Self-Care for Families and Clinicians Who Work

with People Living with Symptoms of Mental Illness

THE GOOD AND noble people in relationships with individuals who experience symptoms of severe mental illness (SMI) struggle. Think about it. If you did not care and did not have high expectations for this person, then his or her living a low quality of life with a lot of dysphoric emotions would be OK with you. Social isolation, psychological suffering, poor self-care, lack of employment and education, and alienation of family members, friends, clinicians, and community establishments through bizarre behaviors, substance misuse, and even violence are *not* acceptable to you, nor should they ever be.

Good, noble, and visionary mental health clinicians struggle to fit in with complacent colleagues who follow the mainstream mental health treatment philosophy. Here, we see outcomes that include individuals with mental illness whose spirit, cognitive capacity, and life status are withering away down *The River* of an isolated, emotionally numb, physically unhealthy lifestyle of simply going through the motions of living. This oppressive *River* of mainstream mental health treatment is not suitable for any human being. And, is it really working? Look at the expansive statistics of homelessness, adolescents and adults who increasingly turn to substances and other behaviors as a way of coping, and the rapid swelling of the population in jails and prisons in the United States. Disability (as a result of mental illness) payroll is also rising drastically.

Good, noble, and visionary mental health clinicians do not identify with nor experience personal rewards in a broken mezzo and macro system. The visionary clinician frequently witnesses transgressions, and the resulting emotional reactions and spiritual deterioration become increasingly difficult to shake off. Things that are witnessed include people in and out of acute and long-term psychiatric hospitalizations without manifesting improvement; short- and long-term negative effects of the overuse of neuroleptic medications, the unequal power differential under which people who need help have no voice, especially when they are treated unjustly, the rippling negative effects of behavioral and chemical addiction, and the frequent attempted and successful suicides as a result of desperation and hopelessness.

Good, noble, and visionary mental health clinicians experience a spiritual and psychological grieving process as it pertains to the enthusiasm with which they entered the human service field. These clinicians struggle to find hopeful and feasible answers from their supervisors, who hold little hope for clients. Frequent are *tongue-in-cheek* comments from inpatient psychiatric professionals: "Oh! I see Nadine is back!" These clinicians struggle to find effective and needed resources when there are so few.

There is always a measure of adjustment to conforming to any new work system. In mainstream mental health treatment, instead of simply learning the logistics of the job, the adjustment often comes in the form of dwindling hope for increased quality of life, expectations for necessary and available resources, and visions for new and feasible inspiration in work environments. In more than an isolated circumstance, as the enthusiastic and visionary student enters her mental health professional internship, the spiritually burnt-out supervisor is personally and unconsciously threatened and begins overly criticizing this optimistic student. A common direction from the supervisor is to tell the student not to spend so much time with a client, suggesting that the clinician is giving too much, enabling the client to become dependent. The intention might consciously be to help the student be successful in the system, but the result is disillusionment and quelling the enthusiasm. Some workers protest and either cause change or leave. For others, burnout is in the foreseeable future. When the system breaks down in this way for clinicians, the clients suffer losses as well, and a cycle of ineffective and uninspired treatment is maintained.

The stories we hear and experience are so complicated and heartbreaking, even to those who are less sensitive. Closely interacting with individuals who live with SMI is hard work, and we must find ways to buffer against the distressing and haunting things people do to each other. To be able to join a person in his distress or even just to hear the stories, as in professional case consultation groups or support groups, and constantly hold hope is an exceptional achievement. To be successful and spiritually full, we must find efficacious ways to be present with clients and then *shake it off* without becoming spiritually burnt out, psychologically hardened, and interpersonally guarded.

This clinical work with people who experience symptoms of SMI can be challenging and difficult to maintain, as the recovery path is rarely in straight and rising succession. Fromm-Reichmann (1960) and other substantial clinicians assert how very slow this work is with people with SMI.

Many mental health professionals come with similar personal histories and family situations, where they have witnessed the struggle with symptoms of mental illness and its impact on individuals and families. The good, noble, and visionary mental health clinicians and family members struggle to manage their own countertransference reactions and feelings, such as shame, disappointment, and overcompensation. The struggle is productive, for the opposite of struggle is to deny and submit, which would lead to social and spiritual pandemonium.

This chapter is intended to accurately understand, validate, and intentionally make efforts to maintain mental, physical, and spiritual health among mental health treatment professionals and other people in close relationships with those who experience symptoms of SMI, especially psychosis. I am conscious that in this and the previous chapter, I have diverted from the word "psychosis" to a more inclusive phenomena of SMI. In the last chapter, I was discussing interventions to reach people with all kinds of SMI symptoms that go beyond psychosis, including addiction, depression, and social disruptions, such as violence. In this chapter, self-understanding and effective interventions are offered for those who are in close relationship with people with SMI, including psychosis and beyond.

SELF-CARE TIPS

The following pages are filled with concrete interventions for the maintenance of physical, mental, and spiritual health for any person who is in close relationship with individuals who experience symptoms of SMI. Do not be discouraged by the simplicity or seemingly far-reaching interventions listed here. Consider this chapter as a self-care checklist, and seriously attend to and make room for each topic. Everyone partakes in self-care in his or her own unique pace and manner.

Get Enough Sleep

Each body and brain operates more efficiently and at peak when all its needs are met. Simply put, sleep washes out toxins in the brain that have collected through the day and replenishes necessary neurotransmitters, resulting in the person experiencing a stable sense of pleasurable well-being. Any less, and the person will feel any range of physical illness, impulsivity, and unstable emotions including irritability, depression, and a sense of being overwhelmed. People need approximately 6 to 9 hours of sleep each 24-hour period. If one gets only 4 hours of sleep one night, making up the sleep on another night is nearly impossible. To make up the sleep would require the person to sleep 8 plus 4 hours (= 12 hours) of sleep, but it can be done over a period of time. Demanding responsibilities and the natural circadian rhythm do not naturally allow for sleep to be made up. There is general scientific consensus on the eroding physical effects of sleep deprivation, including overeating and the resulting physical diseases (i.e., diabetes, hypertension, joint dysfunction, etc.), poor response times that are worse than performing under substance (alcohol) influence, and decreased immune function and ability to fight off cancer and other serious diseases. Simply put, to perform at one's peak, a person must get his or her unique amount of sleep.

Busy and demanding schedules keep our brains alert. Bedtime routines that include wind-down rituals are necessary. Here are some simple examples of wind-down rituals: Change into comfortable bedclothes. Consciously let go of the day's worries and emotional reactions by way of meditation, writing, or listening to soft music, such as Native American flutes, Tibetan bowls, or nature sounds, which can be calming and comforting (Siegel, 2007). Eat a light snack, such as fruit or soup. Avoid spicy or heavy carbohydrate foods, as these are stimulating. Soak in a warm bath with soothing essential oils, such as lavender, chamomile, or patchouli. (A word of caution! Essentials oils are concentrated; therefore, only a drop will do. Many of the fragrances are quite strong and may be stimulating or offensive to your senses.) Be sure you are warm or cool enough, altering your clothing and use of blankets, opening or closing windows, and adjusting the thermostat. Do not use electronics 2 hours before closing eyes or in the middle of the night when you cannot fall back to sleep. The blue light in televisions and electronic screens (computers and smartphones, too) are stimulating to the brain, interrupting neurotransmitters. For survival reasons, we are drawn toward moving objects or scenes, which will monopolize our attention and keep us stimulated. Thus, avoiding the use of screens before bedtime is recommended. As one cannot sleep, repeat any of these behaviors. Remember, you do not have to be unconscious to enjoy the benefits of sleep. Quiet rest can cause brain rejuvenation. Additionally, tossing and turning in bed is counterproductive and will often result in the person becoming agitated because he or she cannot fall asleep. Get out of bed and do something either productive to positively expend some energy or something calming. During exceptionally stressful times, when you are experiencing an extended lack of sleep, the temporary use of over-the-counter or prescription sleep medications can be discussed with your physician. A sufficient amount of sleep is necessary for the brain and body to efficiently function.

Eat Nutritiously

Just as proper sleep is essential in peak mental and physical functioning, regular nutritious eating habits are fundamental. Make sure to eat foods that are rich in nutrients. Joel Fuhrman, a medical physician and a nutritionist, in his bestselling books, *Eat to Live* (2011) and *Eat to Live Cookbook* (2014), explains how eating healthy and nutritious foods keep a person thinking more clearly and feeling emotionally stable and physically healthy. Fuhrman emphasizes not to indulge in too much food with carbohydrates, including sugar, bread, and pasta, which make us sluggish, irritable, hungry, and sick. We all know how we feel when we overindulge in the delicious satisfaction of M&M's or the convenience of a Doritos lunch. These overindulgences cause people to put on weight, be irritable, not think clearly, and crave more. Fuhrman (2011) emphasizes eating primarily and daily from the *GBOMBS* categories: Greens, Beans, Onions, Mushrooms, Berries, and Seeds. He asserts that eating several small meals throughout the day is much more sustainable than eating one to three heavy meals, as this latter frequency causes peaks and crashes in sugar levels, which alter thinking and energy levels. He emphasizes that intentional nutritious eating requires prethought and planning. You know when you are going to be hungry about the same times every single day, so plan for and have available the foods that your machine requires for peak performance.

Regularly Meet All of Your Needs in an Intentional,
High-Quality Manner

We are hardwired for mutual human relationships. Visit with your friends and colleagues in a place where you can freely engage in a shared conversation. Do not only plan these visits in loud, busy places, such as a basketball game, music concert, or dance club. Make sure your car is dependable. If you use a computer for your work or daily tasks, make sure it is dependable. If your feet hurt, see a podiatrist and follow the recommendations.

Identify and Plug Energy Drainers

If there is a person or activity in your life that negatively consumes a large portion of your energy, alter, minimize, or stop contact. In one of my several existential crises, on the recommendation of my wise friend, Wanda, I told my husband that I was on an energy budget. I realized I was spending way too much time with people I felt obligated toward, whose company I did not enjoy. Before, during, and after spending time with these people, I felt emotionally and cognitively exhausted, for which I then carried resentment. Additionally, spending my time with such people reduced the already-limited time I had to spend alone or with people in which a mutual enjoyment of each other's company existed. Choose to spend your time with people who are present, get you, and leave you feeling inspired and refreshed. We all have people to whom and responsibilities to which we choose to be obligated. Family members often fall into this category. Here, we focus on the positive rewards (such as fulfilling your family duty) and perform the obligations with joy in our hearts (Tolle, 2018).

Things, as well as people, can be energy drainers. Fix or replace things in your environment that no longer work. Many people come from financial situations and cultures that do not look positively on overindulgence, with frugality and prudence being the primary cultural values. We often use things until they literally fall apart, which causes us to lose time trying to improvise so we can use that thing one more time. Over the next week, make the intention to look around your environment and identify things that are broken. Either fix, discard (by way of donation, recycling, or trash), or replace the things you frequently use. You will notice a profound shift energetically when you clear your physical space, rather than adjusting your life to accommodate the dysfunction.

Now, that said, in our capitalist and consumption-driven Western culture, the spaces where we spend the majority of our time can be overcome with environments that no longer work. How do you feel in your office or workspace? How do you feel in your car? How do you feel in your home? How do you feel when you open your workbag? All too often, these environments reflect our psychology and do not lend to a productive space. In his book *It's All Too Much Workbook: The Tools You Need to Conquer Clutter and Create the Life you Want* (2009), Peter Walsh talks spiritually and practically about clearing the clutter in our living spaces. Now, I have about seven of these *organizing* books. I have to say that Walsh talks about clearing clutter in a motivating, practical, and supportive way that resonated with me. As practical as he is, he surrounds everything with spirituality, which seems to be an irregular characteristic for a professional organizer but very genuine in Walsh's case. Seeing him speak, it is apparent that Walsh is a compassionate person who wants people to reach their potentials.

Walsh (2009) begins with the following guide points:

- Clutter stops us from living in the present.
- Clutter makes us forget what is really important.
- Clutter robs us of real value.
- Clutter steals our space.
- Clutter monopolizes our time.
- Clutter takes over.

- Clutter jeopardizes our relationships.
- Other people's clutter robs us of opportunities that should be ours.
- Clutter denies us peace of mind.
- Clutter erodes our spiritual Selves.

Walsh offers the following steps: (1) think of the purpose of the room; (2) put only the things in there that you need for that purpose, (the tricycle does not belong in the bedroom), make sure those things are in good condition (toss or repair broken items), and consider the number of the things you need and no more (e.g., 10 pairs of cozy socks are not necessary); (3) get rid of everything else by recycling; and (4) enjoy the simplicity of space and peace of organization and intention.

Walsh has many practical ideas. One that I liked is to turn all the hangers of your clothes backward. When you wear something, turn the hanger forward. See how many hangers are not turned at the end of the year. Try the same practice with cookbooks. When you use a cookbook, tag the page. At the end of a year, see how many cookbooks are not tagged. Consider passing on the ones you do not use.

Enjoy the process of letting go, repurposing, and making room for new opportunities that nurture your soul. A note of caution, this letting go process is contagious. You will naturally get into the intellectual practice of evaluating everything and every aspect of your life, which is a life-changing, emotional, and liberating experience.

Develop and Nurture Rich and Rewarding Life Experiences

- Be with inspirational and comforting people with whom you feel good.
- Participate in activities, hobbies, and relationships you enjoy so much that you lose track of time. These activities will also give you natural doses of dopamine, a naturally occurring neurotransmitter responsible for experiencing pleasure.
- Participate in activities that are predictable and you know to be enjoyable. Stay in your comfort zone.
- Get out of your comfort zone. Seek out people, places, and activities you would like to explore.

Be Reflective of Your Feelings That Bring on Strong Reactions

Keep clean your side of the street.

- Own and regulate power struggles with others. Likely, there is a particular person or type of person with whom you find yourself in a power struggle or another nonproductive dynamic. Be reflective about this pattern. Talk to a trusted friend or other guide to get some insight about your part in the interpersonal struggle. Let go of any denial or other face-saving thoughts to which you might cling. Construct and carry out a detailed and intentional plan as to how you want these relationships to go in the future.

- Be assertive when necessary. If someone shortchanges you or overcharges you, let them know. Stand up for yourself with those whose style has exploitative or bullying tones.

- Be flexible when possible. If someone you love (like a family member with mental illness) has a need at an inconvenient time, reconsider your priorities. Sometimes, you will choose to drop everything to help. Sometimes, you will choose to keep your distance and communicate your unavailability. Every person and their situation are unique, and only you know what is best for you.

Take Breaks and Vacations Without Feeling Guilty

- On your break, participate in things that are rejuvenating and soothing. Maybe you want to meet some new people. Maybe you want to isolate. Maybe you want to explore different ethnic restaurants or try a new activity, such as canoeing or hearing a speaker. Participate in the things you know *blow your hair back*, such as a massage, foreign films, being with children, cooking, visiting museums, hiking, or riding your motorcycle, to name a few.

- Take small breaks from hearing the despairing experiences that people experience. It is OK to admit that these experiences can be too much for the mind to bear. Do not sit with these overwhelming stories and feelings alone. Speak with a supervisor or trusted colleague about your reactions to what you see and hear. Getting yourself in a therapeutic relationship to understand and offload the most overwhelming parts of hearing these stories is another necessary self-care activity. Therapy does not have to be with a formal evidence-based modality. Therapy occurs within relieving or healing intentions. Spending time with children can serve these purposes. Doing a focused art form (painting or crafting) or sport (bicycle riding) can be therapeutic. Eastern practices such as acupuncture, meditation, massage, yoga, the use of teas and herbs, and intuitive awareness all have therapeutic actions. You have to find what method most enjoyably and efficiently relieves and heals you.

Exercise Compassion, Especially Toward Yourself

The person who is your client or family member has likely been through some emotionally wrenching experiences. Make every possible effort to be the compassionate helper you imagine you would want for yourself or your loved one when help is needed. In my lifetime of full-time work with people with SMIs in emergency settings, drawing on my compassion, as well as an infinite resource bank, and occasional self-directed humor have been my saving graces. With each and every person with whom I spoke, my compassionate spirit leapt forward and conducted the therapeutic interview.

By My Special Guest

One evening, I came through the main hospital entrance to my usual shift work in emergency department. Immediately, I reacted to the strong stench of old feces, urine, and sweat. Before I deposited my belongings, I asked the triage nurse for some details about this strong odor. She simply pointed to a small interview room where a man was slumped over in a wheelchair. I asked where he was in line to be seen by the medical staff. She gruffly responded, "We will get to him!"

About 20 minutes later, I went back to see where this man was in the triage line. Still, he had not been seen. Upon asking, I was given the message that I, as the social worker, was crossing her line. "There were other, more urgent medical situations ahead of him." Well, realizing that it was, indeed, a Trauma I emergency department, there were likely people experiencing cardiac arrest, gunshots, kidney failure, and other very serious medical situations. After two hours of my own arrival, the triage nurse still had not seen the man in the wheelchair. He was not even in line to be seen by medical staff.

During the months when Chicago felt its harshest and most unforgiving temperatures (February, when the wind chill factor can easily be felt at -25°F), a mobile psychiatric crisis team is sent out to assist those individuals who are not able to find his or her way inside, else one's life will imminently be at risk.

Gerry's history was not all that uncommon. He had a representative payee whose job it was to receive his monthly financial deposits and pay his rent, provide groceries, and perform other essential financial disbursements. Over these harsh weather months, he and his representative payee had somehow been disconnected. With this, Gerry was evicted from his hotel room (SRO) and was literally sitting for several days on a park bench. The bustling Michigan Avenue passersby fed him their restaurant leftovers. He did not leave the bench, even to use the bathroom. His jeans were filled with wet and dry feces. His boots were filled with frozen urine. His extremities were frost bitten. I could not passively allow this man to sit in his own feces for hours in a nationally renowned hospital emergency department without doing something about it.

Seeing that Gerry was being avoided and no one knew the extent of his acute medical needs, I rounded up another mental health worker. We made eye contact and allowed our sense of justice to move us. "Let's roll." Within minutes, we were gowned from head to toe in hospital protective gear. The stench was so severe, that we all had to wear hospital masks with cotton balls of perfume inside. We brought the man into an interview room. Fortunately, he was very cooperative and grateful. He repeatedly told us, "When this is all over, I am going to have a party at my house on Long Island, and you will be my special guests." We later found out that Gerry's family had provided a large trust fund, and he had a trust officer whose task was to manage these funds.

Gerry's jeans, which had to be cut off, were stiff with ice made of hardened feces and urine. His legs were filled with infected sores. His feet were so inflamed, swollen, and red like a tomato, he could not even stand on them. It was necessary to also cut off his urine filled boots. We bathed him again and again. The stench was so offensive that we had to take intermittent breaks and go outside to fully breathe. He continued to say how grateful he was and invited us as his "special guests" to his Long Island mansion.

Just as we were bagging up the washcloths, emptying soap containers, and collecting his clothes—two hours later—the triage nurse and the shift nurse manager busted into the room with an ironic tone that felt as though they were angry at us for cleaning up Gerry. "We were looking all over for this guy! We were just about to do all this. You did not have to do this!" It did not take a rocket scientist to see that these administrative nurses were embarrassed and ashamed for their professional transgression.

Ultimately, Gerry was admitted first to a general medical unit and then transferred to a transitional housing and treatment facility. It was our strong sense of compassion and doing right by this vulnerable man that allowed us to make our way through this unimaginable (on several levels) situation. Had I been angry and resentful about having to clean up this man, all of us would have had a very negative experience. Compassion and humanity motivated our work with Gerry.

Allow Your Intuition to Give You Useful Information and Guide Your Steps

Some people would say, "Trust your gut." Others would say, "Use your good clinical judgment." All these methods are ways in which your wise mind receives and communicates the most accurate and useful information. Sometimes, I sense what to pay attention to, important information on which to focus, or innovative ideas. Sometimes, we get information about potential dangers and needs or explanations.

Sometimes, current symptoms give clues about a person's likely trauma history. Paying attention to your active intuition can save yours and others' lives.

Allow Yourself to Be Curious

In our Western society and even in our professional lives, we are often discouraged from getting too close and asking too many questions, as this may be negatively perceived as being *nosey*, snooping, or meddlesome. Remember, people who experience symptoms of psychosis are often socially marginalized and have very few trustworthy people with whom to talk. The person is seeking support and intervention from you. You can preface your questioning with statements, such as "I know this is a sensitive topic . . . ," or "I'll bet that lots of people in your situation would turn to marijuana. Is this something you are doing?"

The more information you have will help you to more accurately assist the person in his or her situation. If your authenticity and genuine desire for the individual's well-being are being considered and your tone is respectful, the person will often, but not always, drop their guard.

Communicate Commitment and Repair When There Is Tension in the Relationship

People tend to bring to a relationship personal baggage or relevant issues that collide with the personal experiences of the other person. When these conflicts happen, repairing and recommitting to the relationship is essential for successful therapeutic work.

You Do Not Want to Work with Me Either!

Jessie is a 27-year-old female who was self-referred to a mental health and addiction treatment facility. She had a lifetime of sexual abuse and abandonment. She had alienated all family, except her grandmother. She carried a haughty tone with all residents and staff, except Brianne, who had a motherly demeanor—forgiving but firm. Brianne accepted another work position and was leaving the facility, causing Jessie to need to transfer therapists. Joyce would be Jessie's new therapist. Jessie's attitude was described as negative, hostile, and isolative. She often sat in groups alone with arms crossed and frequently rolled eyes. The following conversation occurred:

JOYCE: When we are together, I notice an attitude that is getting in the way of our work. Do you feel it?

JESSIE: (with arms crossed) Hmmmmmm (suggesting yes, but I don't give a damn).

JOYCE: Can we talk about this together?

JESSIE: (screaming) You said you were going to be my new therapist as you were walking down the hall! You said this in front of everyone!

JOYCE: Jessie, did you feel like my introduction to you was not sensitive and that I might not really want to work with you? Did my introduction feel as though I was sharing your business with everyone?

JESSIE: YES! No one really wants to work with me anyway! You are starting out disrespecting me, too!

JOYCE: I can see that you are feeling very sensitive about your work with your therapist, and you would have preferred if I had introduced myself in private so that we could have talked about it, which would have respected your privacy.

JESSIE: (more quietly but still emotional, now crying) Ya.

JOYCE: (looking in Jessie's eyes, handing her tissue) Jessie, I apologize for the way I introduced myself to you. I was excited to work with you and wanted to tell you this news as soon as I saw you. I can see how you thought this way was not taking our work seriously. I also see that you are a very private person, and I will be sure to respect your privacy in our work together. Do you think we can work together? To do good work, we need a partnership. Is this something you are interested in?

JESSIE: (slowing down crying, sitting up straighter, and wiping her own tears) Yes.

JOYCE: Great! I am looking forward to our work together! (In their first private session, Jessie and Joyce had a conversation about what each would need from each other to work together. These points were written down and referred to from time to time in their work together.)

Remember, this person has likely had multiple experiences that include social marginalization or rejection, especially when help is most needed. As you sense that miscommunication or a power struggle has occurred, as soon as possible, recognize it, identify it with the person, make attempts to repair (aka, apologize, construct mutual strategies for better results), and restate your commitment to the helping/supportive relationship (i.e., "I am here for you. Can we try again?").

Trust in the Person's Rational Side, as Well as the Spiritual Side

All people, whether living with a mental illness or not, have some sense of spirituality about them and seek the following:

- Connection with others;
- Forgiving/absolving/cleansing experiences;
- Blissful and peak experiences;

- Inspiration and support for personal growth;
- Explanations that are bigger than the self;
- A sense of accomplishment, mastery, and power.

While some communications are bizarre and difficult to decipher, equally, some communications are factual and straightforward.

Increase the Capacity to Tolerate Primitive Affect

People who have psychotic experiences are in touch with primitive and strong emotions. If the intention is to help, we must hear and be able to tolerate these expressions. I want to acknowledge again the extreme and unthinkable experiences that people have, often at the hands of others and, many times, trusted others. While we do not want to force people to talk about these experiences if they do not want to, we do want to be available and be able to handle the short- and long-term emotional reactions.

The process of developing the capacity to tolerate primitive affect is a delicate one, as a particular amount of distance is required. If too much distance occurs, coldness may be perceived. If too much closeness occurs, burnout or overdependence are risked. Interpersonal closeness and distance are both necessary for effective work with people who live with psychotic experiences.

> If the staff can cope with the anxiety generated in them and can convey their willingness to understand the patients, a sense of containment develops and the anxiety is gradually relieved. Containment is not, however, a passive phenomenon, and the patient has to feel understood to feel contained. He may then come to believe that someone can enter into his experience and share some of his suffering without themselves collapsing. (Jackson & Williams, 1994, p. xiii)

In his book *Unimaginable Storms*, Murray Jackson shares edited process recordings of therapeutic conversations with people who experience psychosis. He points out the range in which people respond to their treatment. As a result of the psychodynamic interpretive therapeutic work, many show a lasting transformation, others show little to no change, and others relapse quickly as the therapeutic support is terminated. This slow, tedious, and potentially unsustainable work causes the clinician to question his or her efforts. In one Greek myth, Sisyphus, a king, was doomed to the pattern of pushing a heavy rock up a hill, only to have it immediately roll back down. Faced with such continuous disappointments, the existential philosopher Camus (1942) asserted, we have three reactionary options:

1. Discover the meaninglessness of this pattern, stop trying, and walk away;
2. Acknowledge and accept the never-ending pattern that is devoid of purpose, and go through the motions;
3. Keep trying, and look outside the situation to a higher power for inspiration and hope for change.

We see this range of adaptation with staff members who are faced with making the change from the authoritarian medical model to the collaborative and hopeful recovery model in working with people with symptoms of mental illnesses:

1. Some do not believe in the principles and decide to walk away and resign. (If the person does not believe in the hope and feasibility of increasing quality of life, walking away is a desired response.)
2. Some give a nod to recovery model principles and go through the motions, but they are emotionally, interpersonally, and intellectually dissociated, thus, going through the motions of daily work.
3. Some seek additional education and training to be able to identify and practice more humane and accurate therapeutic principles and strategies. Individuals in the third group are more likely to be present, effective, and hopeful in their work, enjoying more personal reward.

Clients who work with this third group of clinicians are more likely to be more stable, having reduced psychiatric hospitalizations, using less street drugs, experiencing fewer medical and mental health crises, having fewer interactions with the criminal justice system, having a wider social support network, and enjoying employment or education. Jackson shares his ideas of psychotherapeutic principles with people who live with psychotic experiences in his book, *Weathering the Storm: Psychotherapy for Psychosis* (Jackson, 2001).

We Are Hardwired for Interpersonal Closeness, and People Who Have Psychotic Experiences Want and Need This, Too

Clinicians are often oversocialized to be a *blank screen*. This means that the clinician is interpersonally distant and guarded and offers little to no interpersonal interaction to the client. The therapeutic purpose of being a blank screen is so that the clinician's identity does not impact the client's identity or reactions, keeping clear the pathway for the client's authentic development of self. However, with little to nothing to go on, an environment is created in which self-depreciating material festers, especially among people who have experiences of repeated interpersonal rejection or trauma.

I Love You

I hung up the phone at my office desk in a residential treatment facility. My client Darrisha had walked in just as I said, "Goodbye. I love you!" Darrisha was beside herself with disbelief and anger. She shot me a look that was piercing and left the office. I went to her room to repair any transgression on my part, but first, I had to ask her what just happened, for I did not know what her assumptions were. Fortunately, she agreed to speak with me and asked me who I was just talking with on the phone. Since I had been trained to be that blank screen, I responded, "Who could you imagine that I was speaking with?" She slammed the door in my face and would not speak to me for several days. When she had cooled off a bit, I discovered that Darrisha thought I was speaking with a client and had wondered why I had not ever ended our conversation with an "I love you." Her anger had served to defend her ideal sense of self that knew she was deserving of my love. The interaction would have gone much differently if I had simply answered that it was my mother I was speaking with on the phone.

Because of the social marginalization and lack of trusted people to interact with, people with psychotic experiences see mental health treatment as a medium for regular and therapeutically intimate interactions. The client is expected to reveal everything about his or her most inner thoughts. Being so blank is often experienced as being sterile and withholding, at the least.

One day, a colleague and I were discussing her client who has psychotic experiences. At one point in the conversation, the clinician alarmingly stopped and asked, "Wait, did my client have that dream or did I?" This level of psychological merging is, at times, necessary to truly understand the experiences of another. Sometimes, it is useful to first accurately and deeply understand these experiences so we have the opportunity to relieve and heal. Many times, we do not know what is happening or why. We must have a developing capacity to tolerate lack of control and not knowing. Healing can and does occur even when past trauma is not consciously known or discussed. A strong sense of patience and humility are required for this healing process to occur.

Fearlessly and Realistically Acknowledge the Depth of the Lived Experience Details

Allow yourself to go through an authentic and comprehensive grieving process that begins with identification of the genuine issues. This necessary process is alive from the time your loved one has entered a pattern of living with symptoms of mental illness. Those around the person with mental illness will go through these classic stages of grief reactions. Because of the unthinkable trauma that surrounds mental illness, the grief process will be categorized as *complicated grief,* which means grief reactions may be prolonged and intense. Additional risk factors for complicated grief include being female, high stress, low social support, previous symptoms of mood disorder, insecure attachments, an intimate and dependent relationship with the individual with a new onset of symptoms, or death (APA, 2013).

Stages of Grief

Shock/Denial. Some of the stories we hear and the behaviors we see are unimaginable and shocking. Denial reactions are common in the initial grief stage of shock.

Bargaining. In reaction to these shocking stories and experiences, people often offer bargaining beliefs and behaviors. "My son's psychotic reaction was because someone slipped a drug into his drink." Since many cultures believe that an omnipotent God caused this psychotic behavior, "He, too, can take away this illness." Many families will oblige the individual with psychotic experiences to go to church daily or wear religious icons, such as a rosary or a saint card.

Anger. Anger is a difficult reaction to a loved one experiencing symptoms of SMI. This reaction is common and understandable. Some people blame themselves for the illness. "I was a rotten parent. This is all my fault." Staying stuck in anger can potentially have destructive effects on the self and others, including partners, other children, colleagues, and friends.

Depression. Depression is the beginning of acceptance. Depression is a form of submission to helplessness. When control is relinquished, adjustment to the present can begin. Those who have vulnerabilities to mental and physical illnesses should seek support and guidance to prevent a downward spiral.

Acceptance. To experience true acceptance is to allow for embracing reality, and the healing can now begin. Acceptance means no illusional untruths but knowing and radically embracing the situation. With radical acceptance, the person has no need to blame others or use other defensive coping behaviors. With radical acceptance, we can now decide how to understand the origin of the mental illness and what interventions are feasible, available, and necessary.

Some people find traveling through this grieving process easier with social support. Others feel the need to do this grieving process in private. Every individual's methods of coping should be respected. The trick is not to get stuck at any one place. Any stage other than *acceptance* can be difficult for the individual and everyone around him or her to live with. Whereas it is important to remain positive and supportive to the individual with symptoms of mental illness, your life and health depends on your authentic emotional reactions and the life-giving behaviors that maintain you.

At some points in the process, you may decide to keep your situation a secret from people, even those in your inner circle. I encourage you to find and develop a supportive network with whom you can talk, even just to generally let your situation be known. You can talk to strangers at a support group or on Internet chat rooms or to trusted people within the fabric of your lives. At the very least, you will receive emotional validation, support, and clarity, and these feelings will keep you afloat. One day, you will be able to return these mutually supportive favors, if not to those very individuals and, possibly, to others who are also traveling this journey. Some formal support groups are available and listed in Appendix B of this book. You are encouraged to resist the impact of stigma and seek and use available healing resources around you.

You are encouraged to take what you need and leave the rest. No one person or group has all the answers, and many individuals and groups can provide various insightful perspectives. You are encouraged to hear from a variety of perspectives and see which ones most resonate with you, keeping in mind that some will not resonate with you.

- The NAMI conducts a free 12-week evidence-based, educational, and supportive course for families and significant others to help to (1) understand, (2) cope, and (3) hold hope with/for a family member who experiences symptoms of mental illness. Trained family members teach the program. The NAMI website lists the following topics that are covered in this program (see Appendix B; Additionally, this program is also available in Spanish and other languages in some states):
  - How to manage crises, solve problems, and communicate effectively;
  - Taking care of yourself and managing your stress;
  - Developing the confidence and stamina to provide support with compassion;
  - Finding and using local supports and services;
  - Staying up-to-date with information on mental health conditions and how they affect the brain;
  - Current treatments, including evidence-based therapies, medications, and side effects;
  - The impact of mental illness on the entire family.
- William McFarlane (2004), in his book *Multi-Family Groups in the Treatment of Severe Psychiatric Disorders*, provides the theoretical and step-by-step curriculum by which mental health treatment professionals can construct an evidence-based healing network with families with a member who lives with SMI. It is noteworthy that while this curriculum is intended to be time-limited, at the beginning and ending of every session, social time is built

into every agenda so families can naturally and authentically build mutually supportive relationships that extend beyond the group. Finally, McFarlane's book discusses the unique applications and contexts of multifamily groups with specific symptoms of mental illnesses, including bipolar illness, depressive disorder, borderline personality disorder, obsessive-compulsive disorder, and chronic medical disorders.

There is a wide range of supportive and inspirational groups for individuals who live with mental illnesses. Some are scientific and tout evidence-based practices, some are antipsychiatry, some are philosophical, anthropological, or historical in nature, some are narratives from psychiatric survivors, and others are clinical-skills focused. Again, each person is encouraged to explore with open eyes, watching for a group whose members and mission inspires and supports your beliefs and situation. No one can tell you what is right for you. Only you can decide for yourself. Additionally, many of these groups and links (see Appendix B) provide a list of practitioners who do not fully buy into mainstream mental health treatment.

FINAL THOUGHTS

In recognizing how good and noble clinicians, family members, and loved ones struggle for survival when finding themselves swimming upstream in the mainstream public mental health treatment delivery system, self-care tips become essential in maintaining the emotional presence and stamina required to be effective. While each person will choose which of these self-preserving practices best resonates with him, survival and positive living requires frequent and regular practice of several of these efforts.

Summary of Unit III

ARMED WITH THE information about the nature of standardized treatment and the underpinnings of where psychosis may originate, this unit continued the discussion by providing an understanding of how to create the change required in working with people living with psychosis. The efforts of the antipsychiatry movement support the notion that more ethical treatment is needed, and understanding the objectives of compassionate work helps to bridge the divide between what this movement calls for and how we might accomplish fulfilling that desire. The goal of intentional mental health treatment is to accurately address the distress experienced by this population, and supporting these individuals on their journey through psychosis, as well as ourselves, as we fastidiously work to understand them, creates an open and caring environment where real progress can be accomplished.

UNIT IV

Where Do We Go from Here?

13

Conclusions and Future Remarks

EXPLORING MAINSTREAM MENTAL health treatment in the United States uncovers shocking and unthinkable stories of iatrogenic traumatic experiences that are all too commonly true. Given what we have discovered, we then grapple with essential questions. What does this all mean for attaining recovery and a high quality of life for people living with mental illness? Whom does this revealed information best serve going forward? Whom these realities do not serve is obvious; the short answer is everyone financially, socially, and spiritually. Finally, what must be done, by way of short-term interventions and long-term planning, to enable individuals and families who live with severe mental illness (SMI) to embrace philosophies and standards of care that would result in creating a self-determined life worth living for all people? Furthermore, how can access to sustainable quality mental health treatment be made available to all people, not excluding anyone, as is done now, based on income, sexual orientation, ethnicity, age, symptom severity, or religion.

WHERE WE HAVE BEEN

A long list of historical books, museums, and documentaries provide testimonies from people with mental illnesses. Repeatedly, then and now, people with symptoms of SMI report feeling reduced to a psychiatric diagnosis and forced into traditional treatments, which are experienced as traumatic, even torturous, and result in increased stress and anxiety levels, other psychiatric conditions, and physical illnesses. Other patients who helplessly witnessed these treatments experienced similar terror. While mental health laws and basic civil rights have abolished the more acute and permanently altering interventions, contemporary handling/control of people with SMI includes forced psychiatric treatments that result in iatrogenic trauma, including forced medication that significantly reduces emotional experiences, energy, and the ability to impact one's own world; physical restraints; mandated segregation from society; and solitary confinement.

Furthermore, and at the point of no return, newspaper front-page headlines too often read something in the way of "Police Kills Mentally Ill Person." The conclusion in almost every one of these cases is something akin to "officer shooting in the line of duty." Police forces are not being adequately trained to appropriately manage individuals who are in an active state of emotional dysregulation and experiencing positive symptoms of psychosis. In turn, the bullet becomes the preferred method of managing extreme symptoms of mental illness.

WHEN A RADICAL CHANGE WAS RECOGNIZED
BY THE GENERAL PUBLIC

Throughout history, people who live with symptoms of mental illnesses and their advocates have publically put their personal testimonies of mental health treatment (or trauma, as it were) forth to federal, state, local, agency, and individual legislative bodies. However, stigma, prejudice, and extremely inhumane conditions have systematically disenfranchised, disempowered, and discredited these individuals who live with mental illness. In fact, the practice of eugenics in the form of coerced or compulsory sterilization of those with "undesirable" human traits—especially the poor, Blacks, Native Americans, Hispanics, and the mentally ill—was endorsed by the US federal government until 1974, evidenced by using government dollars to pay for these surgeries. Prior to 1974, many individuals were threatened that their government benefits (i.e., welfare) would be discontinued if they did not consent to the surgery, some were not told of the "added" procedure that was performed during other medical procedures such as birth or appendectomy. Many had not given informed consent, especially as informed consent guidelines were not published until September 3, 1973. Even after the new guidelines were published and a moratorium was asserted, many women were sterilized, signing the consent (which required a 72-hour waiting period) the day of Cesarean section delivery and under the influence of anesthesia; during painful labor; or even signing the day after the sterilization surgery took place (Lawrence, 2000). The US Supreme Court spoke of "sterilization as a small 'sacrifice' that the unfit should make for the national good" (Whitaker, 2010, p. 60). Between the years 1907 and 1963, more than 64,000 men and women were forcibly sterilized under such US eugenics laws (Reilly, 1997). Most of these surgeries were performed on disabled people who lived in institutions and on women.

Since the 1800s, when the United States first saw the establishment of mental hospitals, people and groups such as Dorothea Dix, Clifford Beers, the Mental Hygiene Movement, Quakers, and other reform workers, publicized deplorable treatment conditions and demanded that human rights be upheld for people who experience symptoms of mental illnesses. Over time, pockets of mental health treatment conditions improved, new buildings were constructed, and relevant laws were revised and established through these humanitarian reform efforts.

People once considered "mental patients" and their supporters and advocates organized what we now know as the antipsychiatry movement. This historical consumer-run movement continues in a variety of formal and informal arenas today. Over the years, many theorists, psychiatrists, philosophers, and survivors have initiated public protests, debates, and formal and informal conferences in an effort to expose legitimized and systematic abuses, torture, financial profiteering, marginalization, and oppression toward people who experience symptoms of psychosis. The antipsychiatry movement has its pros and cons. Followers of the movement, being extreme in their conclusions, may exclude themselves from an effective intervention. Is there a middle ground where people's personal experiences can be heard and honored and effective interventions accessed?

Since the 1980s, people with experiences in the mental health treatment system have demanded that recovery be a choice, not a mandate. After all, people do have a right to be different. Leaders in the recovery movement have demanded that the individual be empowered to identify and prioritize the issues addressed. People are demanding a choice of how to solve problems and treat symptoms deemed distressing. The issue of medication is raised: to use or not to use, which medications to use, and proper medication dosage.

Mainstream mental health treatment delivery has left people who access this kind of help suffering, oppressed, and hopeless. We are seeing increasing numbers of individuals with mental illness enrolled on Social Supplemental Income (SSI) and Social Supplemental Disability Income (SSDI), experiencing pervasive drug and behavioral addiction, and contemplating suicide.

Psychotic symptoms, especially positive ones, are not going away. In fact, as Western society becomes more competitive, fast-paced, focused on instant gratification, and computerized, people with symptoms of mental illness may feel more stigmatized, isolated, and marginalized, thus increasing psychotic symptoms. Humane and effective treatments are, and will be, desperately needed to accurately understand and effectively communicate with people who are actively experiencing symptoms of psychosis.

WHO IS IMPACTED BY THIS INFORMATION?

Through reading the information presented in this book, people living with mental illness and consuming mainstream mental health treatment may see their personal experiences of iatrogenic trauma resulting from this treatment validated. In recognizing that their experiences are part of the cultural fabric of mental health treatment, rather than isolated experiences, they may find more confidence in their belief in the unjustness of mainstream mental health treatment and in taking the necessary steps to be involved in the management of their symptoms of psychosis. Some of these individuals may hear or respond to the call to advocate for more effective, just, and compassionate mental health treatment for others.

Families have the potential for more accurate and detailed insight into the experiences of the individual who experiences symptoms of mental illness and resistance to treatment. Additionally, supportive people may now have information to confidently access other (not alternative) methods, not just medication and social skills groups, to manage positive symptoms of psychosis and other symptoms of mental illness.

Clinicians who rely on accurate listening and the therapeutic relationship, not solely on medications as treatment of psychosis, no longer have to *whisper* about these exchanges and their successes. In the context of *Listening with Psychotic Ears*, clinicians can openly discuss, with specific terminology, these situations and their interventions in case consultations, supervision, and other brainstorming conversations where healing results are sought. The intentions that motivated the writing of this book included validating the experiences of people who experience psychosis and giving a voice with new language to those who must rely on these skills.

When mental health treatment is mentioned, the focus of the conversation quickly turns to psychotropic medication: identifying which one to prescribe and how to get the person to be compliant. While psychotropic medications can be humane and show effective results in the short term—if given at accurate dosages, including low doses—they take time to work. Whereas it is doubtful that this information will be accessed by clinicians who solely rely on medications for intervention, the information is available and leads to positive results for many professionals, families, peer workers, and friends of individuals who experience positive symptoms of psychosis and for the individuals themselves. This book is not intended to convert clinicians who only rely on psychotropic medications, but rather to add to their set of effective and humane skills for healing the distress of psychosis.

The mainstream mental health treatment delivery system is no longer efficient in healing symptoms of mental illness. The services and delivery styles that are available are not decreasing symptoms of mental illness; in fact, mental illness is on the rise. Mainstream mental health treatment today is often just moving people along without seeing many positive results. In attempts to see better results, we can no longer afford to *move the furniture around in the room* of the mental health system. The foundation consisting of effective, humane, and sustainable mental health treatment delivery must be reenvisioned and rebuilt. Many aspects can be salvaged and others repurposed. We must rethink how mental healthcare is accessed and delivered. That said, the ultimate purpose of mental health services in our civilized society is the increased quality of life for all people who live with mental illnesses.

Finally, mainstream healthcare is recognizing that mental health and physical health are intertwined. As physical health improves, so does mental health. As mental health improves, the person is less dependent on external things for security and checking out by way of behavioral and chemical addictions. As mental health improves, physical health follows. The healthcare industry is reorganizing so that these two aspects of health sustainability can be intertwined.

The Affordable Care Act is but one needed policy with the intention of making more access to physical and mental healthcare for all people, especially people with low incomes, a reality. In the United States, this population includes an overrepresentation of people of color. The inclusion of evidence-based practices will confront implicit racism, sexism, ageism, and classism, and diverse populations will have more access than ever to effective, humane, and sustainable healthcare treatment options.

In this day, evidence-based practice is heavily relied on to guide mental health treatment interventions. Lots of government dollars are spent in training and supervising mental health clinicians in the evidence-based theories and intervention skills. The use of evidence-based practices is necessary and should be used, especially where rates of recovery are low and unchanging. However, this pendulum swing toward evidence-based practices does not allow for much inclusion of authentic engagement skills and effective qualitative interpretive skills. Additionally, many evidence-based practices are time-limited, and people who experience symptoms of mental illness need extended care that spans over a lifetime.

Listening with Psychotic Ears provides the tools to communicate with persons who are actively experiencing psychosis in real time, yielding immediate and lasting quality-of-life improvements. *Listening with Psychotic Ears* helps people who experience psychosis feel cared for and connected with, despite their difficulty with verbal expression. This experience, in turn, reduces isolation and symptoms of anxiety and can immediately reduce symptoms of psychosis, including hallucinations, delusions, and difficulty processing and expressing information.

The benefits of the *Listening with Psychotic Ears* philosophy and skills extend beyond quick symptom reduction. This practice holds the promise of returning dignity to marginalized populations, enabling affected families to come closer together, contributing to the destigmatization of mental illness, and creating an environment for a person to meaningfully participate in his or her life. From an administrative and societal perspective, the monetary benefits of this philosophy are also great. If we can adopt more effective treatments, there is less dysfunction in the world; as people have more stability in their lives, they have reduced needs for expensive healthcare, including medications and inpatient hospitalizations. As we understand and use more effective treatments, rates of suicide decrease, physical health is improved, the use of social services with the highest impact on government and taxpayer funds, including emergency rooms and disability benefits, is reduced, and people are able to get back to more productive lives. In essence, the industries that will not benefit from *Learning with Psychotic Ears* are pharmaceutical companies, healthcare, and detention centers, including jails, prisons, and long-term psychiatric facilities, because the overreliance on these industries to pick up the pieces will diminish, creating a less profitable reality for them.

Recovery is a choice. The method by which an individual pursues recovery is also a choice. A person could choose one or a combination of recovery methods. This person might find a psychiatrist with whom they can collaboratively decide on which medications and doses provide the most symptom reduction with the least amount of side effects. They might find validation, relief, inspiration, and liberation with a psychotherapist who engages in conversation. He or she might join a grassroots psychiatric survivor group that promotes human rights in mental health treatment. He or she might engage in Eastern practices and focus on intentions, chakras, a collective conscious, herbs, meditations, poses, and breathing. They might pick up a hobby, such as roller derby, allowing for a new spiritual focus and a new identity. He or she might join a peer-run group where he or she can find a place in wellness activities, give trainings, participate in advocacy, supervise peer-run support groups in mental health agencies, and more.

High-profile celebrities and athletes who have resources to choose recovery methods are coming forth to share their stories. They tell that recovery from mental illness is possible. These testimonies are intended to bring about sustainable healing from symptoms of mental illness and wipe out stigma for people who live with mental illnesses.

Paulo Freire was an activist who educated, empowered, and advocated for the transformation of disenfranchised people in disenfranchised countries, especially in

Brazil, Bolivia, and Chile (www.freire.org). He encouraged people to talk so they could agree on what was being done to them and have a choice about what to do about it.

For me, working with people who experience symptoms of psychosis is a deeply meaningful experience. I have been working with people with psychotic experiences since I was 15 years old, which is most of my life. Over these years, I saw the themes discussed in this book. Then, I was able to look at literature dating back over 100 years to 1910. Now, we can incorporate what we know about the brain to give words to and expand on the neurological experiences. We have evidence-based practices and practice-based evidence to give us options in our clinical toolbox of accurate understanding and effective communication for the healing of psychosis and other symptoms of mental illnesses. With the philosophy and skills of *Listening with Psychotic Ears*, we now have the opportunity to really hear what people experiencing psychosis are saying and help them with their range of feelings and unique situations. By changing the culture toward valuing all lives, regardless of circumstance, we move away from the myth that this population is worthless—a myth that society has allowed itself to be talked into. If we can get back to valuing all people, then we will value their experiences and communications and improve their quality of life.

- Able Child: Parents for a Label & Drug Free Education—www.ablechild.org
- Alternative to Meds Center—www.alternativetomeds.com
- The Antipsychiatry Coalition—www.antipsychiatry.org
- Beyond Meds: Alternatives to Psychiatry: Interdisciplinary & Integral Holistic Well-Being—www.beyondmeds.com
- Bibliography of First-Person Madness Narratives—http://www.isps-us.org/pdf/Bibliography_4th_edition.pdf
- Center for the Human Rights of Users and Survivors of Psychiatry—http://www.chrusp.org/
- The Coalition for the Abolition of Electroshock in Texas—www.endofshock.com
- European Network on Training, Evaluation and Research in Mental Health (ENTER)—www.entermentalhealth.net
- Freedom Center—www.freedom-center.org
- Free Psychiatric News—www.freepsychiatricnews.com
- Foundation for Excellence in Mental Health Care—http://www.mentalhealthexcellence.org/
- Hearing Voices Network—http://www.hearing-voices.org/
  USA—http://www.hearingvoicesusa.org/
- International Early Psychosis Association—www.iepa.org.au
- The International Hearing Voices Network—www.intervoiceonline.org
- International Network for Training, Education, and Research into Hearing Voices (INTERVOICE)—www.intervoiceonline.org

- International Network Toward Alternatives and Recovery (INTAR)—www.intar.org
- International Society for Psychological and Social Approaches to Psychosis (ISPS)—http://www.isps-us.org/
- Life Center for a New Tomorrow Residential Center—www.lifecenterforanewtomorrow.com
- Mad in America: Science, Psychiatry, and Community—http://www.madinamerica.com/
- Mind Freedom—http://www.mindfreedom.org/
- Natural Health News & Self-Reliance—www.naturalnews.org
- National Mental Health Self-Help Clearinghouse—www.mhselfhelp.org
- NYC Parachute Project—http://www.nyc.gov/html/doh/html/mental/parachute.shtml
- Oikos Work Camps and Volunteer Programs in Italy—www.oikos.org
- Project Return Peer Support Network—http://prpsn.org/
- ProPublica: Journalism in the Public Interest—www.propublica.org
- Psychiatric Survivor Archives of Toronto—http://www.psychiatricsurvivorarchives.com/
- The Saks Institute for Mental Health Law, Politics, and Ethics—http://weblaw.usc.edu/centers/saks/
- Soteria: Schizophrenia without Antipsychotic Drugs & the Legacy of Loren Mosher—www.moshersoteria.com
- The Thomas Scasz MD Cybercenter for Liberty and Responsibility—www.szasz.com
- US Food and Drug Administration—http://www.fda.gov/Safety/MedWatch/
- World Network of Users and Survivors of Psychiatry (WNUSP) http://www.wnusp.net/

WEBSITE RESOURCES BY CHAPTER

CHAPTER 3

- "Bedlam," by Albert Q. Maisel in *Life Magazine*:
  http://mn.gov/mnddc/parallels2/prologue/6a-bedlam/6a-bedlam.html
- Howard Dully's story:
  http://www.npr.org/2005/11/16/5014080/my-lobotomy-howard-dullys-journey
- "Bibliography of First Person Narratives of Madness," by the International Society for Psychological and Social Approaches to Psychosis (ISPS):
  http://www.isps-us.org/pdf/Bibliography_4th_edition.pdf

CHAPTER 4

- Loren Mosher's resignation letter to the APA:
  http://www.moshersoteria.com/articles/resignation-from-apa/

CHAPTER 5

- The York Retreat at Lamel Hill, York, England:
  http://www.theretreatyork.org.uk/
- *The Red Book*, by Carl Jung
  http://philemonfoundation.org/wp-content/uploads/2014/11/RedBookPreview_optimized.pdf

- The Carl Jung Institutes and U.S. locations:
  http://www.jung.org
  Boston: http://www.cgjungboston.com
  Chicago: http://www.jungchicago.org
  Los Angeles: http://www.junginla.org
  New York: http://www.cgjungny.org
  San Francisco: http://www.sfjung.org
- William Alanson White Institute, New York, NY
  www.wawhite.org
- The Resident, by Dominic Harris—survivor stories from Kingsley Hall.
  http://www.dominicharris.co.uk/the_residents.html
- News story about Ronald David Laing's death:
  http://www.dailymail.co.uk/news/article-1021176/Son-RD-Laing--psychiatrist-blamed-madness-poor-parenting--dead-tent-vodka-bottle.html
- Interview with John Weir Perry by Jeff Mishlove about visionaries:
  http://spiritualrecoveries.blogspot.com/2006/05/dr-john-weir-perry-far-side-of-madness.html
- Soteria House:
  www.moshersoteria.com
  http://www.ciompi.com/en/soteria.html
- Mind Freedom International:
  www.mindfreedom.org
- Christina Grof bio:
  http://www.holotropic.com/bio-christina-grof.shtml
- Video of Stanislav Grof describing holotropic breathwork:
  http://www.youtube.com/watch?v=qCzG9QsM-Pw
- Stanislav Grof website:
  http://www.stanislavgrof.com
- The Spiritual Emergence Network:
  www.spiritualemergence.com
- Dr. Oliver Sacks, Ted Talk:
  http://www.youtube.com/watch?v=SgOTaXhbqPQ
- *Hearing Distressing Voices Toolkit*, by Patricia Deegan:
  http://store.patdeegan.com/collections/toolkits/products/hearing-distressing-voices-toolkit
  or
  www.patdeegan.com
- Mary Ellen Copeland's Copeland Center for Wellness and Recovery
  https://copelandcenter.com/
- Gould Farm
  http://www.gouldfarm.org/about-us

- Openbaar Psychiatrisch Zorgcentrum in Geel, Belgium
  http://www.opzgeel.be/en/home/htm/intro.asp
- Daniel Mackler's documentaries about open dialogue treatment (ODT):
  www.wildtruth.net

CHAPTER 6

- Hearing Voices Network:
  http://www.hearing-voices.org

CHAPTER 7

- Map of the brain:
  http://science.education.nih.gov/supplements/nih2/addiction/images/guide/fig1-2.jpg
- Empathy book instructional videos:
  https://www.youtube.com/watch?v=ruzGK8ySayo
- Video examples of Wernicke's aphasia:
  https://www.youtube.com/watch?v=aVhYN7NTIKU
  https://www.youtube.com/watch?v=dKTdMV6cOZw
- Brain Gym:
  www.braingym.org
- Strategies for improving memory:
  http://www.discovery.com/tv-shows/curiosity/topics/10-ways-to-improve-memory.htm

CHAPTER 8

- National Empowerment Center:
  http://www.power2u.org/recovery-stories.html
- *Madness Network News* (*MNN*) newsletter:
  madnessnetworknews.com
- *On Our Own: Patient Controlled Alternatives to the Mental Health System*, by Judi Chamberlain:
  http://www.power2u.org/articles/recovery/confessions.html
- National Mental Health Consumer's Self-Help Clearinghouse (NMHCSC):
  www.mhselfhelp.org
- World Network of Users and Survivors of Psychiatry (WNUSP):
  www.wnusp.net
- Metropolitan State Hospital lawsuit:
  http://www.justice.gov/crt/about/spl/documents/metro_hosp_findlet.pdf
- Where's the Evidence documentary video:
  https://vimeo.com/117465548
- International Hearing Voices Network:
  www.intervoiceonline.org

CHAPTER 9

- Photographs from *Artistry of the Mentally Ill*, by Hans Prinzhorn:
  http://digi.ub.uni-heidelberg.de/diglit/prinzhorn1922/0012/scroll?sid=8068ad7b8fe7doc8a7195ebb9fd3797f
- *You and Me*, by Debbie Sesula:
  http://www.power2u.org/articles/empower/you_and_me.html
- Agnes's Jacket in the Hans Prinzhorn collection:
  http://ridiculouslyinteresting.com/2011/09/06/agnes-richters-embroidered-straightjacket/
- Fernando Oresete Nannette, images from the Volterra "Ferri" unit:
  http://www.contemporart.eu/oreste-fernando-nannetti/
- Novel by Anonymous, Chongqing, China:
  http://indulgy.com/post/PafHehm7U1/an-anonymous-authors-novel-written-on-the-wall
- Glide Memorial Church
  www.glide.org

CHAPTER 11

- Mental Health America's Village of Long Beach
  http://www.mhala.org/mha-village.htm
- Harm Reduction: *Insight* CNN documentary:
  https://www.youtube.com/watch?v=BvFjY1mJIng
- Harm Reduction Coalition:
  www.harmreduction.org
- The Linehan Institute:
  www.behavioraltech.org

CHAPTER 12

- National Alliance of Mental Illness (NAMI):
  http://www.nami.org/familytofamily

REFERENCES

Abi-Dargham, A., Gil, R., Krystal, J., Baldwin, R. M., Seibyl, J. P., Bowers, M., . . . Laruelle, M. (1998). Increased striatal dopamine transmission in schizophrenia: confirmation in a second cohort. *American Journal of Psychiatry, 155*(6), 761–767.

Adams, J., & Drake, R. (2006). Shared decision-making and evidence-based practice. *Community Mental Health Journal, 42,* 87–105.

Adriano, F., Caltagirone, C., & Spalletta, G. (2012). Hippocampal volume reduction in first-episode and chronic schizophrenia: a review and meta-analysis. *The Neuroscientist, 18*(2), 180–200.

Agartz, I., Andersson, J., & Skare, S. (2001). Abnormal brain white matter in schizophrenia: A diffusion tensor imaging study. *Clinical Neuroscience and Neuropathology, 12,* 2251–2254.

Ainsworth, M. D., Blehar, M, Waters, E, & Wall, S. (1978). *Patterns of attachment: A psychological study of the strange situation.* Hillsdale, NJ: Erlbaum.

Akutagawa, R. (1918). The spider's thread. *Akai Tori.* Tōkyō: Nihon Kindai Bungakkan, Shōwa.

Allen, J. G., & Coyne, L. (1995). Dissociation and vulnerability to psychotic experience: The Dissociative Experiences Scale and the MMPI-2. *Journal of Nervous and Mental Disease, 183*(10), 615–622.

Allen, J., Coyne, L., & Console, D. (1996). Dissociation contributes to anxiety and psychoticism on the Brief Symptom Inventory. *Journal of Nervous and Mental Disease, 184,* 639–641.

Allen, J., Coyne, L., & Console, D. (1997). Dissociative detachment relates to psychotic symptoms and personality decompensation. *Comprehensive Psychiatry, 38,* 327–334.

Almeida, O. (2011). Smoking causes brain cell loss and cognitive decline. *NeuroImage.* Retrieved April 1, 2018. http://www.news.uwa.edu.au/201102093273/business-and-industry/smoking-causes-brain-cell-loss-and-cognitive-decline

Alvir, J., Lieberman, J., Safferman, A., Schwimmer, J., & Schaaf, J. (1993). Clozapine-induced agranulocytosis: Incidence and risk factors in the United States. *New England Journal of Medicine, 329*, 162–167.

Amenson, C. (1998). *Schizophrenia: A Family Education Curriculum.* Pasadena, CA: Pacific Clinics Institute.

American Foundation for Suicide Prevention. (2015). *Facts and figures.* Retrieved from https://www.afsp.org/understanding-suicide/facts-and-figureshttps://www.afsp.org/understanding-suicide/facts-and-figures

American Psychiatric Association. (2008). *Annual meeting program: Full disclosure index.* Washington, DC: Author.

American Psychiatric Association (1980–2011). Annual Reports of the Treasurer 1980–2011. *American Journal of Psychiatry.*

American Psychiatric Association. (2011). Pharmaceutical revenue. *American Psychiatric Association.*

American Psychiatric Association. (2013). *Diagnostic and statistical manual of mental disorders: DSM-5.* Washington, DC: *American Psychiatric Association.*

Andreasen, N. (1979). Thought, language, and communication disorders: II. Diagnostic significance. *Archives of General Psychiatry, 36*, 1315–1321.

Andreasen, N., O'Leary, D., Flam, M., Nopouls, P., Watkins, G. L., Boles Ponto, L., & Hichwa, R. (1997). Hypofrontality in schizophrenia: Distributed dysfunctional circuits in neuroleptic-naïve patients. *Lancet, 349*, 1730–1734.

Anglin, D. M., & Malaspina, D. (2008). Ethnicity effects on clinical diagnoses compared to best-estimate research diagnoses in patients with psychosis: A retrospective medical chart review. *Journal of Clinical Psychiatry, 69*, 941–945.

Ansorge, M., Zhou, M., Lira, A., Hen, R., & Gingrich., J. (2004). Early-Life Blockade of the 5-HT Transporter Alters Emotional Behavior in Adult Mice. *Science, 306*(5697), 879–881.

Arundine, M., Aarts, M., Lau, A., & Tymianski, M. (2004). Vulnerability of central neurons to secondary insults after in vitro mechanical stretch. *Journal of Neuroscience, 24*, 8106–8123.

Baare, W. F. C., van Oel, C., Hulshoff Pol, H., Schnack, H., Durston, S., Sitskoorn, M., & Kahn, R. (2001). Volumes of Brain Structures in Twins Discordant for Schizophrenia. *Archives of General Psychiatry, 58*(1), 33–40.

Barr, C., Mednick, S., & Munk-Jorgensen. P. (1990). Exposure to Influenza Epidemics During Gestation and Adult Schizophrenia: A 40-Year Study. *Archives of General Psychiatry, 47*(9), 869–874.

Baumeister, A., & Francis, J. (2002). Historical development of the dopamine hypothesis of schizophrenia. *Journal of the History of the Neurosciences, 11*, 265–277.

Beck, J., & Van der Kolk, B. (1987). Reports of childhood incest and current behavior of chronically hospitalized psychotic women. *American Journal of Psychiatry, 144*, 1474–1476.

Beckett, S. (1954). *Waiting for Godot: A tragicomedy in two acts.* New York, NY: Grove Press.

Beebe, G. (1975). Follow-up studies of World War II and Korean War prisoners: II. Morbidity, disability, and maladjustments. *American Journal of Epidemiology, 101*, 400–422.

Beers, C. (1903). *A mind that found itself.* New York: Longmans, Green, and Co.

Berdoy, M., Webster, J., & Macdonald, D. (1995). Parasite-altered behaviour: Is the effect of *Toxoplasma gondii* on *Rattus norvegicus* specific? *Parasitology, 111*, 403–409.

Berenbaum, H. (1999). Peculiarity and reported childhood maltreatment. *Psychiatry, 62*, 21–35.

Berrios, G. (1999). Falret, Séglas, Morselli, and Masselon, and the "language of the insane": A conceptual history. *Brain Language, 69,* 56–75.

Berrios, G. (2009). On alterations in the form of speech and on the formation of new words and expressions of madness by L. Snell (1852). *History of Psychiatry, 20,* 480–496.

Bishop, K. M., & Wahlsten, D. (1997). Sex differences in the human corpus callosum: Myth or reality? *Neuroscience and Biobehavioral Reviews, 21,* 581–601.

Bleuler, M. (1978). *The schizophrenia disorders: Long-term patient and family studies.* New Haven, CT, US: Yale University Press.

Blow, F., Zeber, J., McCarthy, J., Valenstein, M., Gillon, L., & Bingham, C. R. (2004). Ethnicity and diagnostic patterns in veterans with psychoses. *Social Psychiatry and Psychiatric Epidemiology, 39,* 841–851. http://www.ncbi.nlm.nih.gov/pubmed/?term=Bingham CR%5BAuthor%5D&cauthor=true&cauthor_uid=15669666

Bockoven, J. S., & Solomon, H. C. (1975). Comparison of two five-year follow-up studies: 1947 to 1952 and 1967 to 1972. *The American Journal of Psychiatry, 132*(8), 796–801.

Bola, J. (2005). Medication-free research in early episode schizophrenia: Evidence of long-term harm? *Schizophrenia Bulletin, 32,* 288–296.

Bola, J., & Mosher, L. (2003). Treatment of acute psychosis without neuroleptics. *Journal of Nervous and Mental Disease, 191,* 219–229.

Borgwardt, S., Picchioni, M., Ettinger, U., Toulopoulou, T., Murray, R., & McGuire, P. (2010). Regional gray matter volume in Monozygotic twins concordant and discordant for schizophrenia. *Biological Psychiatry, 67*(10), 956–964.

Bowers, M. (1974). Central dopamine turnover in schizophrenic syndromes. *Archives of General Psychiatry, 31,* 50–54.

Bowlby, J. (1979). *The making and breaking of affectional bonds.* Tavistock Publications Limited.

Bowman, J. (2014). *Temporal lobe epilepsy.* http://www.healthline.com/health/temporal-lobe-epilepsy#Overview1

Brand, B. L., Myrick, A. C., Loewenstein, R. J., Classen, C.C., Pain, C., Lanius, R., . . . Putnam F.W. (2012). A survey of practices and recommended treatment interventions among expert therapists treating patients with dissociative identity disorder and dissociative disorder not otherwise specified. *Psychological Trauma, 4,* 490–500.

Brekke, J., Ell, K., & Palinkas, L. (2007). Translational science at the National Institute of Mental Health: Can social work take its rightful place? *Research on Social Work Practice, 17,* 123–133.

Briere, J. (2004). *Psychological assessment of adult posttraumatic states: Phenomenology, diagnosis, and measurement* (2nd ed.). Washington, DC, US: American Psychological Association.

Bromet, E. J., Kotov, R., Fochtmann, L. J., Carlson, G., Tanenberg-Karant, M., Ruggero, C., & Chang, S. (2011). Diagnostic shifts during the decade following first admission for psychosis. *American Journal of Psychiatry, 168,* 1186–1194.

Brown, A. (2005). Oliver Sacks Profile: Seeing double. *The Guardian.* March 4, 2005.

Brown, A., Schaefer, C., Quesenberry, C., Liu, L., Babulas, V., & Susser, E. (2005). Maternal exposure to toxoplasmosis and risk of schizophrenia in adult offspring. *American Journal of Psychiatry, 162,* 767–773.

Brown, A., Begg, M., Gravenstein, S., Schaefer, C., Wyatt, R., Bresnahan, M., Babulas, V., & Susser, E. (2004). Serologic Evidence of Prenatal Influenza in the Etiology of Schizophrenia. *Archives of General Psychiatry, 61*(8), 774–780.

Brown G. G., & Thompson W. K. (2010). Functional Brain Imaging in Schizophrenia: Selected Results and Methods. In: N. Swerdlow (Ed.), *Behavioral Neurobiology of Schizophrenia and Its Treatment. Current Topics in Behavioral Neurosciences, vol 4*. Springer, Berlin, Heidelberg.

Bruch, H. (1982). Personal reminiscences of Frieda Fromm-Reichmann. *Psychiatry, 45*, 98–102.

Buka, S., Tsuang, M., & Lipsett, L. (1993). Pregnancy/delivery complications and psychiatric diagnosis: A prospective study. *Archives of General Psychiatry, 50*, 151–156.

Burt, D., Creese, I., & Snyder, S. (1977). Antischizophrenic drugs: Chronic treatment elevates dopamine receptor binding in brains. *Science, 196*, 326–327.

Busine, L., Brand-Blaussen, B., & Douglas, C. (1998). *Beyond reason: Art and psychosis works from the Prinzhorn collection*. Berkeley, CA: University of California Press.

Butler, R. W., Meuser, K. T., Sprock, J., & Braff, D. L. (1996). Positive symptoms of psychosis in posttraumatic stress disorder. *Biological Psychiatry, 15*, 839–844.

Camus, A. (1942). *The Myth of Sisyphus*. Penguin Books.

Cannon, T. (1997). On the nature and mechanisms of obstetric influences in schizophrenia: A review and synthesis of epidemiologic studies. *International Review of Psychiatry, 9*(4), 387–397.

Carey, B. (2008, July 12). Psychiatric group faces scrutiny over drug industry ties. *New York Times*.

Cardno, A. G., & Gottesman, I. (2000). Twin studies of schizophrenia: From bow-and-arrow concordances to star wars Mx and functional genomics. *American Journal of Medical Genetics, 97*, 12–17.

Carpenter, W. (1977). Treatment of acute psychosis without neuroleptics. *American Journal of Psychiatry, 134*, 14–20.

Carpenter, W. T., McGlashan, T. H., & Straus, J. S. (1977). The Treatment of Acute Schizophrenia Without Drugs: An Investigation of Some Current Assumptions. *American Journal of Psychiatry, 134*(1), 14–20.

Case, B., Bertollo, D., Laska, E., Price, L., Siegel, C., Olfson, M., & Marcus, S. (2013). Declining use of electroconvulsive therapy in United States general hospitals. *Biological Psychiatry, 73*, 19–20.

Casslon, A. (1988). The current status of the dopamine hypothesis of schizophrenia. *Neuropsychopharmacology, 1*, 179–183.

Castrogiovanni, P., Iapichino, S., Pacchierotti, C., & Pieraccini, F. (1998). Season of birth in Psychiatry. *Neuropsychobiology, 37*, 175–181.

Centers for Disease Control and Prevention, National Center for Injury Prevention and Control. NCHS Data Brief, No. 168, October 2014. US Department of Health and Human Services Centers for Disease Control and Prevention National Center for Health Statistics Mortality in the United States. 2012. Jiaquan Xu, M.D.; Kenneth D. Kochanek, M.A.; Sherry L. Murphy, B.S.; Elizabeth Arias, Ph.D.

Chamberlain, J. (1978). *On our own: Patient-controlled alternatives to the mental health system*. Portland, OR: Hawthorn Books.

Chamberlain, J. (2013). *Confessions of a Non-compliant Patient. National Empowerment Center* (http://www.power2u.org/articles/recovery/confessions.html).

Charles, C., Gafni, A., & Whelan, T. (1997). Shared decision-making in the medical encounter: What does it mean? (Or it takes at least two to tango). *Social Science and Medicine, 44*, 651–661.

Charles, C., & DeMaio, S. (1993). Lay participation in health care decision making: a conceptual framework. *J Health Polit Policy Law, 18*(4), 881–904.

Chochinov, H., Wilson, K., Enns, M., & Lander, S. (1998). Depression, hopelessness, and suicidal ideation in the terminally ill. *Psychosomatics, 39,* 366–370.

Chouinard, G., & Jones, B. (1980). Neuroleptically-induced supersensitivity psychosis. *American Journal of Psychiatry, 137,* 16–20.

Cirino, P., & Willcutt, Erik. (2017). An introduction to the special issue: Contributions of executive function to academic skills. *Journal of Learning Disabilities, 50*(4), 355–358.

Cohen, J., Mannarino, A., Deblinger, E. (Eds.) (2012). *Trauma-focused CBT for children and adolescents: Treatment applications.* New York, NY: Guilford Press.

Cohen, R. (Producer). (1975). *Hurry tomorrow* [Motion picture]. United States: Richard Cohen Films.

Cohen, R. A. (1982). Notes on the life and work of Frieda Fromm-Reichmann. *Psychiatry, 45,* 90–98.

Coll, J., Weiss, E., & Exum, H. A. (2010). *A civilian counselor's primer to counseling veterans* (2nd ed.). Ronkonkoma, NY: Linus Publications.

Copeland, M. E. (2012). *Facilitator training manual: Mental health recovery including WRAP.* Advocates for Human Potential, Inc.

Corina, D. P., Vaid, J., & Bellugi, U. (1992). The linguistic basis of left hemisphere specialization. *Science, 255,* 1258–1260.

Cosgrove, L. (2006). Financial ties between DSM-IV panel members and the pharmaceutical industry. *Psychotherapy Psychosomatics, 75,* 154–160.

Cosgrove, L. (2012). A comparison of DSM-IV and DSM-5 panel members' financial associations with industry. *PLoS Med, 9*(3).

Cozolino, L. (2010). *The neuroscience of psychotherapy: Healing the social brain* (2nd ed.). Norton.

Cullberg, J. (2006). *Psychosis: An Integrative Perspective.* Routledge.

Dalai Lama. Compassion and the individual. http://www.dalailama.com/messages/compassion

Dalman, C., Allebeck, P., Cullberg, J., Grunewald, C., & Koster. M. (1999). Obstetric complications and the risk of schizophrenia: a longitudinal study of a national birth cohort. *Archives of General Psychiatry, 56*(3), 234–240.

Darabont, F. (1994). *The Shawshank redemption.* Directed by Frank Darabont.

Darves-Bornoz, J., Lempérière, T., Degiovanni, A., & Gaillard, P. (1995). Sexual victimization in women with schizophrenia and bipolar disorder. *Social Psychiatry Psychiatr Epidemiol, 30,* 78–84.

Davidson, J., & Smith, R. (1990). Traumatic experiences is psychiatric outpatients. *Journal of Traumatic Stress, 3,* 459–475.

Davidson, L., Chinman, M., Sells, D., & Rowe, M. (2006). Peer support among adults with serious mental illness: A report from the field. *Schizophr Bull, 32,* 443–450. 2.

Davis, L., Suris, A., Lambert, M., Heimberg, C., & Petty, F. (1997). Post-traumatic stress disorder and serotonin: New directions for research and treatment. *Journal of Psychiatry Neuroscience, 22*(3), 18–26.

De Belis, M., Keshavan, M., Clark, D., Casey, B., Giedd, J., Boring, A., . . . Ryan, N. (1999). Developmental traumatology: Part II. Brain development. *Biological Psychiatry, 45,* 1271–1284.

Deegan, P. (2018). The Recovery Library. https://www.recoverylibrary.com/

DeSisto, M., Harding, R., McCormick, T., Ashikaga, T., & Brooks, G. (1995). The Maine and Vermont three-decade studies of serious mental illness: I: Matched comparison of cross-sectional outcome. *British Journal of Psychiatry,* Sept. *167,* 331–338.

Devinsky, O. (2000). Right Cerebral Hemisphere Dominance for a Sense of Corporeal and Emotional Self. *Epilepsy & Behavior, 1*(1), 60–73.

Dierks, T., Linden, D., Jandl, M., Formisano, E. Goebel, R., Lanfermann, H., & Singer, W. (1999). Activation of Heschl's Gyrus during auditory hallucinations. *Cell Press, 22,* 615–621.

Dix, D. (1824). *Conversations on common things.* Boston: Munroe & Francis.

Dix, D. (1843). *Memorial to the legislature of Massachusetts.* Boston: Munroe & Francis.

Dix, D. (2006). "I tell what I have seen": The reports of asylum reformer Dorothea Dix. *American Journal of Public Health, 96,* 622–624.

Driesen, N. R., & Raz, N. (1995). The influence of sex, age, and handedness on corpus callosum morphology: A meta-analysis. *Psychobiology, 23,* 240–247.

Dully, H., & Fleming, C. (2007). *My lobotomy: A memoir.* Three Rivers Press.

Dunn, S. (2002). *"I have softening of the brain and I will soon be dead": Understanding acute psychotic decompensation from the patient's perspective.* Doctoral dissertation. Loyola University of Chicago.

Eitenger, L., & Grunfeld, B. (1966). Psychosis among refugees in Norway. *Acta Psychiatr Scand, 42,* 315–328.

Elbogen, E., Wagner, R., Fuller, S., Calhoun, P., Kinneer, P., Mid-Atlantic Mental Illness Research, Education, and Clinical Center Workgroup, & Beckham, J. (2010). Correlates of anger and hostility in Iraq and Afghanistan war veterans. *American Journal of Psychiatry, 167,* 1051–1058.

Ellason, J., & Ross, C. (1997). Two-year follow-up of inpatients with dissociative identity disorder. *American Journal of Psychiatry, 154,* 832–839.

Epstein, N. (2008). Uncle Xenon: The element of Oliver Sacks. *Moment Magazine.* No. *BMJ, 336,* 1405.

Fava, G. (2008). Should the drug industry work with key opinion leaders? No. *BMJ, 336,* 1405.

Feist, J. (1994). *Theories of personality* (3rd ed.). Fort Worth, TX: Harcourt Brace College Publishers.

Fisher, D. (2006). Recovery from schizophrenia: From seclusion to empowerment. *Medscape.* www.medscape.com/viewarticle/523539

Ford, H. (n.d.). Henry Ford quotes. *Quotes.net.* Retrieved September 20, 2016, from http://www.quotes.net/quote/6037

Fowler, D. (2000). Psychological formulation for early episodes of psychosis: A cognitive model. In M. Birchwood, D. Fowler, & C. Jackson (Eds), *Early intervention in psychosis* (pp. 101–127). New York, NY: John Wiley.

Frank, E., Kupfer, D., Thase, M., Mallinger, A., Swartz, H., Fagiolini, A., . . . Monk, T. (2005). Two-year outcomes for interpersonal and social rhythm therapy in individuals with bipolar I disorder. *Archives of General Psychiatry, 62,* 996–1004.

Frankl (1959). *Man's Search for Meaning.* Beacon Press.

Freud, S. (1913). *The interpretation of dreams* (3rd ed.). New York: Macmillan.

Freud, S. (1914/1925). On narcissism: An introduction. In J. Strachey et al. (Trans.), *The Standard Edition of the Complete Psychological Works of Sigmund Freud, Collected Papers* (Vol. 4, pp. 30–59). London: Hogarth Press.

Freud, S. (1925). *Collected Papers.* London: Hogarth Press.

Freudenreich, O., Schulz, S., & Goff, D. (2009). Initial medical work-up of first-episode psychosis: A conceptual review. *Early Interv Psychiatry, 3,* 10–18.

Friedman, R. A. (2006). Violence and mental illness: How strong is the link? *New England Journal of Medicine, 355,* 2064–2066.

Friedman, S., & Harrison, G. (1984). Sexual histories, attitudes and behaviour of schizophrenic and normal women. *Arch Sex Behav,13,* 555–567.

Frith, C., & Corcoran, R. (1996). Exploring theory of mind in people with schizophrenia. *Psychological Medicine, 26,* 521–530.

Fromm-Reichmann, F. (1948). *Notes on the development of treatment of schizophrenics by psychoanalytic psychotherapy.* Basic Books.

Fromm-Reichmann, F. (1950/1960). *Principles of intensive psychotherapy.* Chicago, IL: University of Chicago Press.

Fromm-Reichmann, F. (1952). Some Aspects of Psychoanalytic Psychotherapy with Schizophrenics. In E. B. Brody & F. C. Redlich (Eds.), *Monograph series on schizophrenia, no. 3. Psychotherapy with schizophrenics* (pp. 89–111). Madison, CT, US: International Universities Press, Inc.

Fromm-Reichman, F. (1954). The academic lecture of psychotherapy of schizophrenia. *American Journal of Psychiatry, 111,* 410–419.

Fromm-Reichmann, F. (1974). *Psychoanalysis and psychotherapy selected papers.* Chicago: University of Chicago Press.

Fuhrman, J. (2011). Eat to live: The Amazing Nutrient-Rich Program for Fast and Sustained Weight Loss. Little, Brown, and Company.

Gabbard, G. O. (2014). *Gabbard's treatment for psychiatric disorders* (5th ed.). Washington D.C.: American Psychiatric Association Publications.

Gardos, G., & Cole, J. (1977). Maintenance antipsychotic therapy: Is the cure worse than the disease? *American Journal of Psychiatry, 133,* 32–36.

Gerhart, U., & Marley, J. (2010). *Caring for the chronically mentally ill* (2nd ed.). Independence, KY: Brooks Cole.

Gillon, R. (1994). Medical ethics: Four principles plus attention to scope. *British Medical Journal, 309*(6948), 184–188.

"Mission and Values." Our Mission—GLIDE, www.glide.org/mission

Goff, D., Brotman, A., Kindlon, D., Waites, M., & Amico, E. (1991). Self-reports of childhood abuse in chronically psychotic patients. *Psychiatry Research, 37,* 73–80.

Goffman, E. (1961). *Asylum: Essays on the social situation of mental patients and other inmates.* New York, NY: Anchor/Doubleday.

Goldstein, E. (1995). Ego psychology and social work practice. (2nd ed.) New York, NY: Free Press.

Goldstein, J. (2009). Geel, Belgium: A model of "community recovery." Samford University Psychology Department. http://faculty.samford.edu/~jlgoldst/

Gottesman, I. (1990). *Schizophrenia genesis: The origins of madness.* New York, NY: W. H. Freeman.

Gottesman. I. (1991). *Schizophrenia Genesis.* W.H. Freeman, New York.

Gottesman, I. I., & Shields, J. (1982). *Schizophrenia: The Epigenetic Puzzle.* Wiley, New York.

Graf, P., & Schacter, D. L. (1985). Implicit and explicit memory for new associations in normal and amnesic subjects. *Journal of Experimental Psychology, 11,* 501–518.

Greenfield, S., Stratowski, S., Tohen, M., Batson, S., & Kolbrener, M. (1994). Childhood abuse in first-episode psychosis. *British Journal of Psychiatry, 164,* 831–834.

Gregory Zilboorg. (1941). *A History of Medical Psychology.* W.W. Norton, 261.

Grillon, C., Southwick, S. M., & Charney, D. S. (1996). The psychobiological basis of post traumatic stress syndrome. *Molecular Psychiatry, 1,* 278–297.

Grimby, A. (1993). Bereavement among elderly people: Grief reactions, post-bereavement hallucinations and quality of life. *Acta Psychiatrica Scandinavica, 87,* 72–80.

Grof, S. (1988). *The adventure of self-discovery: Dimensions of consciousness and new perspectives in psychotherapy and inner exploration.* Albany, NY: State University of New York.

Grof, S., & Grof, C. (Eds.). (1989). *Spiritual emergency: When personal transformation becomes a crisis.* Los Angeles, CA: Tarcher.

Gunawardana, L., Zammie, L., Lewis, G., Gunnell, D., Hollis, Wolke, D., & Harrison, G. (2011). Examining the association between maternal analgesic use during pregnancy and risk of psychotic symptoms during adolescence. *Schizophrenia Research, 126,* 220–225.

Gunst, V. K. (1982). Memoirs—professional and personal: A decade with Frieda Fromm-Reichmann. F. *Psychiatry, 45,* 107–115.

Hamann, J., & Heres, S. (2014). Adapting shared decision making for individuals with severe mental illness. *Psychiatric Services, 65,* 1483–1486.

Haracz, J. (1982). The dopamine hypothesis: An overview of studies with schizophrenic patients. *Schizophrenia Bulletin, 8,* 438–458.

Harding, C., Brooks, G., Ashika, T., Strauss, J., & Breier. (1987). The Vermont longitudinal study of person with severe mental illness. *American Journal of Psychiatry, 144,* 727–734.

Harding, C., & Zahniser, J. (1994). Empirical correction of seven myths about schizophrenia with implications for treatment, *Acta Psychiatrica Scandinavica, 384,* 14–16.

Harm Reduction Coalition. (n.d.). Principles of Harm reduction. Retrieved from http://harmreduction.org/about-us/principles-of-harm-reduction/

Harris, Dominic. (2012). The residents: Stories of Kingsley Hall, East London, 1965–1970 and the experimental community of RD Laing. Dominic Harris Publisher.

Harrison. P. J. (1995). On the neuropathology of schizophrenia and its dementia: Neurodevelopmental, neurodegenerative, or both? *Neurodegeneration, 4,* 1–12.

Hartz, S., Carlos, P., Medeiros, H., Cavazos-Rehg, P., Sobell, J., Knowles, J., Bierut, L., & Pato, M. (2014). The Genomic Psychiatry Cohort Consortium: Comorbidity of severe psychotic disorders with measures of substance use. *JAMA Psychiatry, 71,* 248–254. Retrieved from http://archpsyc.jamanetwork.com/article.aspx?articleid=1790914#Abstract

Hatfield, B., Huxley, P., & Mohamad, H. (1992). Accommodation and employment: A survey into the circumstances and expressed needs of users of mental health services in a northern town. *British Journal of Social Work, 22,* 60–73.

Havens, L. (1996). *A safe place: Laying the groundwork of psychotherapy.* Cambridge, MA: Harvard University Press.

Hawn Foundation. (2011). *The MindUP Curriculum: Grades PreK–2: Brain-focused strategies for learning—and living.* New York, NY: Scholastic Teaching Resources.

Hayman, R. (1999). *A Life of Jung.* New York: W.W. Norton & Co, Inc.

Healey, D. (2002). *The creation of psychopharmacology.* Cambridge, MA: Harvard University Press.

Healey, E. C., Mallard, A. R., 3rd, & Adams, M. R. (1976). Factors contributing to the reduction of stuttering during singing. *Journal of Speech and Hearing Research, 19,* 475–480.

Hearing Voices Network. About Us. http://www.hearingvoicesusa.org/about-us

Heins, T., Gray, A., & Tennant, M. (1990). Persisting hallucinations following childhood sexual abuse. *Australia and New Zealand Journal of Psychiatry, 24,* 561–565.

Heston, L. L. (1966). Psychiatric disorders in foster home reared children of schizophrenic mothers. *British Journal of Psychiatry, 112,* 819–825.

Hewitt, J., & Coffey, M. (2005). Therapeutic working relationships with people with schizophrenia: Literature review. *Journal of Advanced Nursing, 52,* 561–570.

Hiday, V., Swartz, M., Swanson, J., Borum, R., & Wagner, H. R. (1999). Criminal victimization of persons with severe mental illness. *Psychiatric Services, 50,* 62–68.

Hiroeh, U., Appleby, L., Mortensen, P. B., & Dunn, G. (2001). Death by homicide, suicide, and other unnatural causes in people with mental illness: A population-based study. *Lancet, 358,* 2110–2112.

Hirsch, S. (1974). *Madness network news reader.* San Francisco: Glide Publications.

Hoff, S. G. (1982). Frieda Fromm-Reichmann: The early years. *Psychiatry, 45,* 115–120.

Holmes, T. H., & Rahe, R. H. (1967). The Social Readjustment Rating Scale. *Journal of Psychosom Res, 11,* 213–218.

Honing, A. M. (1988). Cumulative traumata as contributors to chronicity in schizophrenia. *Bulletin of Menninger Clinics, 52,* 423–434.

Honig, A., Romme, M. A., Ensink, B. J., Escher, S. D., Pennings, M. H., & deVries, M. W. (1998). Auditory hallucinations: A comparison between patients and nonpatients. *Journal of Nervous and Mental Disease, 186,* 646–651.

Hopper, K., & Wanderling, J. (2000). Revisiting the developed versus developing country distinction in course and outcome in schizophrenia: Results from ISoS, the WHO collaborative follow up project. *Schizophrenia Bulletin, 26*(4), 835–846.

Hornstein, G. (2005). *To redeem a person is to redeem the world.* New York: Other Press.

Hornstein, G. (2012). *Agnes's jacket: A psychologist's search for the meaning of madness.* Harlan, IA: Rodale Books.

Howes, O., & Kapur, S. (2009). The dopamine hypothesis of schizophrenia: Version III—The final common pathway. *Schizophrenia Bulletin, 35,* 549–562.

Hull, C. L. (1933). *Hypnosis and suggestibility.* New York, NY: Appleton Century.

Hutchings, P., & Dutton, M. (1993). Sexual assault history in a community mental health centre clinical population. *Community Mental Journal, 29,* 59–63.

Huttunen, M. O. (1989). Maternal Stress during Pregnancy and the Behavior of the Offspring. In: S. Doxiadis & S. Stewart (Eds.), *Early Influences Shaping the Individual* (pp. 175–182).

Hyman, S. (1996). Initiation and adaptation: A paradigm for understanding psychotropic drug action. *American Journal of Psychiatry, 153,* 151–161.

Hynd, G., Hall, J., Novey, E., Eliopulos, D., Black, K., Gonzalez, J., . . . Cohen, M. (1995). Dyslexia and corpus callosum morphology. *Archives of Neurology, 52,* 32–38.

Innocenti, G. M., Ansermet, F., & Parnas, J. (2003). Schizophrenia, neurodevelopment and corpus callosum. *Mol Psychiatry, 8*(3), 261–274.

Insel, T. (2013). Director's blog: Transforming diagnosis. April 29, 2013. http://www.nimh.nih.gov/about/director/2013/transforming-diagnosis.shtml

Jacobson, A., & Richardson, B. (1987). Assault experience of 100 psychiatric inpatients: Evidence of the need for routine enquiry. *American Journal of Psychiatry, 144,* 908–913.

Jacobson, N., & Greenley, D. (2001). What is recovery? A conceptual model and explication. *Psychiatric Services, 52,* 482–485.

Jackson, M. (2001). *Weathering the storm: Psychotherapy for psychosis.* New York: Routledge.

Jackson, M., & Williams, P. (1994). *Unimaginable storms: A search for meaning in psychosis.* London: Karnac Books.

Janet, P. (1893). L'amnésie continue [Continuous amnesia]. *Annual Review of Genetics Science, 4,* 167–179.

Job, D., Whalley, H., Johnstone, E., & Lawrie, S. (2005). Grey matter changes over time in high risk subjects developing schizophrenia. *NeuroImage, 25,* 1023–1030.

Jung, C. (1963/1989/1995). Memories, dreams, reflections. London: Fontana Press.

Jung, C. (1968). *Man and his symbols.* Dell.

Jung, C. (1995). *Memories, dreams, reflections.* London: Fontana Press.

Jung, C. (2009). *The red book* (S. Shamdasani, Ed.). New York, NY: W.W. Norton & Co.

Kahneman, D., & Tyersky, A. (1979). Prospect theory: An analysis of decision under risk. *Econometrica, 47,* 263–291.

Kanter, J. (1990). Community-based management of psychotic clients: The contributions of D. W. and Clare Winnicott. *Clinical Social Work Journal, 18,* 23–24.

Kantrowitz, J., & Javitt, D. (2010). N-methyl-d-aspartate (NMDA) receptor dysfunction or dysregulation: The final common pathway on the road to schizophrenia? *Brain Research Bulletin, 83,* 108–121.

Kellner, C. (2015). Contemporary ECT for depression, Part 1: Practice update. *Psychiatric Times.* http://www.psychiatrictimes.com/authors/charles-h-kellner-md

Kelly, T. M. (2012). Akutagawa Ryûnosuke's "The spider thread": Translation and commentary. Edogawa University. Retrieved January 12, 2012. http://www1.edogawa-u.ac.jp/~tmkelly/research_spider.html

Kendler, K., Gruenberg, A., & Tsuang, M. (1985). Psychiatric Illness in First-degree Relatives of Schizophrenic and Surgical Control Patients: A Family Study Using DSM-III Criteria. *Archives of General Psychiatry, 42*(8), 770–779.

Kendler, K. S., Gruenberg, A. M., & Kinney, D. K. (1994). Independent diagnoses of adoptees and relatives as defined by DSMIII criteria, in the provincial and national samples of the Danish adoption study of schizophrenia. *Archives of General Psychiatry, 51,* 456–468.

Kendler, K., & Robinette, C. (1983). *Schizophrenia in the National Academy of Sciences National Research Council Twin Registry: A 16 year update. American F Psychiatry, 140,* 1551–1563.

Kessler, R. (1996). *The sins of the father: Joseph P. Kennedy and the dynasty he founded.* New York, NY: Warner Books, 1996.

Kety, S. (1983). Mental illness in the biological and adoptive relatives of schizophrenic adoptees, findings relevant to genetic and environmental factors in etiology. *American F Psychiatry, 140,* 720–727.

Kievit, J., Nooij, M. A., & Stiggelbout, A. M. (2001). Stability of patients' preferences for chemotherapy: The impact of experience. *Medical Decision Making, 21,* 295–306.

Kingdon, D. G., & Turkington, D. (1999). Cognitive-behavioural therapy of schizophrenia. In T. Wykes, N. Tarrier, & S. Lewis (Eds.), *Outcome and innovation in the psychological treatment of schizophrenia* (pp. 59–79). London: Wiley.

Kinzie, J., & Boehnlein, J. (1989). Posttraumatic stress among Cambodian refugees. *Journal of Traumatic Stress, 2,* 185–198.

Klein, H., Zellermayer, J., & Shanan, J. (1963). Former concentration camp inmates on a psychiatric ward. *Archives of General Psychiatry, 8,* 334–342.

Kolb, B., & Whishaw, I. (2003). *Fundamentals of human neuropsychology.* New York, NY: Worth Publishers.

Kraepelin, E. (1908). Zur Entartungsfrage. Zentralblatt für Nervenheilkunde und Psychiatrie, 31: 745–51; reprinted in Burgmair et al., 2006: 61–70. Liepzig.

Kubota, M., Nakazaki, S., Hirei, S., Seiki, N., & Yamaura, A. (2001). Alcohol consumption and frontal lobe shrinkage of 1432 non-alcoholic subjects. *J Neurol Neurosurg Psychiatry, 71*(1), 104–106.

Laing, R. D. (1965). *The divided self: An existential study in sanity and madness.* New York: Penguin Books.

Landsman, N. C. (2001). *Nation and province in the first British empire.* Lewisberg, PA: Bucknell University Press.

Lapidus, K., Kopell B., Ben-Haim S, Rezai A., & Goodman W. (2013). History of psychosurgery: A psychiatrist's perspective. *World Neurosurg, 80*(3-4).

Larkin, W., & Morrison, A. (2015). *Trauma and psychosis: New directions for theory and therapy.* Routledge.

Lasko, N. B., Gurvits, T. V., Kuhne, A. A., Orr, S. P., & Pitman, R. K. (1994). Aggression and its correlates in Vietnam veterans with and without chronic posttraumatic stress disorder. *Computers in Psychology, 35,* 373–381.

Lawrence, J. (2000). The Indian Health Service and the sterilization of Native American women. *American Indian Quarterly, 24* (pp. 400–419). University of Nebraska Press. https://muse.jhu.edu/article/200/pdf

Lee, T., Seeman, P., Tourtelloute, W., Farley, I., & Hornykeiwicz, O. (1978). Binding of ³H-neuroleptics and ³H-apomorphine in schizophrenic brains. *Nature, 274,* 897–900.

Lehman, A. F. (1995). Vocational rehabilitation in schizophrenia. *Schizophr Bull, 21,* 645–656.

Lenzer, J. (2004, August 21). Obituary: Loren Mosher. *British Medical Journal, 329,* 463.

Lessig, L. (2014). What an originalist would understand "corruption" to mean. *California Law Review, 102,* 1–24.

Leo, R., & Del Regno, P. (2000). Atypical antipsychotic use in the treatment of psychosis in primary care. *Prim Care Companion J Clin Psychiatry, 2,* 194–204.

Levitin, D. J. (2006). This is your brain on music: The science of a human obsession. Plume/Penguin.

Lewis, G., David, A., Andréasson, S., & Alleback, P. (1992). Schizophrenia and city life. *Lancet, 340,* 137–140.

Lewis, C., Levinson, D., Wise, L., DeLisi, L., Straub, R., Hovatta, I., . . . Gurling, H. M. D. (2003). Genome scan meta-analysis of schizophrenia and biolar disorder: Part III. Schizophrenia. *American Journal of Human Genetics, 73,* 34–48.

Lewis, S. (2007). *Fast facts: Schizophrenia* (2nd ed.). Abingdon, England: Health Press Limited.

Lewontin, R. (1993). *The doctrine of DNA: Biology as ideology.* London: Penguin Books.

Lim, K., Hedehus, M., Moseley, M., de Crespingy, A., Sullivan, E., & Pfefferbaum, A. (1999). *Archives of General Psychiatry, 56,* 367–374.

Limosin, Rouillon, Payan, Cohen, & Strub, (2003). Prenatal exposure to influenza as a risk factor for adult schizophrenia. *Acta Psychiatr Scand, 107*(5), 331–335.

Lindemann, E. (1944). The symptomatology and management of acute grief. *American Journal of Psychiatry, 101,* 141–148.

Lindstrom, L. H., Gefvert, O., Hagberg, G., Lundberg, T., Bergstrom, M., Hartvig, P., & Långström B. (1999). Increased dopamine synthesis rate in medial prefrontal cortex and striatum in schizophrenia indicated by L-(ß-11C) DOPA and PET. *Biological Psychiatry, 46,* 681–688.

Linehan. M. (1993/2014). *Cognitive-behavioral treatment of borderline personality disorder.* New York: Guilford Press.

Linehan, M. (2014). *Dialectical behavioral skills training workbook* (2nd ed.). New York: Guilford Press. The Linehan Institute.

Link, B., Phelan, J., Bresnahan, M., Stueve, A., & Pescosolido, B. (1999). Public conceptions of mental illness: Labels, causes, dangerousness, and social distance. *American Journal of Public Health, 89,* 1328–1333.

Little, M. (1985). Winnicott working in areas where psychotic anxieties predominate. *Free Associations, 3,* 9–42.

Livingston, R. (1987). Sexually and physically abused children. *Journal of the American Academy of Child and Adolescent Psychiatry, 26,* 413–415.

Lynn, S. J., Berg, J., Lilienfeld, S. O., Merckelbach, H., Giesbrecht, T., Accardi, M., & Cleere, C. (2012). Dissociative disorders. In M. Hersen, D. C. Beidel (Eds.), *Adult psychopathology and diagnosis* (pp. 497–538). Hoboken, NJ: Wiley.

Loomes, G., & Sugden, R. (1982). Regret theory: An alternative theory of rational choice under uncertainty. *Economics Journal, 92,* 805–824.

Lopez-Munoz, F., Bhatara, V. S., Alamo, C., & Cuenca, E. (2004). [Historical approach to reserpine discovery and its introduction in psychiatry] [Article in Spanish] *Actas Esp Psiquiatr, 32,* 387–395. Full text in English and Spanish. http://www.arsxxi.com/Revistas/mostrararticulo. php?idarticulo=411106110

MacKay, A., Iversen, L., Rossor, M., Spokes, E., Bird, E., Arregui, A., . . . Snyder, S. (1982). Increased brain dopamine and dopamine receptors in schizophrenia. *Archives of General Psychiatry, 39,* 991–997.

Mackler, D. (2000a). *Healing homes* [video file]. https://www.youtube.com/watch?v= JV4NTEp8S2Q

Mackler, D. (2000b). *Open dialogue* [video file]. https://www.youtube.com/watch?v= HDVhZHJagfQ

Mackler, D. (2000c). *Take these broken wings* [video file]. https://www.youtube.com/watch?v= EPfKc-TknWU

Maguire, E. A., Gadian, D. G., Johnsrude, I. S., Good, C. D., Ashburner, J., Frackowiak, R. S. J., & Frith, C. D. (2000). Navigation-related structural change in the hippocampi of taxi drivers. *Proceedings of the National Academy of Sciences of the United States of America, 97,* 4398–4403.

Maher, B. A. (1974). Delusional thinking and perceptual disorder. *Journal of Individual Psychology, 30*(1), 98–113.

Maisel, A. (1946). Bedlam 1946: Most mental hospitals are a shame and a disgrace. *Life Magazine.* May 6, 1946.

Mamah, D., Wang, L., Barch, D., de Erausquin, G. A., Gado, M., & Csernansky, J. G. (2007). Structural analysis of the basal ganglia in schizophrenia. *Schizophrenia Research, 89*(1–3), 59–71. http://www.ncbi.nlm.nih.gov/entrez/eutils/elink.fcgi?dbfrom=pubmed&retmode=ref& cmd=prlinks&id=17071057

Manon, P. (2010). From a patient's perspective: Clifford Whittingham Beers' work to reform mental health services. *American Journal of Public Health, 100*, 2356–2357.

Marner, L., Nyengaard, J., Tang, Y., & Pakkenberg, B. (2003). Marked loss of myelinated nerve fibers in the human brain with age. *Journal of Comparative Neurology, 462*, 144–152.

Marshall, P. (1990). Director. *Awakenings* [video file]. Chatsworth, CA: Distributed by Image Entertainment.

Martinot, J. (1990). Striatal D2 dopaminergic receptor assessed with positron emission tomography and bromospiperone in untreated schizophrenic patients. *American Journal of Psychiatry, 147*, 44–50.

Masters, K. J. (1995). Environmental trauma in psychosis. *Journal of the American Academy of Child and Adolescent Psychiatry, 34*, 1258.

Maté, G. (2010). *In the realm of the Hungry Ghost*. Berkeley, CA: North Atlantic Books.

Mathews, S. (1979). A non-neuroleptic treatment for schizophrenia. *Schizophrenia Bulletin, 5*, 322–332.

Matthews, S., Roper, M., Mosher, L., et al. (1979). A controlled trial of social intervention in the families of schizophrenic patients. *British Journal of* Psychiatry, *141*, 121–134.

McFarlane, W. (2004). *Multifamily groups in the treatment of severe psychiatric disorders*. New York: Guilford Press.

McGrath, J., Saha, S., Chant, D., & Welham, J. (2008). Schizophrenia: A concise overview of incidence, prevalence, and mortality. *Epidemiol Rev, 30*, 67–76.

McGuffin, P., & Owen, M. (1995). Genetic basis of schizophrenia. *Lancet, 346*, 678.

McKinnon, B. (1986). The movement. *Phoenix Rising, 6*, 7.

McKnight, W. (2015, September 2). Data grow in support of ECT for depression. *Clinical Psychiatry News Digital Network*. https://www.mdedge.com/clinicalpsychiatrynews/article/102398/depression/data-grow-support-ect-depression

McNeil, T. F. (1988). A prospective study of postpartum psychoses in a high-risk group. *Acta Psychiatrica Scandinavica, 77*(6), 645–653.

Mead S. (2003). Defining peer support. http://www. intentionalpeersupport.org/documents/DefiningPeerSupport.pdf

Mechanic, D. (2008). *Mental health and social policy: Beyond managed care* (5th ed.). Boston, MA: Pearson.

Mednick, S. A., Machon, R. A., Huttunen, M. O., & Bonett, D. (1988). Adult schizophrenia following prenatal exposure to an influenza epidemic. *Archives of General Psychiatry, 45*(2), 189–192.

Meldrum, M. (2003). *Where's the evidence? A challenge to psychiatric authority*. Vimeo. https://vimeo.com/117465548

Menniger, K., Mayman, M., & Pruyser, P. (1963). *The vital balance: The life process in mental health & illness*. New York: Viking Adult Press.

Merikangas, K. R., Akiskal, H. S., Angst, J., Greenberg, P. E., Hirschfeld, R. M., Petukhova, M., & Kessler, R. C. (2007). Lifetime and 12-month prevalence of bipolar spectrum disorder in the National Comorbidity Survey replication. *Archives of General Psychiatry, 64*, 543–552.

Mezzich, J. (2007). The dialogal basis of our profession: Psychiatry with the Person. *World Psychiatry, 6*, 129–130.

Miller, G. (2004). *R. D. Laing*. Edinburgh: Edinburgh University Press.

Miller, W., & Rollnick, S. (2012). *Motivational interviewing: Helping people change* (3rd ed.). New York: Guilford Press.

Minkoff, Kenneth. (date?) *Dual Diagnosis*. [video file].

Minsky, R. (1996) *Psychoanalysis and gender*: An introductory reader. Routledge.

Monnig, A., Tonigan, J. S., Yeo, R., Thoma, R., & McCrady, B. (2013). White matter volume in alcohol use disorders: A meta-analysis. *Addiction Biology, 18,* 581–592.

Morgan, M. (2003). Prospective analysis of premature mortality in schizophrenia in relation to health service engagement. *Psychiatry Research, 117,* 127–135.

Morrison, A. (2001). The interpretation of intrusions in psychosis: an integrative cognitive approach to hallucinations and delusions. *Behavioural and Cognitive Psychotherapy, 29,* 257–276.

Morrison, A., Frame, L., & Larkin, W. (2003). Relationships between trauma and psychosis: A review and integration. *British Journal of Clinical Psychology* (2003), *42,* 331–353.

Mortensen, P., Pederson, C., Westergaard, T., Wohlfahrt, J., Ewald, H., Mors, O., . . . Melbye, M. (1999). Effects of family history and place and season of birth on the risk of schizophrenia. *New England Journal of Medicine, 340,* 603–608.

Mosher, L. (1998). Letter of resignation to the American Psychiatric Association. http://www.moshersoteria.com/articles/resignation-from-apa/.

Mosher, L. (1999). Soteria and other alternatives to acute psychiatric hospitalization: A personal and professional review. *Journal of Nervous and Mental Disease, 187,* 142–149.

Mosher, L. (2004). *Soteria: Through madness to deliverance*. Bloomington, IN: Xlibris.

Mosher, L., & Burti, L. (1989). *Community mental health: Principles and practice*. New York: W.W. Norton & Co.

Mosher, L., & Menn, A. (1978). Community residential treatment for schizophrenia: Two-year follow-up data. *Hospital and Community Psychiatry, 29,* 715–723.

Mosher, L., Menn, A., & Matthews, S. (1975). Evaluation of a homebased treatment for schizophrenics. *American Journal of Orthopsychiatry, 45,* 455–467.

Mosher, L., Vallone, R., & Menn, A. (1990). *The treatment of acute psychosis without neuroleptics: New data from the Soteria project*. Lecture presented at the Annual Meeting of the American Psychiatric Association, New York.

Mueser, K., Goodman, L., Trumbetta, S., Rosenberg, S., Osher, F., Vidaver, R., Auciello, P., Foy D. (1998). Trauma and posttraumatic stress disorder in severe mental illness. *Journal of Consult Clinical Psychology, 66,* 493–499.

Murray, R., Jones, P., O'Callaghan, E., Takei N., & Sham, P. (1992). Genes, viruses and neurodevelopmental schizophrenia. *Journal of Psychiatric Research, 26*(4), 225–235.

Nasrallah, H. A. (1985). Cerebral Basis of Psychopathology. *American Journal of Psychiatry, 142*(5), 645-a-646.

National Alliance on Mental Illness. (NAMI). *Family to family program*. http://www.nami.org/familytofamily

Naz, B., Bromet E., & Mojtabai R. (2003). Distinguishing between first-admission schizophreniform disorder and schizophrenia. *Schizophr Res, 62*(1–2), 51–58.

Nelson, G., Lord, J., & Ochocka, J. (2001). *Shifting the paradigm in community mental health: Towards empowerment and community*. Buffalo: University of Toronto Press.

Neria, Y., Bromet, E., Sievers, S., Lavelle, J., & Fochtmann, L. (2002). Trauma exposure and posttraumatic stress disorder in psychosis: Findings from a first-admission cohort. *J Consult Clin Psychology, 70,* 246–251.

Nestler, E., & Hyman, S. (2002). *Molecular Neuropharmacology.* New York: McGraw Hill. p. 392.

New York Times. (2005, September 7). The former First Lady Barbara Bush calls evacuees better off. http://www.nytimes.com/2005/09/07/national/nationalspecial/07barbara.html?_r=0

Noble, L. M., & Douglas, B. C. (2004). What users and relatives want from mental health. *Current Opinion in Psychiatry, 17,* 289–296.

NPR. (2005, November 16). My lobotomy. *All Things Considered.* http://www.npr.org/2005/11/16/5014080/my-lobotomy-howard-dullys-journey

O'Donnell, K., O'Connor, T. G., & Glover, V. (2009). Prenatal Stress and Neurodevelopment of the Child: Focus on the HPA Axis and Role of the Placenta. *Dev Neurosci, 31,* 285–292.

Olsen, M. (2014). The promise of open dialogue. *Mad in America: Science, Psychiatry, and Community.* January 1, 2014. http://www.madinamerica.com/2014/01/promise-open-dialogue-response-marvin-ross/http://www.madinamerica.com/2014/01/promise-open- dialogue-response-marvin-ross/

Oruc, L. & Bell, P. (1995). Multiple rape trauma followed by delusional parasitosis: A case from the Bosnian war. *Schizophrenia Research, 16,* 173–174.

Palmer, B. A., Pankratz, S., & Bostwick, J. M. (2005). The lifetime risk of suicide in schizophrenia. *Archives of General Psychiatry, 62,* 247–253.

Pandya, A., & Jän Myrick, K. (2013). Wellness and recovery programs: A model of self-advocacy for people living with mental illness. *Journal of Psychiatric Practice, 19,* 242–246.

Perälä, J., Suvisaari, J., Saarni, S. I., Kuoppasalmi, K., Isometsä, E., Pirkola, S., . . . Lönnqvist, J. (2007). Lifetime prevalence of psychotic and bipolar I disorders in a general population. *Archives of General Psychiatry, 64,* 19–28.

Perry, C., & Lawrence, J. R. (1984). Mental processing outside of awareness: The contributions of Freud and Janet. In K. S. Bowers & D. Meichenbaum (Eds.), *The unconscious reconsidered* (pp. 9–48). New York, NY: Wiley.

Perry, J. W. (1952). *The self in psychotic process: Its symbolization in schizophrenia.* Putnam, CT: Spring Publications.

Perry, J. W. (1974). *The far side of madness.* Putnam, CT: Spring Publications.

Perry, J. W. (1998). *Trials of a visionary mind.* Albany, NY: State University of New York Press.

Plyer, A. (2014). *Facts for features: Katrina impact.* The Data Center. http://www.datacenterresearch.org/data-resources/katrina/facts-for-impact/

Pollack, G. (1981). Report of the treasurer. *American Journal of Psychiatry, 138.*

Polsky, D., Mandelblatt, J., Weeks, J., Venditti, L., Hwang, Y., Glick, H., . . . Schulman, K. (2003). Economic evaluation of breast cancer treatment: Considering the value of patient choice. *Journal of Clinical Oncology, 21,* 1139–1146.

Post, R. (1975). Cerebrospinal fluid amine metabolites in acute schizophrenia. *Archives of General Psychiatry, 32,* 1063–1068.

Prein.R. (1971). Discontinuation of chemotherapy for chronic schizophrenics. *Hospital and Community Psychiatry, 22,* 20–23.

Prinzhorn, H. (1922). *Artistry of the mentally ill: A contribution to the psychology and psychopathology of configuration.* New York: Springer. (2nd ed. published in 1972.)

Prochaska, J., & DiClemente, C. (1986). Toward a comprehensive model of change. *Treating Addictive Behaviors, 13*, 3–27.

Rappaport, M. (1978). Are there schizophrenics for whom drugs may be unnecessary or contraindicated? *International Pharmacopsychiatry, 13*, 100–111.

Raunch, S. I., & Savage, C. R. (1997). Neuroimaging and neuropsychology of the striatum: Bridging basic science and clinical practice. *Psychiatric Clinics of North America, 20*, 741–768.

Raune, D., Kuipers, E., & Bebbington, P. (1999). Psycho-social stress and delusional and verbal and auditory hallucinatory themes in first episode psychosis: Implications for early intervention. Presented to the Third International Conference of Psychological Treatments for Schizophrenia. Oxford, England.

Read, J. (1997). Child abuse and psychosis: A literature review and implications for professional practice. *Prof Psychol Res Pr, 28*, 448–456.

Read, J. (2006). Breaking the silence: Learning why, when, and hot to ask about trauma and how to respond to disclosures. In W. Larking & A. P. Morrison (Eds.) *Trauma and psychosis: New directions for theory and therapy*. New York: Routledge.

Read, J., Agar, K., Argyle, & Aderhold, (2003). Sexual and physical abuse during childhood and adulthood as predictors of hallucinations, delusions and thought disorder. *Psychol Psychother, 76*(Pt 1), 1–22.

Read J., & Argyle N. (1999). Hallucinations, delusions and thought disorders among adult psychiatric inpatients with a history of child abuse. *Psychiatr Serv, 50*, 1467–1472.

Read, J., & Fraser, A. (1998). Abuse histories of psychiatric inpatients: To ask or not to ask? *Psychiatric Services, 49*, 355–359.

Read, J., Hammersley, P., Rudegeair, T. (2007). Why, when, and how to ask about child abuse. *Advances in Psychiatric Treatment, 13*, 101–110.

Read, J., Perry, B., Moskowitz, A., & Connolly, J. (2001). The contribution of early traumatic events to schizophrenia in some patients: A traumagenic neurodevelopmental model. *Psychiatry: Interpersonal and Biological Processes, 64*, 319–345.

Read, J., & Ross, C. (2011). Psychological trauma and psychosis: Another reason why people diagnosed schizophrenic must be offered psychological therapies. *Journal of the American Academy of Psychoanalysis and Dynamic Psychiatry, 31*, 247–268.

Read, J., van Os, J., Morrison, A., & Ross C. (2005). Childhood trauma, psychosis and schizophrenia: A literature review with theoretical and clinical implications. *Acta Psychiatr Scand, 112*, 330–350.

Reaume G. (2002). Lunatic to patient to person: Nomenclature in psychiatric history and the influence of patients' activism in North America. *Int J Law Psychiatry, 25*, 405–426.

Reaume, G. (2008, July). A history of psychiatric survivor pride day during the 1990s. *Consumer/Survivor Information Resource Centre Bulletin*.

Reilly, P. (1991). *The Surgical Solution: A History of Involuntary Sterilization in the United States*. The Quarterly Review of Biology, June 1987; 62(2).

Reaume, G. (2008). A History of Psychiatric Survivor Pride Day During the 1990s. *Mad Pride*, Issue Bulletin *374*, July 14.

Reilly, P. (1991). *The surgical solution: A history of involuntary sterilization in the United States*. Baltimore, MD: John Hopkins University Press.

Rhodes, J., & Jakes, S. (2009). *Narrative CBT for psychosis*. New York: Routledge.

Ridgeway P, Rapp C. (1998). *The active ingredients in achieving competitive employment for people with psychiatric disabilities: A research synthesis.* Critical Ingredients series. Lawrence, KS: Commission on Mental Health and Developmental Disabilities.

Robertson, J. (1952). *A two year old goes to hospital.* http://www.robertsonfilms.info

Robinson, P. Asylum. (1972). Peter Robinson Films, Surveillance Films. Kino Video. [video file].

Rodman, R. (2004). *Winnicott: His life and work.* Boston, MA: Da Capo Lifelong Books.

Rogers, L. (2011). *The ice pick lobotomist: Dr. Walter Freeman.* Retrieved July 11, 2011. https://lisawallerrogers.com/2009/01/16/266/

Romme, M. (2011–2018). Hearing Voices Network USA: About Us. http://www.hearingvoicesusa.org/about-us

Romme, M., & Escher, (1989). Hearing Voices. *Schizophr Bulletin, 15,* 209–216.

Roosens, E., & Van de Walle, L. (2007). *Geel revisited after centuries of mental rehabilitation.* Antwerp: Garant.

Rosenhan, D. L. (1973). On being sane in insane places. *Science, 179,* 250–258.

Rosenthal, D., Wender, P. H., Kety, S. S., Schulsinger, F., Welner, J., & Ostergaard, L. (1968). Schizophrenics' offspring reared in adoptive homes. In D. Rosenthal & S. S. Kety (Eds.), *The transmission of schizophrenia.* Oxford: Pergamon Press.

Ross, C., Anderson, G., & Clark, P. (1994). Childhood abuse and the positive symptoms of schizophrenia. *Hospital and Community Psychiatry, 45,* 489–491.

Ross, C., & Joshi, (1992). Paranormal experiences in the general population. *J Nerv Ment Dis, 180,* 357–361; discussion 362–368.

Ross, M. (2013). Don't be too quick to praise this new treatment. *HuffingtonPost.* November 11, 2013. http://www.huffingtonpost.ca/marvin-ross/schizophrenia-treatment_b_4254350.htm

Rothman, K., & Michels, K. (1994). The continuing unethical use of placebo controls. *N Engl J Med, 331,* 394–398.

Rush, B. (1812). *Medical inquiries and observations upon the diseases of the mind.* Philadelphia: Kimber and Richardson.

Sacks, O. (1973). *Awakenings.* New York City: Vintage.

Sacks, O. (2013). *Hallucinations.* New York City: Vintage.

Sacks, O. (September 18, 2009) Ted Talk. http://www.youtube.com/watch?v=SgOTaXhbqPQ

Saks, E. (2008). *The center cannot hold: My journey with madness.* New York: Hachette Book Group.

Sansonnet-Hayden, H., Haley, G., Marriage, K., & Fine, S. (1987). Sexual abuse and psychopathology in hospitalized adolescents. *Journal of the American Academy of Child and Adolescent Psychiatry, 26,* 753–757.

Saulny, S. (2007, March 18). At housing project, both fear and renewal. *New York Times.* Retrieved from http://www.nytimes.com

Schacter, D. (1987). Implicit memory: History and current status. *Journal of Experimental Psychology, 13,* 501–518.

Schiffer, F., Teicher, M. H., & Papanicolaou, A. C. (1995). Evoked potential evidence for right brain activity during the recall of traumatic memories. *Journal of Neuropsychiatry Clinical Neuroscience, 7*(2), 169–175.

Schmajuk, N. (2001). Hippocampal dysfunction in schizophrenia. *Hippocampus, 11*(5), 599–613.

Scott & Hicks. (1996). Shine Fine Line Films. [motion picture].

Searles, H. (1979). *Countertransference and related subjects: Selected papers.* Madison, CT: International Universities Press.

Seeman, P. (2011). Schizophrenia diagnosis and treatment. *CNS Neuroscience and Therapeitu023, 17*(2), 81–82.

Seikkula, J., Alakare, B., & Aaltonen, J. (2000). Two-year follow-up on open dialogue treatment in first episode psychosis: Need for hospitalization and neuroleptic medication decreases. *Social and Clinical Psychiatry, 10,* 20–29.

Seikkula, J., Alakare, B., Aaltonen, J., Holma, J., Rasinkangas, A., & Lehtinen, V. (2003). Open dialogue approach: Treatment principles and preliminary results of a two-year follow-up on first episode schizophrenia. *Ethical Human Sciences and Services, 5,* 163–182.

Seikkula, J., Aaltonen, J., Alakare, B., Haarakangas, K., Keränen, J., & Lehtinen, K. (2006). Five-year experience of first-episode nonaffective psychosis in open-dialogue approach: Treatment principles, follow-up outcomes, and two case studies. *Psychotherapy Research, 16,* 214–228.

Sekar, A., Bialas, A., de Rivera, H., Davis, A., Hammond, T., Kamitaki, N., . . . McCarroll, S., (2016). Schizophrenia risk from complex variation of complement component 4. *Nature, 530,* 177–183.

Semrad, E. (1955). Psychotherapy of psychosis: An attempt at a working formulation of some of the clinical psychopathological factors observed in schizophrenic patients. *Journal of Clinical and Experimental Psychopathology, 16,* 10–21.

Sesula, D. (2013). *You and me.* National Empowerment Center. http://www.power2u.org/articles/empower/you_and_me.html

Sabshin, M. (2008). *Changing American Psychiatry: A personal perspective.* Washington, D.C.: American Psychiatric Association.

Shalin, D. (2010). *Erving Goffman as a pioneer in self-ethnography? The "Insanity of Place" revisited.* Paper presented at Annual Meeting of the American Sociological Association, Atlanta, August 14, 2010.

Shaner, A., & Eth, S. (1989). Can schizophrenia cause posttraumatic stress disorder. *American Journal of Psychotherapy, 43,* 588–597.

Shenton, M., Kikinis, R., Rerenc, J., Pollak, S., LeMay, M., Wible, C., . . . McCarley, R. (1992). Abnormalities of the left temporal lobe and thought disorder in schizophrenia—A quantitative magnetic resonance imaging study. *New England Journal of Medicine, 327,* 604–12.

Shepherd, G., Murray, A., &Muijen, M. (1994). *Relative values: The different views of users, family carers and professionals on services for people with schizophrenia.* London: Sainsbury Centre for Mental Health.

Short, S., Lubach, G., Karasin, A., Olsen, C., Styner, M., Knickmeyer, R., Gilmore, J., & Coe, C. (2010). Maternal influenza infection during pregnancy impacts postnatal brain development in the rhesus monkey. *Biological Psychiatry, 67,* 965–973.

Shorter, E. (1998). *A history of psychiatry: From the era of the asylum to the age of prozac.* Hoboken, NJ: Wiley.

Shumway, M., Saunders, T., Shern, D., Pines, E., Downs, A., Burbine, T., & Beller, J. (2003). Preferences for schizophrenia treatment outcomes among public policy makers, consumers, families, and providers. *Psychiatric Services, 54,* 1124–1128.

Siegel, D. (2007). *The mindful brain: Reflection and attunement in the cultivation of well-being.* W.W. Norton & Company.

Siegel, D. (2009). Tedx. The Power of Mindsight. Retrieved March 18, 2018. http://drdansiegel. com/about/audio_video_clips/

Siegel, D. (2010). *Wheel of awareness meditation.* http://drdansiegel.com/resources/wheel_of_ awareness/audio/

Siegel, D. (2010a). *The mindful therapist: A clinician's guide to mindsight and neural integration.* New York: W.W. Norton & Co.

Siegel, D. (2010b). *Mindsight: The new science of personal transformation.* New York: Bantam Books.

Silberman, E., & Weingartner, H. (1986). Hemispheric lateralization of functions related to emo- tion. *Brain and Cognition, 5,* 322–353.

Silverman, E. (2008). Grassley probes psychiatrists over ties to pharma. July 11, 2008. Pharmalot.com. https://tmap.wordpress.com/2008/07/11/grassley-probes-psychiatrists-over-ties-to-pharma/

Soares, J. C., & Innis, R. B. (1999). Neurochemical brain imaging investigations of schizophrenia. *Biol Psychiatry, 46*(5), 600–615.

Sommer, R. (1959). Patients who grow old in a mental hospital. *Geriatrics, 14,* 586–587.

Spiegel, D., Loewenstein, R. J., Lewis-Fernández, R., Sar, V., Simeon, D., Vermetten, E., Cardena, E., & Dell, P. (2011). Dissociative disorders in DSM-5. *Depress Anxiety, 28,* 824–852.

Strakowski, S. M., McElroy, S. L., Keck, P. E., Jr., & West, S. A. (1996). Racial influence on diag- nosis in psychotic mania. *Journal of Affective Disorders, 39,* 157–162.

Stanton, A. H. (1982). Frieda Fromm-Reichmann, MD: Her impact on American psychiatry. *Psychiatry, 45,* 121–127.

Steele, C. J., Bailey, J. A., Zatorre, R. J., & Penhune, V. B. (2013). Early musical training and white matter plasticity in the corpus callosum: Evidence for a sensitive period. *Journal of Neuroscience, 33,* 1282–1290.

Stevens, G., & Gardner, S. (1982). *The women of psychology: Vol. I. Pioneers and innovators.* Cambridge, MA: Schenkman.

Stewart, M., & Brown, J. (2001). Patient-centredness in medicine. In G. Elwyn, & A. Edwards (Eds.), Evidence-based patient choice: Inevitable or impossible? Oxford University Press, New York. Stewart, M. A

Stromgen, E. (1994). Recent history of European psychiatry ideas, developments and personalities: The annual Eliot Slater Lecture. *Am F Med Genet, 54,* 405–410.

Stuart, H. (2003). Violence and mental illness: an overview. *World Psychiatry, 2,* 121–124.

Sullivan, H. S. (1947). Therapeutic investigations in schizophrenia. *Journal for the Study of Interpersonal Processes, 10,* 121–125.

Sullivan, H. S. (1955). *The psychiatric interview.* London: Tavistock Publications.

Sullivan, H. S. (1968). *The interpersonal theory of psychiatry.* New York: W.W. Norton & Co.

Sullivan, P. F. (2005). The genetics of schizophrenia. *PLoS Med, 2,* e212. doi:10.1371/journal. pmed.0020212

Susser, E., Brown, A., & Matte, T. (1999). Prenatal Factors and Adult Mental and Physical Health. *The Canadian Journal of Psychiatry, 44*(4), 326–334.

Susser, E., & Wanderling, J. (1994). Epidemiology of nonaffective acute remitting psychosis vs schizophrenia: Sex and sociocultural setting. *Archives of General Psychiatry, 51,* 294–301.

Takagi, T., Jin, W., Taya, K., Watanabe, G., Mori, K., & Ishii, S. (2006). Schnurri-2 mutant mice are hypersensitive to stress and hyperactive. *Brain Res, 1108,* 88–97.

Tausk, V. (1933). On the origin of the influencing machine in schizophrenia. *Psychoanalytic Quarterly, 2,* 519–556. Reprint *Journal of Psychotherapy Practice and Research, 1* (Spring 1992).

Terr, L. (1991). Childhood traumas: An outline and overview. *American Journal of Psychiatry, 148,* 10–20.

Tienari, P. (1992). Implications of adoption studies on schizophrenia. *The British Journal of Psychiatry, 161*(Suppl 18), 52–58.

Tiihonen, J., Wahlbeck, K., Lönnqvist, J., Klaukka, T., Ioannidis, J. P., Volavka, J., & Haukka, J. (2006). Effectiveness of antipsychotic treatments in a nationwide cohort of patients in community care after first hospitalisation due to schizophrenia and schizoaffective disorder: Observational follow-up study. *BMJ, 333,* 224.

Tolle, E. (2018). Audio recording. www.eckharttolletv.com/

Torrey, E., & Yolken. (2003). Toxoplasma gondii and schizophrenia. *Emerg Infect Dis, 9,* 1375–1380.

Tuke, S. (1813/1996). *Description of the retreat.* London: Process Press.

Ursuliak, Z., Milliken, H., & Morgan, N. (2015). Wellness program for people with early psychosis: Promoting skills and attitudes for recovery. *Psychiatric Services, 66,* 105.

van Eck, M., Berkhof, H., Nicolson, N., & Sulon, J. (1996). The effects of perceived stress, traits, mood states, and stressful daily events on salivary cortisol. *Psychosomatic Medicine, 58,* 447–458.

van Os & Selten. (1998). Prenatal exposure to maternal stress and subsequent schizophrenia. The May 1940 invasion of The Netherlands. *Br J Psychiatry, 172,* 324–326.

von Baeyer, V. (1977). On the pathogenic significance of extreme psychosocial stress in the development of endogenous psychosis. *Nervenarzt, 48,* 471–477.

Vujanovic, A., Youngwirth, N., Johnson, K., & Zvolensky, M. (2009). Mindfulness-based acceptance and posttraumatic stress symptoms among trauma-exposed adults without Axis-I psychopathology. *Journal of Anxiety Disorders, 23,* 297–303.

Walker, E., & Diforio, D. (1997). Schizophrenia: A neural diathesis-stress model. *Psychological Review, 104,* 667–685.

Walsh, J. (2011). Therapeutic communication with psychotic clients. *Clinical Social Work Journal, 39,* 1–8.

Walsh, R. (2011). Lifestyle and mental health. *American Psychologist, 66*(7), 579–592.

Walsh, P. (2009). *It's All Too Much Workbook: The Tools You Need to Conquer Clutter and Create the Life You Want.* New York: Free Press.

Webster, J., Kaushik, M., Bristow, G., & McConkey, G. (2013). *Toxoplasma gondii* infection, from predation to schizophrenia: Can animal behaviour help us understand human behavior? *Journal of Experimental Biology, 216,* 99–112.

Weiden, P., & Havens, L. (1994). Psychotherapeutic management techniques in the treatment of outpatients with schizophrenia. *Hospital and Community Psychiatry, 45,* 549–555.

Weigert, E. V. (1959). Foreword. In F. Fromm-Reichmann, *Psychoanalysis and psychotherapy.* Chicago: The University of Chicago Press.

Weiner, D. B. (1992). Philippe Pinel's "Memoir on Madness" of December 11, 1794: A fundamental text of modern psychiatry. *American Journal of Psychiatry, 149,* 725–732.

Wender, P. H., Rosenthal, D., Kety, S. S., Schulsinger, F., & Welner, J. (1974). Cross-fostering: A research strategy for clarifying the role of genetic and experimental factors in the etiology of schizophrenia. *Archives of General Psychiatry, 30,* 121–128.

Wexler, B. E., & Heninger, G. R. (1979). Alterations in cerebral laterality during acute psychotic illness. *Archives of General Psychiatry, 36,* 278–284.

Whitaker, R. (2010). *Mad in America: Bad science, bad medicine, and the enduring mistreatment of the mentally ill.* New York: Basic Books.

Whitaker, R. (2011). *Anatomy of an epidemic: Magic bullets, psychiatric drugs, and the astonishing rise of mental illness in America.* New York, NY: Broadway Paperbacks.

Whitaker, R., & Cosgrove, L. (2015). *Psychiatry under the influence: Institutional corruption, social injury, and prescriptions for reform.* London: Palgrave Macmillan.

White, M. (2007). *Maps of narrative practice.* New York, NY: W. W. Norton.

White, M., & Epston, D. (1990). *Narrative means to therapeutic ends.* New York, NY: W.W. Norton.

Wilker, D. (2009). A crisis in medical professionalism. In D. Arnold (Ed.), *Ethics and the business of biomedicine.* New York, NY: Cambridge University Press.

Williams, M., & Williams, P. (1994). *Unimaginable storms: A search for meaning in psychosis.* London: Karnac Books.

Willis, T. (1684). *The Practice of Physick: Two Discourses Concerning the Soul of Brutes.* (Classic)

Wilson, H. (1982). *Deinstitutionalized residential care for the mentally disordered. The Soteria House approach.* New York, NY: Grune & Stratton.

Winnicott, D. W. (1955/1975). A case managed at home. In *Through paediatrics to psycho-analysis.* London: Hogarth Press.

Winnicott, D. W. (1963/1965). The mentally ill in your caseload (MPFE). In *Maturational processes and the facilitating environment: Studies in the theory of emotional development.* London: Hogarth Press.

Winnicott, D. W. (1964). *The child, the family, and the outside world.* London: Penguin.

Winnicott, D. W. (1965a). *Maturational processes and the facilitating environment: Studies in the theory of emotional development.* London: Hogarth Press.

Winnicott, D. W. (1965b). The prize of mental health (unpublished manuscript).

Winnicott, D. W. (1971). *Playing and reality.* London: Tavistock.

Witelson, S. (1985). The brain connection: The corpus callosum is larger in left-handers. *Science, 229,* 665–668.

Wolf, J. A., Stys, P. K., Lusardi, T., Meaney, D., & Smith, D. H. (2001). Traumatic axonal injury induces calcium influx modulated by tetrodotoxin-sensitive sodium channels. *Journal of Neuroscience, 21,* 1923–1930.

World Health Organization. (1973). *The International Pilot Study of Schizophrenia.* Geneva: World Health Organization Press. Volume 1.

World Health Organization. (2017). *International Classification of Diseases, 10th Revision, Clinical Modification (ICD-10-CM).* Retrieved March 19, 2018. Wyatt,R. J. (1997). Research in schizophrenia and the discontinuation of antipsychotic medications. *Schizophrenia Bulletin, 23,* 3–9.

Yan, J. (2010, June 18). New guidelines govern APA's relations with industry. *Psychiatric News.*

Yang, Y., & Raine, A. (2009). Prefrontal structural and functional brain imaging findings in antisocial, violent, and psychopathic individuals: A meta-analysis. *Psychiatry Research, 174,* 81–88.

Zemeckis, R. (2000). *Cast away* [motion picture].

Zilboorg, G. (1941). *A history of medical psychology.* W.W. Norton, 261.

Zinman, S. (2015). History of the consumer/survivor movement. Retrieved March 17, 2017. https://na4ps.files.wordpress.com/2015/09/history-of-movement_zinman-bluebird.pdf (slide 35).

Zubin, J., & Spring, B. (1977). Vulnerability; a new view of Schizophrenia. *Journal of Abnormal Psychology, 86,* 103–126.